W9-CAT-324

Lippincott's Review Series

Mental Health and Psychiatric Nursing

Third Edition

Ann Isaacs, RN, CS, MSN
Professor
Luzerne County Community College
Nanticoke, Pennsylvania

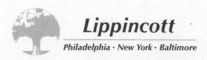

Lippincott
Philadelphia · New York · Baltimore

Acquisitions Editor: Jennifer Brogan
Developmental Editors: Danielle DiPalma/Beth Goldner
Assistant Editor: Hilarie Surrena
Senior Project Editor: Tom Gibbons
Senior Production Manager: Helen Ewan
Production Coordinator: Pat McCloskey
Assistant Art Director: Doug Smock
Manufacturing Manager: William Alberti
Indexer: Nancy Newman

Library of Congress Cataloging in Publications Data
Isaacs, Ann.
    Mental health and psychiatric nursing / Ann Isaacs.—3rd ed.
       p. ; cm.—(Lippincott's review series)
    Includes bibliographical references and index.
    ISBN 0-7817-2188-1 (pbk. : alk. paper)
     1. Psychiatric nursing—Examinations, questions, etc. I. Title. II. Series.
    [DNLM: 1. Mental Health—Examination Questions. 2. Psychiatric
    Nursing—Examination Questions. WY 18.2 I74m 2000]
    RC440.L57 2000
    6109.73'68'076—dc21   00-027375

9 8 7 6 5 4 3

Dedication

To my husband Bob, my sons Jeff and Dennis, and grandson Taylor—
thank you for your love and support.
To all my LCCC students, past, present, and future—thank you.

Acknowledgment

I would like to thank Beth Goldner and the staff at Lippincott Williams &
Wilkins for their careful editing. Their contribution was invaluable. I
would also like to thank my typist Maria Choman, for her hard work.

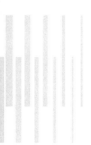

Introduction

Lippincott's Review Series is designed to help you in your study of the key subject areas in nursing. The series consists of six books, one in each core nursing subject area:

Medical-Surgical Nursing   Mental Health and Psychiatric Nursing
Pediatric Nursing   Pathophysiology
Maternal-Newborn Nursing   Fluids and Electrolytes

Lippincott's Review Series was planned and developed in response to your requests for comprehensive outline review books that address each major subject area and also contain a self-test mechanism. These books meet the need for strong and weak areas of knowledge. Each book is a complete source for review and self-assessment of a single core subject—all six together provide an excellent comprehensive review of entry-level nursing.

Each book is all-inclusive of the content addressed in major textbooks. The content outline review uses a consistent nursing process format throughout and addresses nursing care for well and ill clients. Also included are necessary teaching and other concepts such as pharmacology. Special features include:

- **Nursing process overview sections** ⊕ review each step of the nursing process for the system or group of disorders in discussion. These reviews improve your ability to apply principles to practice by highlighting common assessment findings, diagnoses, goals, interventions, and outcomes.
- **Nursing Alerts** 🖐 are fundamental guidelines you can follow to ensure safe and effective care.
- **Drug charts** provide quick reference for medications that are commonly used in treating the disorders discussed within a given chapter. The drug classification, indications, and selected nursing interventions are provided.
- **Client and family teaching boxes** detail health teaching information, which may be applied in the clinical setting.

- **Chapter study questions** help you chart your progress through each chapter. Answer keys are provided with rationales for correct and incorrect responses.
- **Comprehensive examination** mimics the NCLEX and allows you to assess your strengths and weaknesses. An answer key is provided with rationales for correct and incorrect responses.
- **Accompanying CD-ROM** provides 200 additional NCLEX-style questions so you can practice computer adaptive test-taking skills. Answers are provided with rationales for correct and incorrect responses.

You can use the books in this series in several different ways. Overall, you can use them as subject reviews to augment general study throughout your basic nursing program and as a review to prepare for the National Council Licensure Examination (NCLEX-RN). How you use each book depends on your individual needs and preferences and on whether you review each chapter systematically or concentrate only on those chapters whose subject areas are particularly problematic or challenging. You may instead choose to use the comprehensive examination as a self-assessment opportunity to evaluate your knowledge base before you review the content outline. Likewise, you can use the study questions for pre- or post-testing after study, followed by the comprehensive examination as a means of evaluating your knowledge and competencies of an entire subject area. Regardless of how you use the books, one of the strengths of the series is the self-assessment opportunity it offers in addition to guidance in studying and reviewing content. The chapter study questions and comprehensive examination questions have been carefully developed to cover all topics in the outline review.

Unlike the NCLEX examination that tests the cumulative knowledge needed for safe practice by an entry-level nurse, these practice tests systematically evaluate the knowledge base that serves as the building block for the entire nursing educational process. In this way, you can prepare for the NCLEX examination throughout your course of study. Good study habits throughout your educational program are not only the best way to ensure ongoing success, but also will prove the most beneficial way to prepare for the licensing examination.

Keep in mind that these books are not intended to replace formal learning. They cannot substitute for textbook reading, discussion with instructors, or class attendance. Every effort has been made to provide accurate and current information, but class attendance and interaction with an instructor will provide invaluable information not found in books. Used correctly, these books will help you increase understanding, improve comprehension, evaluate strengths and weakness in areas of knowledge, increase productive study time, and, as a result, help you improve your grades.

MONEY BACK GUARANTEE—Lippincott's Review Series will help you study more effectively during coursework throughout your educational program, and help you prepare for quizzes and test, including the NCLEX exam. If you buy and use any of the six volumes in Lippincott's Review Series and fail the NCLEX exam, simply send us verification of your exam results and your copy of the review book to the address below. We will promptly send you a check for our suggested list price.

Lippincott's Review Series
Marketing Department
Lippincott Williams & Wilkins
530 Walnut Street
Philadelphia, PA 19106

Contents

1
Introduction to Mental Health and Psychiatric Nursing   1

2
Conceptual Frameworks for Psychiatric Care   19

3
Stress, Anxiety, and Anxiety-Related Disorders   37

4
The Mind–Body Continuum: Common Disorders   59

5
Personality Disorders   81

6
Mood Disorders and Suicidal Behavior   97

7
Schizophrenic Disorders   119

8
Substance-Related Disorders   137

9
Physical Abuse, Sexual Abuse, and Family Violence   161

10
Childhood and Adolescent Psychiatric Disorders   179

11
Cognitive Impairment Disorders   197

12
Treatment Modalities: Crisis Intervention   215

13
Treatment Modalities: Group Therapy   227

14
Treatment Modalities: Family Therapy   237

15
Treatment Modalities: Somatic Therapies   249

Comprehensive Test Questions   280

Answer Key   295

Bibliography   310

Index   314

1 Introduction to Mental Health and Psychiatric Nursing

I. **Evolution of Mental Health Treatment**

A. **Pre-1960. Mental health treatment was provided in large mental hospitals (state or private) that were usually located away from well-populated areas.**

1. A client's length of stay was usually prolonged, and there were few mechanisms for follow-up care after discharge.
2. Clients became dependent and institutionalized; they were not active participants in their health care and treatment.
3. Family members were not considered part of the treatment team.

B. **1960 to 1970. The Civil Rights movement of the 1960s was a catalyst for focusing on the rights of the mentally ill.**

1. The **Community Mental Health Centers Act (1963)** dramatically affected delivery of mental health services.
2. Because of this Act, focus and funding for treatment shifted from large mental hospitals to newly established community mental health centers and included the following services:
   a. **Emergency care:** immediate assessment and initiation of appropriate treatment
   b. **24-hour inpatient care:** hospital-based care for symptom stabilization (ie, short-term care)
   c. **Partial hospitalization:** treatment programs for individuals requiring daily support but not 24-hour hospital care. Clients come for 6 to 8 hours per day and participate in a variety of therapies (eg, group or individual therapy, social skills training).
   d. **Outpatient care:** assessment, psychotherapeutic support, and medication management. Clients come for 1 to 2 hours per week.
   e. **Consultation and education:** outreach programs for community groups on mental health topics, for example, training for police on handling rape trauma, training for employers on assisting employees with an alcohol problem.

C. 1970 to 1980. Treatment shifts from long-term hospital care to shorter inpatient stays, followed by community-based treatment after discharge.

1. Client populations decreased in large mental hospitals, and many hospitals closed.
2. Community mental health centers were often unable to provide services for the resulting greater numbers of clients.
3. Homelessness became a problem for people with persistent chronic mental illness who lacked family resources and adequate social support.

D. 1980 to 1990. The high cost of health care and need for cost containment became national focus.

1. Managed care systems evolved, arranging relationships between payers, providers, and consumers of health care.
    a. These systems monitor distribution of services, actions by providers, and outcomes of treatment.
    b. The goal of managed care is to decrease cost while promoting quality of service.
    c. The relationship between provider and user of services is no longer primary. The managers and insurers of health care monitor the relationship between the provider and the consumer of health care.
2. Types of managed care systems include:
    a. **Health maintenance organizations (HMOs),** which offer a preset fee for clients in a particular population in exchange for delivery of health care services (by a provider) during a given time period
    b. **Independent practice organizations,** in which groups of health care providers contract with HMOs
    c. **Preferred provider organizations,** in which provider groups are approved by a particular HMO to provide services to its client population

E. 1990 to present. There were significant changes in delivery of mental health treatment.

1. Managed care incorporates new structures and services.
    a. **Case management.** A case manager is assigned to coordinate services for individual clients and collaborates with a multidisciplinary team.
    b. **Critical pathways and care maps.** Clinical management tools designate the organization, sequence, and timing of interventions provided by a treatment team for an identified client disorder.
    c. **Population-based community care.** Primary preventive services are provided and focused on (rather than only illness-based care). It includes identification of high-risk groups and education for lifestyle changes to prevent illness.
2. **Alternative settings** provide treatment in the least restrictive setting. Community care and treatment are aimed at tertiary prevention, which is designed to reduce severity of mental health problem and help the person live at the highest functioning capacity possible. Alternative treatment settings are as follows.
    a. **Mental health centers** and community crisis centers

b. **Short-term inpatient psychiatric units** located in community hospitals

c. **Partial hospitalization** and day-care programs

d. **Residential treatment programs** in halfway houses, board-and-care homes, and foster homes

e. **Mobile crisis units** and homeless shelters

f. **Clubhouse programs** offering transitional services to promote independent community living

g. **Prisons**

h. **Nursing homes**

3. **Americans with Disabilities Act (1990)** helps to ensure that people with disabilities, including a mental illness, can fully participate in the economic and social mainstream of society.

4. **Growth of consumer movement**

a. Organizations, such as the National Alliance of the Mentally Ill, remove the stigma of mental illness and provide local community support for people with mental illness and their families.

b. Organizations lobby to increase funding for research and treatment of mental illness.

5. **Knowledge of brain structure and function**

a. The 1990s are considered the "Decade of the Brain" because of the profound growth of knowledge about the workings of the brain.

b. Along with progress in genetics, the resulting knowledge has reshaped the understanding of causes and treatment of mental illness.

II. History of Psychiatric Nursing

A. **Key figures**

1. **Florence Nightingale (1859)** was the founder of modern nursing and author of the first nursing text, *Notes on Nursing.*

2. **Harriet Baily (1920)** wrote the first psychiatric nursing textbook, *Nursing in Mental Diseases.*

3. **Hildegarde Peplau (1952)** wrote *Interpersonal Relations in Nursing,* a landmark book that described a framework for psychiatric nursing practice. Her emphasis on nurse-patient relationships and theoretical constructs to explain patient problems provided the foundation for psychiatric nursing practice.

B. **Nursing organizations provided leadership for development of psychiatric nursing.**

1. **National League for Nursing (NLN), 1937.** The NLN recommended the inclusion of mental health and psychiatric nursing in nursing school curricula.

2. **American Nurses Association (ANA), 1958**

a. The ANA established the **Conference Group on Psychiatric Nursing.** This group worked to define the practice of psychiatric-mental health nursing.

    b. In 1973, the ANA was the first to publish standards of mental health and psychiatric nursing practice; revised standards were published in 1982 and 1994.

III. Current Psychiatric and Mental Health Nursing Practice

In 1994, the Coalition of Psychiatric Nursing Organizations and the ANA jointly published a description of two levels of practice, the generalist and the specialist.

A. Psychiatric-Mental Health Nurse Generalist

    1. Education required is a baccalaureate degree in nursing.

    2. Certification is a formal process regulated by the American Nurses Credentialing Center (ANCC) that validates clinical competence. Designation following certification is *RN,C.*

    3. Functions

        a. A generalist works with individuals, families, groups, and the community to assess mental health needs, develop diagnoses, and plan, implement, and evaluate nursing care.

        b. The psychiatric-mental health generalist uses interventions that include health promotion and maintenance; intake screening and evaluation; case management; provision of a therapeutic environment (ie, milieu therapy); teaching clients and assisting them with self-care activities; administering and monitoring psychobiological treatment regimens; crisis intervention and counseling; and outreach activities in home and community.

    4. Practice settings. Generalists practice in traditional hospital settings, home health agencies, employee assistance programs, mental health clinics, HMOs, primary care centers, homeless clinics, senior centers, emergency and crisis centers, daycare centers, schools, and prisons.

B. Psychiatric-Mental Health Nurse Specialist

    1. Education required is a master's degree in psychiatric–mental health nursing.

        a. **Psychiatric nurse practitioner.** This specialist is an advanced practice RN (APN or APRN) who provides primary care. Individual states have nursing practice acts that govern the scope of practice, including prescriptive authority.

        b. **Clinical nurse specialist (CNS).** This is a master's-prepared RN who provides direct care as a therapist or indirect care as a consultant, educator, or researcher.

    2. Certification is a formal process validating clinical competence by the ANCC. Advanced practice mental health nurses may also become certified as clinical specialists. The designation is *RN, CS,* and it applies to both psychiatric nurse practitioners and clinical nurse specialists.

    3. Functions

        a. The specialist performs all functions of a generalist.

        b. The specialist provides primary mental health care, including prescription of psychoactive medication and ordering of appropriate diagnostic tests according to state nursing regulations.

    c. The specialist analyzes the health needs of both individuals and populations and designs programs that target at-risk groups and cultural and environmental factors that foster health and prevent mental illness.

  4. Practice settings. The specialist may practice in those settings described for the generalist as well as solo and group practice, contracts with employee assistance programs, HMOs, preferred provider organizations, and other settings where services are delivered.

IV. Therapeutic Relationships

A. Definition. A therapeutic relationship is a nurse-client interaction that is directed toward enhancing the client's well being. The client may be an individual, a family, a group, or a community.

B. Elements of the therapeutic relationship

  1. Contract. The time, place, and purpose of meetings as well as conditions for termination are established between the nurse and client.

  2. Boundaries. The therapeutic nature of the relationship (as opposed to a social relationship) is established.

    a. Roles of participants are clearly defined.

    b. The nurse is defined as a professional helper.

    c. The client's needs and problems are the focus of the interaction.

  3. Confidentiality. This is a basic condition of the therapeutic relationship and needs to be maintained by nurse.

    a. The nurse shares client information only with professional staff who need to know.

    b. The nurse obtains the client's written permission to share information with any others outside treatment team.

  4. Therapeutic nurse behaviors are the consistent practice, by the nurse, of the following items:

    a. Self-awareness

    b. Genuine, warm, and respectful behavior

    c. Empathy (Table 1-1)

    d. Cultural sensitivity

    e. Collaborative goal setting

    f. Responsible, ethical practice

C. Phases of the therapeutic relationship

  1. Orientation (assessment and analysis)

    a. The nurse establishes trust with the client.

    b. The nurse assesses the client (Table 1-2).

    c. A nursing diagnosis is formulated.

    d. Priorities of the client's problems are identified.

    e. The nurse and client establish mutually agreed-on goals.

  2. Working phase

    a. The nurse plans outcomes and related interventions to assist client to meet goals.

TABLE 1-1
Empathic Nurse Behaviors

VERBAL BEHAVIORS	NONVERBAL BEHAVIORS
• Asking open-ended questions • Focusing on client feelings • Paraphrasing client comments to check perceptions • Seeking clarification • Communicating nurse's understanding of client feelings and perceptions	• Fully attending to client • Using warm vocal tone • Relaxed, unhurried manner • Leaning forward slightly in an open body posture • Nodding head periodically • Smiling periodically • Synchronizing movements with those of client • Maintaining eye contact (Note: Some cultures are not comfortable with direct eye contact; nurse respects cultural differences)

Definition: **Empathy** *is the emotional and intellectual ability to identify and understand another's feelings and perspective from an objective stance (Morse, 1992).*

    b. The nurse facilitates the client's expression of problems, thoughts, and feelings.

    c. The nurse uses the problem-solving approach in collaboration with the client to resolve problems.

    d. The nurse encourages and teaches coping measures to the client.

    e. The nurse encourages the client to practice adaptive behaviors and evaluates the effectiveness of these efforts.

3. Termination (evaluation)

    a. The nurse evaluates outcomes, reassessing the problems, goals, and interventions, if necessary.

    b. The nurse and client express feelings about termination.

    c. The nurse observes the client for regressive behaviors.

    d. The nurse evaluates the entire nurse-client relationship.

V. Therapeutic Communication

A. Definition. Therapeutic communication is composed of verbal and nonverbal techniques that the nurse uses to focus on the client's needs.

    1. Basic elements of a completed interaction

      a. **Sender:** originator of the message

      b. **Message:** information transmitted; may have both latent and manifest content

      c. **Receiver:** recipient of the message

      d. **Feedback:** receiver's response to the message, indicating understanding

TABLE 1-2
Nursing Assessment of the Psychiatric Client

AREA TO ASSESS	SPECIFIC DATA COLLECTION
1. Client-identifying data	1. Name, address, phone number, date of birth, marital status, education and employment, emergency contact person, primary care provider, type of housing (independent or assisted living)
2. Physical assessment, past medical history	2. Allergies, vital signs, weight, nutritional/diet history, sexual orientation and reproductive history, head-to-toe or body systems assessment as required by client status or agency protocol, major illness and surgeries, medications used
3. Past psychiatric history	3. First occurrence (date, duration), hospitalizations, treatments, community follow-up care, case manager or primary therapist
4. Substance use	4. Determine use of any drugs (name, route, length of time used, amount and frequency of use, history of withdrawal symptoms)
5. Current problem and stressors	5. Client's own words to describe problem; include developmental/situational stressors related to current problem.
6. Family and cultural data	6. Names, ages of significant others, characteristics of relationships, family history of mental illness. Cultural groups, cultural beliefs about health and illness, specific health practices, identification of cultural health practitioner, spiritual beliefs and religious affiliation.
7. Mental status examination	7. Use of standard mental status examination or agency protocol. Includes appearance, behavior, attention and orientation, use of language and speech patterns, cognitive processes, memory and general intellectual functioning, mood and affect, thought patterns and content, degree of insight.

2. **Nonverbal aspects** of therapeutic communication
   a. **Kinetics** are body movements, such as gestures, facial expressions, and other mannerisms (see Table 1-2).
   b. **Proxemics** are the physical spaces between communicators (eg, intimate space, up to 18 inches; personal space, 18 inches to 4 feet; social-consultative space, 9 to 12 feet; and public space, more than 12 feet). Therapeutic communication generally takes place in personal space.
   c. **Touch** can be used in therapeutic communication, but it should be done in a deliberate manner with the nurse analyzing the client's condition and the client's likely response. Touch can be inappropriate in some situations and with some clients (eg, with a client who is suspicious and mistrust-

ful, with a client who is a victim of abuse, with a client who has tenuous ego boundaries, with a client whose culture prohibits or restricts touch).

    d. **Silence** can be a powerful tool for therapeutic communication. It may facilitate the client's expression of thoughts and feelings.

    e. **Paralanguage** is the voice quality (tone, inflection) or how a message is delivered. The nurse should moderate voice quality according to the message being given to the client.

3. Therapeutic communication techniques

    a. **Offering oneself.** The nurse should be available to listen to the client.

    b. **Asking open-ended questions.** The nurse should ask neutral questions that encourage the client to express concerns (eg, "How are things going today?").

    c. **Providing opening remarks** or general statements based on assessment of the client (eg, "I noticed that you seem to be anxious today.")

    d. **Restating.** The nurse should repeat to the client the main content of the communication (eg, "You've told me about how the accident has affected every area of your life...").

    e. **Reflecting.** The nurse directs feelings and questions back to the client to encourage elaboration (eg, "You're feeling really sad since you've been unable to go back to work.").

    f. **Focusing.** The nurse asks goal-directed questions to help the client focus on a specific area of concern (eg, "Let's talk about your difficulty with your father.").

    g. **Encouraging elaboration.** The nurse helps the client describe more fully the concerns or problems under discussion (eg, "Tell me more about that.").

    h. **Seeking clarification.** The nurse helps the client put unclear thoughts or ideas into words (eg, "Do you mean that you become more anxious each time you leave your house?").

    i. **Giving information.** The nurse shares with the client information relevant to her health care and well being (eg, "I have a card describing your medication that I'll review with you.").

    j. **Examining alternatives.** The nurse helps the client explore options (eg, "Have you thought about requesting an extension on that deadline?").

    k. **Using silence.** The nurse allows periodic pauses to give nurse and client time to reflect.

    l. **Summarizing.** The nurse highlights important points of the discussion (eg, "We've talked about your mother's illness, your relationship with your husband, and your concerns about your children.").

VI. Cultural Considerations in Psychiatric Nursing

A. Definitions

    1. Culture: learned values, beliefs, and norms that are shared within a family, group, community, and nation

    2. Enculturation: the process of learning about one's culture

3. **Ethnicity:** one's sense of belonging to a particular cultural group
4. **Stereotyping:** expecting all persons from a particular group to behave, think, and respond in certain ways based on preconceived ideas
5. **Cultural diversity:** variety of cultural groupings, based not only on race and ethnicity but also on age, gender, socioeconomic status, religion, mental illness, and physically challenged conditions
6. **Culturally competent nursing:** complex interaction of knowledge, skills, and attitudes that enhances cross-cultural interaction and communication (Andrews, 1994)

B. **Cultural issues**
1. **General considerations**
   a. There are more than 100 ethnic groups in the United States.
   b. In 1998, racial and ethnic populations in the United States were 72.9% White, 12.1% Black, 10.7% Hispanic, 3.5% Asian Pacific, and 0.7% Native American.
   c. The fastest-growing ethnic populations in the United States are Hispanic and Asian Pacific Americans (Andrews, 1994).
2. There is no conclusive evidence that mental illness rates vary with race or other intrinsic human characteristics. Research has identified some distinctions, however.
   a. African Americans are more likely to be diagnosed with schizophrenia rather than with affective disorders as compared with Whites. (Caregiver bias may be a factor in this.)
   b. Socioeconomic status is a significant factor in mental illness. Poverty profoundly affects child and adolescent development.
3. Ethnic differences play a role in the efficacy of psychoactive medications. These differences result from both biological as well as nonbiological factors (Mohn, 1998). Research is ongoing.
   a. **Biologic factors:** differences in enzyme activity, which accounts for differences in metabolism and therefore efficacy of psychotropic medications
   b. **Nonbiologic factors:** for example, nutrition and diet may influence the effectiveness of psychotropic medications
4. Currently no single psychotherapy has been studied or cross-validated with relation to ethnic groups.
5. Values and beliefs about health, illness, mental disorders, and acceptable treatments may differ among cultural groups.
   a. Some cultural groups believe mental illness is caused by supernatural factors.
   b. What is considered normal and abnormal may be based on cultural perception.
   c. Some cultural groups use the services of a spiritual healer who usually has a mind-body-spirit approach to care.

C. **Culturally competent nursing**
1. Nurses use the following variables as guidelines in performing a cultural assessment of a client (Giger & Davidhizar, 1991).
   a. Meaning of verbal and nonverbal communication

   b. Space (especially personal space)
   c. Social organization, including particular cultures, defined family group, as well as characteristics of relationships
   d. Concepts of time, including orientation to present and future
   e. Environmental control, including special cultural health practices and beliefs about health and illness
   f. Biologic variations among different groups (eg, increased incidence of hypertension among African Americans, which may influence the type of psychotropic medication prescribed for treatment)
2. Nurses use sensitivity and knowledge, combined with cultural assessment, communication, and other mental health nursing skills to provide care for a culturally diverse population of clients.
3. Nurses who value diversity will help clients reach their full potential, preserving their ways of doing things and helping them change only those patterns that are not helpful. For example, the nurse may work with a spiritual healer and include the healer when planning care for the client who relies on that method of treatment.
4. **Guidelines for relating to clients from diverse cultures** (Giger & Davidhizar, 1991)
   a. The nurse will respect a particular cultural group, including their health practices and beliefs about treatment.
   b. The nurse will assess and analyze her personal beliefs regarding different cultures.
   c. The care plan will be based on the client's communicated needs and cultural background. (Acquire basic knowledge about particular beliefs common to the group you are working with.)
   d. The nurse will modify communication approaches to a particular culture. For example, the nurse may modify the use of direct eye contact with a client from a cultural group in which eye contact is inappropriate.
   e. The nurse will use validation as an important therapeutic technique.
   f. The nurse will use an interpreter if client speaks another language.

VII. Legal and Ethical Issues

A. Federal and state legislation as well as significant case law provides the legal basis for psychiatric practice. The following are selected examples.
   1. **State commitment laws.** Each state has legislation governing the types of admission for psychiatric treatment. Clients are either admitted voluntarily or committed involuntarily.
      a. **Voluntary admission.** The client willingly enters and consents to treatment. Clients retain all of their civil rights and may discontinue treatment whenever they choose. (Some states may require the client to sign a 72-hour notice of intent to leave.) If a treatment team disagrees with a client's decision to discontinue treatment, the client signs a form acknowledging that he has been discharged against medical advice, or the treatment team may decide to seek involuntary commitment of the client.

    b. **Involuntary inpatient commitment.** The client is institutionalized against his own will.

        (1) State law defines persons who can be committed and generally includes a person who poses a threat to self or others; a person who lacks the capacity for meeting basic needs; and a person who is seriously mentally ill but fails to seek treatment.

        (2) Commitment is not permanent and state guidelines provide time limits to types of involuntary commitment, which may include evaluation and emergency care, observation and treatment of treatable mental disorder, and extended or indeterminate care.

    c. **Involuntary outpatient treatment.** This option has been used as deinstitutionalization has progressed. Clients who have been court ordered for this treatment include substance-impaired clients, homeless mentally ill clients, and sex offenders.

    d. **Important note:** Involuntary commitment does not mean that an individual is incompetent. The client retains the right to consent to and refuse treatment.

  2. Examples of selected federal legislation. Clients admitted for psychiatric treatment retain their civil rights. In the case of an emergency, deprivation of liberty under cases of involuntary commitment is covered by state law. Additional legislation affecting client rights includes the following.

    a. **Patient's Bill of Rights** was originally issued in 1973 by the American Hospital Association (AHA). In 1980, the Mental Health Systems Act adopted it into law. These rights include appropriate treatment in the least restrictive setting; the right to participate in the planning of treatment; the right to refuse treatment except in an emergency or as permitted by law; and other more specific rights.

    b. **Americans with Disabilities Act of 1990** ensured that people with a mental illness can fully participate in the economic and social mainstream.

    c. **Social Security Act of 1993** provides a client with the right to an individual treatment plan of care, the right to participate in a plan of care, and the right to refuse treatment.

  3. Case law. In the Tarasoff case (1976), the courts found that a therapist must warn others when a mentally ill client poses a serious danger or threat to them ("duty to warn").

B. Important legal issues affecting psychiatric clients and nurses

  1. Confidentiality. Client information is privileged and must be treated confidentially.

  2. Informed consent. Client must be adequately informed about care and treatment and provide consent for treatment.

  3. Right to refuse treatment. All clients (including those committed involuntarily) have the right to refuse treatment. In emergency situations, a client can be given medication or confined by seclusion or restraints. Institutional guidelines are important in these situations.

  4. Seclusion. Isolating a person in a room where he is physically prevented from leaving requires established institutional guidelines.

5. Restraints. The use of chemical (medication) or mechanical devices to control a client's physical activity. Several organizations have written guidelines regarding restraints. Institutional policies also need to be in place for the use of these measures.

    a. Joint Commission on Accreditation of Healthcare Organizations (JCAHO) updated its guidelines on use of restraints in 1996, and the American Psychiatric Association wrote specific guidelines for the use of restraints in 1994.

    b. Specific guidelines include a physician order (in an emergency, the nurse can initiate restraints but must then obtain an order from the physician); provision for checking on client (eg, every 15 minutes) and loosening restraints (eg, every 15 minutes); provision for client to have fluids, food, and use of bathroom; and careful documentation regarding entire procedure. Principle of using least restrictive means apply in this situation.

6. Incompetence. The court determines client incompetence when her self-management is so impaired that she is at risk for grave harm. This procedure requires the client to have legal representation, and following a determination of incompetence, a legal guardian is appointed.

VIII. Ethical Issues in Nursing Practice

Both nursing and psychiatric nursing are governed by ethical and legal principles.

A. Acts and Ethical Codes

    1. Nurse Practice Acts. Each state defines nursing and describes boundaries and standards of nursing practices.

    2. ANA Code of Ethics for Nurses with Interpretive Statements provides ethical guidelines for nursing practice.

    3. ANA Standards of Psychiatric-Mental Health Clinical Practice provide direction for professional nursing practice and reflect the standards and values of psychiatric nursing.

    4. Transcultural Care Principles, Human Rights, and Ethical Considerations have been identified by Madeline Leininger.

B. Ethical principles applicable to nursing

    1. Autonomy: freedom to make choices about one's life

    2. Beneficence: requires nurse to act in ways that benefit clients

    3. Nonmaleficence: requires nurse to act in manner to avoid causing harm to client

    4. Veracity: practice of telling the truth

    5. Confidentiality: nondisclosure of information with which one is entrusted

    6. Justice: fair, equitable and appropriate treatment

    7. Fidelity: faithfulness and practice of keeping promises

C. Ethical issues in psychiatric nursing

    1. Spirituality

        a. **Definition.** Spirituality is defined as an animating force, life principle, or essence of being that permeates life and is expressed in multifaceted connections with self, other, nature, and God or Life Force (Burkhardt, 1998).

b. Nursing has a holistic body-mind-spirit view of individuals. An ethical appreciation of spiritual aspects of care is important to nursing care.

2. **Complementary and alternative therapies.** Use of complementary and alternative therapies by client, especially when conflicting with recommended medical treatment, can be a source of controversy and requires sensitivity to and respect for issues that are not "either/or" areas. Traditional health care providers may have trouble accepting a client's choice of alternative methods of treatment.

3. **Cultural and value differences between nurse and client.** When the client and nurse come from different cultural backgrounds and beliefs, the nurse has the responsibility to employ culturally sensitive techniques in interaction and treatment.

4. **Autonomy and beneficence issues, especially when dealing with seriously mentally ill client.** It can be particularly difficult for the nurse to handle the conflict between knowing that the treatment—especially medication—will help the client and the client refusing medication.

5. **Decisions about limited health care resources.** Managed care decisions, such as early discharge from treatment before maximum beneficial effects for the client, may cause the nurse to feel a sense of failure and frustration.

6. **Controversial client choices, such as abortion and active euthanasia.** Nurses are often faced with decisions about how to reconcile their own values and beliefs when these values and beliefs conflict with a client's choice.

7. **Decision making regarding use of chemical and mechanical restraints.** Restraining and secluding a client has been used as a method of treatment, rather than as a solution of last resort, when the client's behavior may cause harm to the client or others. Nurses may have strong feelings regarding using or not using restraints, which may differ from institutional and legal guidelines.

STUDY QUESTIONS

1. A nurse employed in a managed care system collaborates with the treatment team in monitoring a client's progress from psychiatric inpatient care to a community-assisted living program. The role of the nurse can best be described as
   (1) advanced practice nurse
   (2) case manager
   (3) nurse manager
   (4) staff nurse

2. When a nurse establishes a therapeutic relationship with a client, which of the following is the primary focus for the client's care?
   (1) the medical diagnosis
   (2) the client's needs and problems
   (3) the nursing diagnosis
   (4) the client's social interaction skills

3. Which of the following is the overall purpose of therapeutic communication?
   (1) to analyze client problems
   (2) to elicit client cooperation
   (3) to facilitate a helping relationship
   (4) to provide emotional support

4. A nurse is fully attentive to a client, seeks clarification of unclear statements, and periodically tells the client about the nurse's perception of client feelings. Which of the following is the nurse demonstrating?
   (1) congruence
   (2) empathy
   (3) reflection
   (4) summarization

5. Which of the following legal-ethical principles would a nurse use when interacting with a client with a psychosis who refuses psychotropic medication?

   (1) autonomy
   (2) confidentiality
   (3) empathy
   (4) fidelity

6. While teaching a client about psychotropic medication, a nurse obtains data related to the client understanding what was taught. Which of the following parts of the communication process is the nurse focusing on?
   (1) feedback
   (2) message
   (3) receiver
   (4) sender

7. A nurse is interacting with a client from a different cultural background. Which of the following implementations would the nurse use to provide sensitive care?
   (1) confronting issues of noncompliance
   (2) use of therapeutic silence
   (3) use of therapeutic touch
   (4) validation of communication

8. Shortly after a voluntary admission to a psychiatric inpatient unit, a client tells the nurse, "I don't know if I should be here. What will my family think?" Using reflection, which of the following is the most appropriate response from the nurse?
   (1) "Your family can visit you here, and they will see that this is a helpful place."
   (2) "You think your family will be upset because you have a psychiatric problem?"
   (3) "There is still a stigma associated with mental illness. Hopefully your family won't feel this way."
   (4) "You are wondering if you made the best decision, and you are concerned about your family's reaction."

9. A nurse is assigned to a client who has a domineering and demanding attitude, similar to the nurse's own mother. The nurse seeks out a colleague to share feelings about this situation. The nurse's action indicates

✓**(1)** appropriate self-awareness
(2) an inability to cope effectively
(3) lack of knowledge about the client's problems
(4) a need to change client assignment

10. After an initial nurse-client interaction, the client asks for the nurse's home phone number, indicating a desire to date the nurse. Which of the following responses is most appropriate?
(1) "I may consider dating you once you are fully recovered."
(2) "I'm sorry, but I already have a special relationship."
(3) "It's against hospital policy for me to date clients."
(4) "This is a professional relationship and we need to stay clear on that."

11. A client hospitalized under an involuntary procedure wants to call a lawyer about a personal matter involving a lawsuit. Which of the following nursing actions would be most appropriate?
✓**(1)** Allow phone call without seeking further information.
(2) Ask client questions about the pending lawsuit.
(3) Call the lawyer and explain that the client is in the hospital.
(4) Tell the client the lawsuit would be best settled after discharge from the hospital.

12. The advanced practice RN (APRN) who provides primary psychiatric care, including writing prescriptions, is legally authorized under which of the following?
(1) ANA Standards of Psychiatric Practice
(2) Certification by the ANCC
(3) Graduation from accredited master's program
✓**(4)** State Nurse Practice Act

13. A client has become increasingly unable to maintain self-care, with worsening symptoms of a chronic mental illness and refusal to accept psychiatric treatment. The community psychiatric nurse explains to the client's family that a legal procedure can be initiated to empower another person to give consent for treatment. Which of the following would a court hearing legally establish about this client?
(1) autonomy
✓**(2)** competence
(3) sanity
(4) rights

14. When initiating mechanical restraint of a client who is acting out and a threat to the safety of self and others, the nurse *must*
(1) inform his or her supervisor of the situation
✓**(2)** obtain a physician order as soon as possible after restraining procedure
(3) refrain from using restraints until physician is consulted
(4) use chemical restraints first

15. A community psychiatric nurse visits a client's home following referral from a case manager who is concerned about the client's increased delusions. A spiritual healer from the family's cultural group is present in the home and indicates the desire to work with the client and family. Which of the following actions would be most appropriate?

(1) The nurse explains that the healer's efforts would be incompatible with psychiatric care.

(2) The nurse proceeds with data collection only after requesting a private interview with the client.

(3) The nurse plans to collaborate with the healer in provision of care to client and family.

(4) The nurse refuses to continue with the client and family and contacts the case manager.

ANSWER KEY

1. The answer is (2). In a managed care system, the case manager is responsible for monitoring and ensuring continuity of care, therefore collaborating with the treatment team. Although they provide different levels of care, both the staff nurse and the advanced practice nurse provide primary care. A staff nurse involves supervision of other nursing personnel.

2. The answer is (2). The nurse establishes the therapeutic relationship, which is a helping relationship, to assist the client in working on his needs and problems. Both medical and nursing diagnosis would be important in understanding the client. However, the nurse provides care for the person, not the diagnosis. Improving social interaction skills may be a focus of nursing intervention, but it is not the purpose of the relationship.

3. The answer is (3). The purpose of therapeutic communication is to foster a helping relationship, so that the client can more effectively cope with problems. The other tasks described are part of the helping relationship but are not the overall purpose.

4. The answer is (2). The nurse's behaviors illustrate empathy. The other answer choice options are examples of therapeutic communication techniques.

5. The answer is (1). Autonomy is the legal right of each individual to make decisions affecting herself. This right applies regardless of the existence of a mental illness, unless a client is declared incompetent. Confidentiality is an important aspect of the nurse-client relationship in which a nurse does not reveal information about the client to people who have no right to know. Empathy is a quality the nurse demonstrates in a therapeutic relationship. Fidelity is an ethical principle of keeping promises.

6. The answer is (1). The communication sequence is complete when the receiver of the message provides feedback regarding the content of the message. The other answer choice options are parts of the communication process, but do not apply to this example.

7. The answer is (4). It is important for the nurse to frequently validate nurse-client communication to prevent cultural misunderstandings. Confronting noncompliance is inappropriate, because the nurse's interpretation of this situation may be quite different from the client's perspective. Therapeutic silence is important; however, validating communication will ensure culturally sensitive care. Touch must be used in a cautious manner when trying to understand a client's probable response. Touch is not appropriate for all clients.

8. The answer is (4). Reflection involves rewording the client's statement to indicate a nurse's understanding of the client's experience.

9. The answer is (1). Self-awareness is important. Analyzing and sharing percep-tions about oneself in relation to a client helps a nurse work through countertrans-ference feelings, which could hinder therapeutic process. Seeking colleague con-sultation regarding difficult interaction does not indicate either poor coping or lack of knowledge. If the consultation with the colleague does not improve the nurse's ability to interact therapeutically with this client, a change of assignment may be indicated.

10. The answer is (4). At the beginning of a nurse-client relationship, it is impor-tant for the nurse to clarify parameters of the relationship and establish clear bound-aries.

11. The answer is (1). The client who is committed under an involuntary proce-dure retains all civil rights, including the right to consult a lawyer and the right to sue. The nurse should not ask the client about the lawsuit, because this is intrusive behavior on the nurse's part. Calling the lawyer and telling the lawyer the patient is in the hospital as well as telling the client the lawsuit would best be settled after discharge from the hospital are responses that violate the client's rights.

12. The answer is (4). The State Nurse Practice Acts provide legal parameters and boundaries for the practice of nursing. ANA Standards provide ethical guidelines for practice. Certification is a credentialing issue but does not provide legal authoriza-tion. An adequate knowledge base is acquired through education but does not establish legal authority.

13. The answer is (2). Competence is a legal issue indicating an *ability* to make decisions for oneself. When a client experiences severe impairments in this area, the court may declare the client incompetent and then appoint a legal guardian who can make decisions regarding the client's care and treatment. Autonomy is the legal *right* of each individual to make decisions affecting himself. When a client becomes so impaired that self-care is not possible, the court may intervene and declare the client incompetent. Clients with a mental illness have a right to make decisions about care unless the court declares that the client is incompetent. A court pro-ceeding is unnecessary to establish client legal rights; they are provided by the Con-stitution.

14. The answer is (2). In an emergency situation, the nurse can initiate restraints for a client, but must obtain the physician's order as soon as possible afterward. The supervisor may be notified, but the nurse *must* obtain an order.

15. The answer is (3). The nurse providing culturally sensitive care will respect client beliefs and collaborate with client, family, and spiritual healer. The other answer choice options are actions that do not indicate understanding and respect for diversity, and therefore they are inappropriate.

2 Conceptual Frameworks for Psychiatric Care

A. Definition. Conceptual frameworks are methods of organizing knowledge that provide a basis for understanding human behavior and the relationship of biologic factors, developmental processes, and environmental influences.

B. Function

1. Conceptual frameworks allow the systematic organization of knowledge, guide data collection, provide explanations for assessed behaviors, guide care plan development, provide rationales for selecting interventions, and determine evaluation criteria for outcome measurement.
2. Conceptual frameworks guide research by providing assumptions to be tested.

C. Examples. The following are selected frameworks used in psychiatric care.

1. **Psychobiology theories**
2. **Developmental theories,** including those of Freud, Sullivan, Erikson, and Piaget
3. **Behavioral theories**
4. **Cognitive theories**
5. **Humanistic theories**

A. Definition. Psychobiology is the scientific study of the relationships among the structure and function of the brain, biochemical and hormonal processes, genetics, environmental experiences, and human behavior.

B. Developments influencing psychobiology

1. **Decade of the brain.** The 1990s saw an explosion of knowledge about brain functioning.
2. **Genetic research** has established a relationship between genetics and mental illnesses, especially schizophrenia and depressive disorders.
3. **Psychopharmacology research.** New drugs were developed that affect brain neurotransmitters and receptor sites.
4. **Technology.** Brain imaging techniques (eg, computed tomography [CT], positron emission tomography [PET], single photon emission computed

tomography, magnetic resonance imaging [MRI]) are used to study individuals with mental illness.

C. **Neuroanatomy and behavior**

1. The **cerebrum** is the most superior part of the brain and is composed of two cerebral hemispheres; each hemisphere is divided into four lobes.

   a. The **frontal lobe** is responsible for higher-order thinking, abstract reasoning, decision making, speech, and voluntary muscle movement. Dysfunction is associated with illogical or psychotic thinking, uninhibited behaviors, and incoherent speech.

   b. The **parietal lobe** is responsible for sensory function and body position information. Dysfunction is associated with impaired spatial ability and body image, as well as self-care deficits.

   c. The **occipital lobe** is responsible for visual function. Dysfunction is associated with visual illusions and hallucinations.

   d. The **temporal lobe** is responsible for judgment, memory, smell, sensory interpretation, and understanding sound. Dysfunction is associated with aggressive and violent behaviors, olfactory and auditory hallucinations, and language abnormalities.

2. The **diencephalon** is embedded in the cerebrum and is superior to the brain stem. It is composed of several structures.

   a. The **thalamus** receives and relays sensory information and plays a role in memory and in regulating mood.

   b. The **hypothalamus** is the main visceral control center of the body and is vitally important to body homeostasis. It regulates the autonomic nervous system; body temperature; food intake; water balance; biologic rhythms and drives; and hormonal output of the anterior pituitary gland.

   c. The **limbic system** comprises the limbic lobe and the numerous structures functioning with it, including the frontal cortex; hypothalamus; amygdala; hippocampus; brain stem; and autonomic nervous system. Called the *emotional brain,* the limbic system regulates emotional responses.

D. **Neurotransmitters and receptor sites**

1. **Neurotransmitters** are chemical messengers that carry an inhibitory or stimulating message from one neuron to another across the space between them **(synapse)**. Many psychiatric disorders are associated with abnormal interactions between neurotransmitter systems.

   a. **Serotonin** is involved in depressive and anxiety disorders, and possibly in eating disorders. Many antidepressants increase levels of serotonin at synapses.

   b. **Dopamine** is involved in schizophrenic disorders. Many antipsychotic medications block dopamine from binding to its receptors.

   c. **Norepinephrine** is a catecholamine neurotransmitter of the sympathetic nervous system, which mediates emergency response. Changes in norepinephrine levels are associated with depressive disorders, including bipolar disorder.

    d. **Gamma-aminobutyric acid (GABA)** is an inhibitory neurotransmitter. Antianxiety drugs increase effects of GABA.

    e. **Acetylcholine** is a major neurotransmitter of the parasympathetic nervous system, which controls muscles, memory, and coordination. Changes in acetylcholine levels are associated with Alzheimer disease.

  2. Receptor sites are channels located on presynaptic and postsynaptic cell membranes. They vary in affinity for their respective neurotransmitters. Receptor subtypes are often located in different brain areas and therefore can mediate different behavioral effects.

    a. Each neurotransmitter can latch onto more than one kind of receptor.

    b. There are 15 different receptors identified for serotonin and 5 different receptors identified for dopamine.

E. Genetics

  1. Multiple genes may interact with other neurobiologic and psychosocial factors in contributing to increased vulnerability to certain mental illness. For example, research has demonstrated a relationship between certain genes and the incidence of bipolar disorder in certain Amish families.

  2. Research on schizophrenia, depression, and Alzheimer's disease has identified a genetic vulnerability for these disorders.

    a. Twin and adoption studies have established data related to genetic transmission of schizophrenia (see Chapter 7) and depression (see Chapter 6) within families with histories of these disorders.

    b. Gene malfunction on certain chromosomes has been identified in depression (see Chapter 6), Alzheimer's disease (see Chapter 11), and schizophrenia (see Chapter 7).

F. Hormonal influences

  1. The **hypothalamic-pituitary-adrenal (HPA) axis** has been found to be hyperactive in individuals with depressive disorders.

  2. An **underactive thyroid gland** is linked to depression.

  3. The **stress response** is a neuroendocrine response that causes significant hormonal releases, which affects multiple body systems and can lead to psychological and physiologic symptoms (see Chapter 3).

G. Biology and environment. Research is ongoing about how an individual's environment affects brain development and functioning.

  1. Early life experiences (eg, physical or psychological abuse) can alter brain structure and affect production of hormones and neurotransmitters, which can be related to symptoms of mental illness in later life.

  2. Severe abuse early in life (eg, physical or sexual abuse in infancy and early childhood) can permanently increase gene expression for corticotropin-releasing factor (CRF) and increase risk for depression in adulthood.

  3. The **Kindling model** proposes that repeated environmental stimuli lead to progressively greater neural responsiveness, which changes brain excitability and therefore behavioral responses over time (Post, 1997). For example, an early life experience can contribute to an initial experience of mental illness, which is hypothesized to increase sensitivity of the brain and thus predispose to later episodes of mental illness, given continued life stressors.

H. Treatment approach in psychobiology framework

1. The psychiatric diagnosis is established according to DSM-IV criteria and laboratory and diagnostic studies (eg, brain imaging).
2. Somatic therapies (eg, pharmacotherapy, electroconvulsive therapy, light therapy) are established treatment methods; psychotherapeutic approaches are also used in conjunction with somatic therapies.

I. Application to nursing. Psychiatric nurses integrate psychobiology and advances in psychopharmacology into practice.

1. The American Nurses Association (ANA) established specific psychopharmacology guidelines for psychiatric-mental health nursing (ANA, 1994).
2. The nurse assesses physiologic, emotional, and behavioral aspects of client functioning.
3. For nurses working in primary prevention, developments in genetic research can enhance the nurse's understanding of at-risk families.
4. Understanding psychobiology helps the nurse teach clients and families about biology of mental illness, symptom recognition, medication management, and relapse prevention.
5. The nurse educated at master's level (APRN) may have primary responsibility for care of the client with mental illness (including prescriptive authority).

III.   Developmental Theories

A. Freudian (psychodynamic) theory focuses on intrapsychic processes and psychosexual development.

1. Freudian theory describes three levels of awareness.
    a. **Conscious:** experiences (eg, memories, feelings, thoughts, and wishes) within an individual's awareness
    b. **Preconscious:** experiences that may be recalled to conscious awareness
    c. **Unconscious:** experiences not available to conscious awareness
2. Freudian theory describes personality structure.
    a. **Id** is the most primitive component and is responsible for instincts and impulses, operating by the pleasure principle and primary-process thought (ie, thinking that is characteristic of infancy, as well as "dream" thinking).
    b. **Ego** is the reality-based "I" component, and validates and tests reality; it operates by secondary-process thought (ie, reality-based thinking), balancing impulses from id and demands from superego.
    c. **Superego** is the component of moral principle, or the conscience; it consists of culturally acquired values, beliefs, and standards of behavior.
3. **Psychodynamics** are assumptions made by Freud and psychoanalysis in general that human behavior—and especially emotional problems—occur because of unconscious conflicts and basic instincts.
    a. **Psychic energy (cathexis)** is a force required for mental functioning, and it arises from drives (ie, instincts).

b. **Instincts (drives)** are inborn psychologic representations or wishes and include self-preservation and preservation of species. Freud postulated that humans have both a life and a death instinct.
c. **Anxiety** is a response to unconscious conflict or a threat to ego.
d. **Defense mechanisms** are mental mechanisms (largely unconscious) that operate in protecting the ego (Table 2-1).

TABLE 2-1
Defense Mechanisms

DEFENSE MECHANISM	DEFINITION	CLINICAL EXAMPLE
Repression	Exclusion of unpleasant or unwanted experiences, emotions, or ideas from conscious awareness	A victim of an automobile accident does not remember anything about the accident.
Projection	Attributing one's own feelings or wishes (which are unacceptable to oneself) to another person	A frightened client lashes out at the nurse, saying the nurse is a timid, fearful person and shouldn't be in the role of nurse.
Reaction formation	Adoption of behavior or feelings that are exactly opposite one's true emotions	A client is angry about the care he is receiving, but behaves in a very ingratiating manner.
Displacement	Transferring emotions associated with a particular person or event to another person, object, or situation that is not as threatening	A client who is angry with the physician becomes verbally abusive to the nurses.
Identification	Adopting the thinking or behavioral patterns of another	A teenager hospitalized for diabetes wants to become a nurse as a result of the experience.
Denial	Refusal to believe or accept an unpleasant reality	A client who drinks alcohol every day and cannot stop fails to acknowledge having a problem.
Isolation	Separation of emotions from precipitating event or situation	A rape victim talks about her rape experience without showing any emotion.
Intellectualization	Use of thinking to avoid experiencing emotions that are unpleasant	A father talks with his child about what love should be like but fails to demonstrate love toward the child.
Rationalization	Attempts to justify one's behavior by presenting reasons that sound logical	A client being treated for a drug addiction claims an inability to stop taking drugs because of a "bad marriage."
Sublimation	Substituting constructive and socially acceptable behavior for strong impulses not acceptable in their original form	A mother who lost a child in a drunk-driving accident joins an organization that works to educate the public about the dangers of drunk driving.

4. **Developmental concepts.** Table 2-2 describes the developmental theories of Freud.
5. **View of mental illness in the Freudian context**
   a. All behavior has meaning, although meaning may be unconscious.
   b. Symptoms of mental illness are caused by unconscious internal conflicts arising from unresolved issues in early childhood. Situations occurring in adulthood that are similar to the conflicts of childhood will precipitate symptoms. For example, an adult who has unresolved conflicts related to toilet training may be vulnerable to situations in adulthood that call for giving oneself or sharing one's possessions. These situations create anxiety that is largely unconscious.
   c. Defenses are fixed at an early development stage.
6. **Treatment in a Freudian context**
   a. There is an insight-oriented focus on interpersonal conflicts, anxiety, defenses, and sexual and aggressive drives.
   b. Unresolved conflicts are brought to a conscious level by various techniques (eg, free association, dream analysis, transference analysis).
   c. Psychoanalytic treatment is often long term and expensive.
7. **Application to nursing**
   a. Working in this framework, nurses should assess the client's anxiety levels and use of defense mechanisms.
   b. Psychodynamic theory can be used to understand a client's behavior and provide developmental perspective of behavior.
   c. **Transference** (client feelings toward a therapist arising from unconscious experiences with early significant others, such as the parents) and **countertransference** (feelings in therapist arising from the therapist's early experiences) can assist a nurse in managing the therapeutic relationship.
B. **Sullivan's (interpersonal) theory** focuses on interaction between an individual and his environment.
   1. According to this theory, personality is shaped through interaction with significant others; the child internalizes approval or disapproval from the parents, and therefore the self is shaped by the parental view of the child. **Self-system** is Sullivan's term conceptualizing the three components of personality.
      a. **"Good-me"** develops in response to behaviors receiving approval by parents or significant others.
      b. **"Bad-me"** develops in response to behaviors receiving disapproval by parents or significant others, and leads to anxiety states.
      c. **"Not-me"** develops in response to behaviors generating extreme anxiety in parents or significant others; these behaviors are denied as being part of oneself.
   2. Anxiety is an interpersonal phenomenon that occurs when one experiences conflict or problems in a significant relationship.
   3. The basic needs of an individual include satisfaction (biologic needs) and security (emotional and social needs).

TABLE 2-2
Developmental Theories

FREUD'S (PSYCHOSEXUAL) THEORY	ERIKSON'S (PSYCHOSOCIAL) THEORY	SULLIVAN'S (INTERPERSONAL) THEORY	PIAGET'S (COGNITIVE) THEORY
Infancy (birth to 18 months). Termed the *oral stage*, the infant learns to deal with anxiety by gratification of oral needs	**Infancy.** Termed *trust versus mistrust*, the infant learns to trust others	**Infancy.** Learn to trust others	**Sensorimotor stage (birth to 18 months).** Learn about self and environment by senses and motor activities
Toddler (18 months to 3 years). Termed the *anal stage*, the toddler learns muscle control and social control	**Toddler.** Termed *autonomy versus shame and doubt*, the toddler learns self-control and beginning of independence	**Childhood (18 months to 6 years).** Accept influence of others	**Preconceptual stage (2 to 4 years.)** Develop language and symbolic play
Preschool (3 to 6 years). Termed the *phallic stage*, the child establishes sexual identity	**Preschool.** Termed *initiative versus guilt*, the child learns assertiveness and one's ability to affect interpersonal environment	**Juvenile (6 to 9 years).** Form peer relationships	**Intuitive stage (4 to 7 years).** Learn to classify and group things; egocentric thinking
School age (6 to 12 years). Termed the *latency stage*, the child establishes same-sex relationships	**School age.** Termed *industry versus inferiority*, the child learns self-confidence by cooperation and competition	**Preadolescence (9 to 12 years).** Form friendship with same-sex peers	**Concrete operations stage (6 to 12 years).** Learn to reason in systematic way
Adolescence (12 to 18 years). Termed the *genital stage*, the adolescent establishes relationships with the opposite sex and finds gratifying work	**Adolescence (12 to 18 years).** Termed *identity versus role diffusion*, the child develops a sense of self.	**Early adolescence (12 to 14 years).** Becoming more independent; begin to establish relationships with opposite sex	**Formal operations stage (12 to 18 years and above).** Learn abstract thinking and conceptual thought
	Young adult (18 to 25 years). Termed *intimacy versus isolation*, the young adult develops intimate relationships	**Late adolescence (14 to 21 years).** Develop enduring relationships with member of opposite sex	
	Middle adult (25 to 55 years). Termed *generativity versus stagnation*, the adult guides others and contributes to society		
	Older adult (55 years to death). Termed *integrity versus despair*, the adult feels satisfied with one's life		

4. **Developmental concepts.** Table 2-2 describes the developmental theories of Sullivan.
5. **View of mental illness in interpersonal context**
   a. Symptoms are related to conflictual or problematic interpersonal relationships (eg, anxiety or depression in the spouse of an alcoholic).
   b. **Causes** of mental illness are related to past relationships, inappropriate communication, and the current relationship crisis.
6. **Treatment in interpersonal context**
   a. Treatment focuses on anxiety and its cause.
   b. Therapist is participant-observer in relationship with client; the role of the therapist is more active than passive when compared with psychoanalytic therapy.
   c. The client is encouraged to verbalize feelings and work on modifying problematic relationships.
7. **Application to nursing**
   a. Hildegarde Peplau, renowned nurse theorist, developed an interpersonal theory of nursing. Peplau's theory holds that the nurse and client participate in and contribute to the relationship and, further, that the relationship itself can be therapeutic.
   b. The nurse uses the nurse-client relationship as a corrective interpersonal experience for client.
   c. The nursing intervention often focuses on "here and now" interpersonal concerns (as opposed to past problems or early relationship issues) and problem solving related to interpersonal issues.
   d. Anxiety intervention is an important nursing function (see Chapter 3).

C. **Erikson's (psychosocial) theory** proposes eight developmental phases (see Table 2-2).
   1. According to Erikson, ego development results from social interaction.
   2. Developmental tasks are sequential and depend on prior successful mastery; an individual who fails to master a developmental task at the appropriate age can return later in life to work on mastery.
   3. Views on mental illness and treatment are similar to Freud's theory.
   4. **Application to nursing**
      a. The nurse assesses a client's psychosocial development according to expected norms for specific age.
      b. The nurse can use knowledge of developmental tasks in selecting appropriate interventions for the client.
      c. The nurse fosters healthy behaviors and encourages hope that relearning is possible. For example, the nurse would establish trust with the client and encourage the client to act autonomously or otherwise adopt the positive behaviors associated with each of the eight life stages.

D. **Piaget's (cognitive) theory** focuses on the innate development of thinking ability from infancy to adulthood (see Table 2-2).
   1. According to Piaget, individuals are born with the tendency to organize and to adapt to their environment.
   2. Piaget does not specifically discuss mental illness and treatment.

3. Application to nursing

a. Understanding the way an individual thinks enables the nurse to communicate in an age-appropriate manner.

b. Nursing interventions can be adapted to the individual's cognitive level. For example, the nurse can use dolls or toy medical equipment to try to explain surgery to a preschool-age child about to undergo surgery.

c. The nurse can select teaching strategies according to the client's age-appropriate cognitive processes.

IV. Behavioral Framework

A. General considerations. The behavioral framework describes a person's functioning in terms of identified behaviors.

1. People learn to be who they are by environmental shaping.

2. Behavior can be observed, described, and recorded.

3. Behavior is subject to reward or punishment.

4. Behavior can be modified by changing one's environment.

B. Classical conditioning (Pavlov's theory). Pavlov was an early theorist who established that learning or conditioning can occur when a stimulus (eg, a bell) is paired with an unconditioned response (eg, a dog salivating in response to the sight of food). In other words, the dog learns to salivate at the bell and no longer needs the sight of food to elicit the response.

1. Conditioned response: pairing of stimulus with response (the bell eventually elicits salivation in the dog)

2. Acquisition: gain of learned response (once a response is learned, it continues)

3. Extinction: loss of learned response

4. Operant conditioning (Skinner's theory)

a. **Positive reinforcement:** reward helps to continue the behavior

b. **Negative reinforcer:** removing undesirable consequences helps to continue the behavior

c. **Positive punishment:** aversive consequences decrease a particular behavior

d. **Negative punishment:** withdrawing reward decreases a particular behavior

C. View of mental illness in behavioral framework context

1. Maladaptive behaviors are learned through classical and operant conditioning; they continue because they are rewarding to the individual.

2. Maladaptive behaviors can be changed, without developing insight into underlying causes, by altering environment.

D. Treatment in behavioral framework context. The behavioral framework is commonly used with clients who have anxiety disorders, substance abuse problems, or other specific behavioral problems.

1. Various behavior modification techniques are used in treatment.

a. **Modeling:** new behaviors are learned by imitating the behavior of another person

   b. **Operant conditioning:** tokens (rewards) are provided for desirable behaviors *(token economy)*

   c. **Systematic desensitization:** gradual confronting of a stimulus that evokes intense anxiety; used especially when a client has a specific phobia. The therapist initially teaches the client how to relax, and then begins with a stimulus that causes mild anxiety. The client learns to invoke the relaxation response when confronted with the stimuli. The process continues until an intensely anxiety-provoking stimulus no longer causes the client to feel anxious.

   d. **Aversive therapy:** unpleasant consequences result from undesirable behavior. It may be used in treatment of paraphilias (eg, electric shocks may be paired with the impulse to humiliate or hurt a nonconsenting sexual partner).

   e. **Biofeedback:** training techniques used to control physiologic responses (eg, the stress response and its physiologic manifestations, such as tachycardia and vasoconstriction of blood vessels leading to hypertension).

   f. **Relaxation techniques:** training techniques used to counteract anxiety symptoms

   g. **Assertiveness training:** training techniques used to overcome passivity or aggression in interpersonal situations

E. Application to nursing

   1. In the behavioral framework, the nurse assesses both adaptive and maladaptive behaviors.

   2. The nurse and client collaborate in identifying behaviors that need to change.

   3. As a member of the treatment team, the nurse uses various behavioral modification techniques.

   4. The nurse uses principles of behavioral theory when teaching the client.

V.   Cognitive Framework

A. General considerations. The cognitive framework focuses on distorted or negative thought patterns that lead to maladaptive or symptomatic feelings and behaviors.

   1. Patterns of thinking are learned, become automatic, and significantly affect a person's feelings and behaviors.

   2. The amount of perceived control over a situation affects how an individual responds to stressors and problems.

    a. **Internal locus of control:** an individual believes in her own power to affect the outcome of a situation

    b. **External locus of control:** the individual believes she is controlled by powerful outside forces

B. View of mental illness in cognitive context

   1. In this framework, it is believed that an individual's distorted thinking leads to and perpetuates maladaptive behaviors.

2. In this framework, it is believed that certain common thought patterns can be identified as misperceptions (Table 2-3).

C. **Treatment in cognitive context**

1. The therapist helps the client develop awareness of negative thinking and recognize the effect of negative thinking on feelings and behaviors.

2. The client is encouraged to practice alternative thought patterns that lead to healthier behaviors.

3. **Types of treatment** in the cognitive framework
   a. **Rational-emotive therapy** (Albert Ellis). The therapist actively disputes a client's irrational beliefs.
   b. **Gestalt therapy** (Fritz Perls). The therapist promotes the client's self-awareness and increased self-responsibility for meeting needs.
   c. **Beck's cognitive therapy** (Aaron Beck). The therapist teaches the client to identify and correct dysfunctional thoughts about the self, the world, and the future.

4. Examples of **cognitive techniques**
   a. **Cognitive restructuring:** teaching the client to change maladaptive beliefs through positive self-statements and refuting irrational beliefs
   b. **Thought stopping:** the client is taught consciously to say "stop" to maladaptive thoughts

D. **Application to nursing**

1. The nurse assesses the client's thought patterns and identifies misperceptions (see Table 2-3).

TABLE 2-3
Cognitive Framework: Common Misperceptions of Thought Patterns

MISPERCEPTION	DEFINITION	CLINICAL EXAMPLE
Arbitrary inference	Holding beliefs in absence of supporting evidence	"I don't care what things you do to help me, I know you dislike me."
Selective abstraction	Concentrating on a single detail while ignoring others	"Look at how fat my thighs are." (Said by person who is underweight.)
Overgeneralization	Making global assumptions based on an isolated incident	"People who are in authority are like my boss—unfair and critical."
Magnification	Greatly exaggerating a situation	"I don't understand this one paragraph—I'll never be able to read this book."
Minimization	Belittling personal ability, action, or response	"I'm a person who has no abilities or good qualities."
Dichotomous thinking	"All or nothing" patterns of thought	"If you don't agree with me on this issue, then you're not my friend."

2. The nurse encourages the client's assumption of responsibility for one's own behaviors and fosters awareness of the effect of negative thinking on feelings about self-image.

3. The nurse uses cognitive techniques in intervention strategies.

VI. Humanistic Framework

A. General considerations. This theory focuses on "here and now"—current behaviors, issues, and problems—as well as spiritual values and meanings.

    1. In this framework, there is a belief that human nature is positive and growth oriented, and existence involves search for meaning and authenticity.

    2. Maslow's theory. Human needs are organized in a hierarchy.

        a. Physiologic needs

        b. Safety and security

        c. Love and belonging

        d. Self-esteem and esteem for others

        e. Self-actualization

B. View of mental illness in humanistic context

    1. The failure to develop one's full potential leads to poor coping.

    2. Lack of self-awareness and unmet needs interfere with feelings of security (self-esteem) as well as with relationships.

    3. Fundamental human anxiety is the fear of death, which leads to existential anxiety (ie, concern about the meaning of one's life).

C. Treatment

    1. Client-centered therapy (Carl Rogers)

        a. Psychotherapy fosters the process of learning to be fully one's own self. Rogers believes that mental illness is a result of the failure to develop oneself fully as a human person.

        b. The therapist is genuine and without facade when relating to the client. The therapist is active and expresses her own feelings and emotions directly and honestly.

        c. The client's behavior changes toward positive self-functioning when the therapist conveys acceptance, respect, and genuine empathy for client.

    2. Existential therapy

        a. This talk therapy focuses on life issues of freedom, helplessness, loss, isolation, aloneness, anxiety, and death.

        b. Through psychotherapy, the client discovers his own meaning of existence.

D. Application to nursing. Humanism establishes a theoretical framework for the caring component of nursing.

    1. Nurse-client relationship is based on positive regard, respect, and empathy.

    2. It is essential for the nurse to analyze herself when working with the psychiatric client.

    3. The nurse assesses the spiritual aspects of the client, including beliefs and values about spirituality or religion, the meaning of one's life, and the meaning of suffering and painful experiences; relationship with a higher being; connection with people, society, and nature; and the importance placed on values such as truth, beauty, love, tolerance, patience, and forgiveness.

4. Through reflective listening and empathic responses, the nurse helps the client gain self-understanding.

5. The nurse advocates the client's freedom to choose alternatives of behaviors in congruence with beliefs about the meaning and value of one's life.

STUDY QUESTIONS

1. A nurse is teaching a client with schizophrenia and his family about treatment for the chemical imbalance associated with this disease. Which of the following neurotransmitters would the nurse identify as being the target for antipsychotic medications?
   (1) acetylcholine
   ✓(2) dopamine
   (3) norepinephrine
   · (4) serotonin

2. A nurse is reviewing the laboratory findings of a client being treated for depression. In which of the following hormones will the nurse look for evidence of alteration?
   (1) testosterone
   (2) insulin
   (3) parathyroid hormone
   ✓(4) thyroid hormone

3. A client diagnosed with cancer does not talk about or acknowledge the diagnosis. Which of the following defense mechanisms is this client using?
   ✓(1) denial
   (2) identification
   (3) projection
   (4) rationalization

4. In planning care for a client, the nurse identifies privileges (eg, telephone privileges, participation in recreational activities) to be used as rewards for desirable behavior. These privileges serve as
   (1) an extinctive response
   (2) operant conditioning
   (3) a behavioral technique
   ✓(4) a positive reinforcer

5. A nurse listens carefully to a client talk about choices and responsibilities in life, and then encourages value clarification of choices to be made. The client discusses the meaning of life in accordance with spiritual values. Which conceptual framework is being used by the nurse?
   (1) behavioral framework
   ✓(2) humanistic framework
   (3) psychodynamic framework
   (4) psychobiologic framework

6. During an assessment, a client tells the nurse, "I don't know what to do. My marriage is terrible, and I just got fired from my job." Which of the following is a client-centered response?
   (1) "Your thoughts are negative right now and this keeps you from making decisions."
   ✓(2) "Things in your life are not working well now and you feel unsure about what to do."
   (3) "Have you considered marriage counseling? Many people have benefitted from this."
   (4) "Other people have difficulties too. Have you thought about joining a support group?"

7. Following Erikson's theory, assessment of an adolescent client for age-appropriate development task work is conducted by asking questions about
   (1) ability to complete tasks
   (2) development of an intimate relationship
   (3) level of trust in others
   ✓(4) self-identity

8. According to Piaget's theory, which of the following is the typical age in which children would be able to participate in a group discussion about the concept of self-esteem?
   (1) 6 to 7 years of age
   (2) 4 to 5 years of age
   (3) 8 to 10 years of age
   ✓(4) 12 to 14 years of age

9. A primary nurse encourages a client to record her ongoing thoughts in a daily diary. The nurse then reviews the diary with the client to identify thought patterns that contribute to feelings of depression and anxiety. Which of the following conceptual frameworks is the nurse using?
   (1) behavioral
   ✓ (2) cognitive
   (3) interpersonal
   (4) psychodynamic

10. A client in a homeless shelter had his possessions stolen while sleeping and now has neither shoes that fit nor a winter coat. The client is well known to the community nurse as having a persistent mental illness, and he tells the nurse that the theft is proof of a FBI plot against him. Which of the following is the priority nursing intervention?
    (1) Discuss the client's feelings about loss.
    (2) Encourage the client to interact with other residents.

    ✓ (3) Obtain appropriate clothing for the client.
    (4) Refer the client for outpatient treatment.

11. A person released from prison for selling narcotics has been rehabilitated and now works for a youth drug prevention agency. This person's current behavior reflects which of the following defense mechanisms?
    (1) denial
    (2) displacement
    (3) identification
    ✓ (4) sublimation

12. A client tells a nurse that because she failed an important test in school, she will never have an opportunity for a good job. Using cognitive theory, the nurse would identify the client's misperception as
    (1) dichotomous thinking
    (2) minimization
    ✓ (3) overgeneralization
    (4) reaction formation

ANSWER KEY

1. The answer is (2). The neurotransmitter dopamine is associated with schizophrenia. In general, antipsychotic medications will block receptor sites for this chemical. The remaining answer choice options are all neurotransmitters, but they are not the targets for antipsychotic medications.

2. The answer is (4). Research has shown that decreased functioning of the thyroid gland is associated with depression. The other hormones have not been associated with depression.

3. The answer is (1). The failure to acknowledge the reality of the diagnosis is an example of the defense mechanism of denial. The other defense mechanisms do not apply to this situation.

4. The answer is (4). In behavioral theory, the use of rewards for desirable behaviors will reinforce those behaviors. The stated examples are positive reinforcers. Extinction refers to stopping undesirable behavior by withholding reinforcers. Operant conditioning is the process used in behavioral change, not the particular reward system. The use of rewards is a behavioral technique; however, this response is not specific enough to answer the question.

5. The answer is (2). Humanistic framework focuses on individual choice and responsibility. Using this framework, the nurse provided client-centered care.

6. The answer is (2). Client-centered responses are based on active listening techniques. In this example, the nurse reflects what the client said. Client-centered responses help the client attain greater self-understanding. The response in **(1)** is incorrect because the nurse is focusing on the client's cognitive processes. The responses in **(3)** and **(4)** are incorrect, because the nurse is ignoring the client's feelings by suggesting that the client discuss them with someone else.

7. The answer is (4). The developmental task of the adolescent is identity versus role diffusion. The nurse is assessing the client's sense of identity by asking how the client views him or herself. Questions relating to **(1)**, **(2)**, and **(3)** would assess other developmental tasks, prior to adolescence **(1, 3)** and the young adult period **(2)**.

8. The answer is (4). Self-esteem is a concept and, according to Piaget, children develop the ability to think in a conceptual manner from 12 years of age to adulthood. The other answer choice options are incorrect because children in these age groups are developmentally unable to use abstract thinking.

9. The answer is (2). The cognitive approach is based on the idea that thoughts influence behavior and feelings. In this example, the client must first identify recurrent thought processes that are related to depression and anxiety. The behavioral approach focuses on identifying and changing particular behaviors by changing the environmental reinforcers that allow symptoms to persist. The interpersonal framework focuses on the client's relationships with significant others and the effects of these relationships on the client's behavior and symptoms. The psychodynamic framework focuses on the role of unconscious processes and the way in which these processes influence the client's behavior or symptoms.

10. The answer is (3). The client's basic needs are not met, because essential items of clothing have been taken. The nurse establishes priorities for intervention based on Maslow's theory of the hierarchy of human needs. The responses of **(1)** and **(4)** would be more appropriate following resolution of the current problem (ie, when client again has appropriate clothing). The response of **(2)** is inappropriate at this time, because the client is experiencing delusional thoughts about others.

11. The answer is (4). Sublimation is the defense mechanism whereby an individual substitutes constructive, socially acceptable behavior for strong impulses that are unacceptable. The other answer choice options are other defense mechanisms not applicable in this situation.

12. The answer is (3). The client is making a global assumption that a good job cannot be attained because of an isolated incident (ie, failing an important test). This is a common misperception as identified by cognitive theory. Answer choice options **(1)** and **(2)** are also misperceptions identified by cognitive theory, but they do not apply to the given example. Answer choice option **(4)** is a defense mechanism.

3
Stress, Anxiety, and Anxiety-Related Disorders

Overview of Stress and Anxiety

A. **Definitions**
1. **Stress** is a stimulus or situation that produces distress and creates physical and psychological demands on a person, requiring coping and adapting.
2. **Anxiety** is characterized by feelings of apprehension, uneasiness, uncertainty, or dread, resulting from real or perceived threat; anxiety is the subjective response to stress.
3. **General adaptation syndrome,** or **Selye's theory,** describes stress as wear and tear on the body occurring regardless of whether the stressor is positive or negative. The body's response is predictable without regard to the particular stressor or cause.
   a. **Alarm reaction** occurs when the sympathetic nervous system and endocrine system react to stress ([eg, the "fight or flight" response] Table 3-1 and Fig. 3-1).
   b. The **stages of resistance** are adaptive responses that attempt to limit the damage of stress.
   c. The **stage of exhaustion** is when physiologic and psychological resources are depleted and the immune system becomes depressed.
B. **Concepts.** Stress and anxiety can motivate and challenge a person as well as cause distress.
1. Both positive and negative transition and changes can be source of stress.
2. **Holmes and Rahe (1967)** developed a numerical scale ranking stressful life events and the amount of distress they cause. According to their research, the greater the number of stressful life events over a given period of time, the more likely the individual is to develop physical or mental illness.
3. Anxiety occurs in degrees of increasing intensity that can affect an individual's ability to function (Fig. 3-2).
4. In the *Diagnostic and Statistical Manual of Mental Disorders,* 4th edition (DSM-IV), psychosocial stressors are rated in terms of severity on Axis IV of the multiaxial system of diagnosing mental illness.
5. A person's response to stress and anxiety depends on, but is not limited to, the following factors:
   a. Age, developmental maturity, or both
   b. Physical and mental health status

TABLE 3-1
Components of the "Fight or Flight" Response

BODY PART OR SYSTEM	ADAPTATION TO STRESS
Hypothalamus	Sympathetic nervous system (SNS) stimulated
SNS	Adrenal medulla stimulated
Adrenal medulla	Epinephrine and norepinephrine released
Eyes	Pupils dilate
Lacrimal glands	Tear secretion increases
Respiratory system	Bronchioles and pulmonary blood vessels dilate; respiratory rate increases
Cardiovascular system	Force of cardiac contraction increases
	Cardiac output increases
	Heart rate increases
	Blood pressure increases
Gastrointestinal system	Gastric motility (stomach and intestines) decreases
	Secretions decrease
	Sphincters contract
Liver	Glycogenolysis (glucose breakdown) and gluconeogenesis (glucose manufactured from other body substances increase)
	Glycogen synthesis decreases
Urinary tract	Ureter motility increases
	Bladder muscle contracts
	Bladder sphincter relaxes
Sweat glands	Secretion increases
Fat cells	Lipolysis initiated

    c. Genetic predisposition (ie, increased sensitivity to stress)
    d. Perceived meaning (stress can be viewed as harmful, threatening, or challenging)
    e. Cultural and spiritual values
    f. Social and environmental supports
    g. Learned coping responses (Display 3-1)

C. Psychobiologic aspects of stress and anxiety

    1. The neurobiologic brain changes involved in the alarm phase of the "fight or flight" response (stimulation of the hypothalamic-pituitary axis) result in cardiovascular, neuromuscular, gastrointestinal, and respiratory system effects (see Table 3-1). The individual is likely to complain of symptoms of tachycardia, headache, diarrhea, nausea, tachypnea.

    2. Neurotransmitter alterations in the brain, especially in the limbic system, have been implicated in stress, anxiety, and some anxiety-related disorders.

        a. **Gamma-aminobutyric acid (GABA)** is an inhibitory neurotransmitter associated with the relaxation response. Because medications used to treat anxiety enhance GABA, it is theorized that a relative deficiency or imbalance in GABA is directly related to the experience of anxiety.

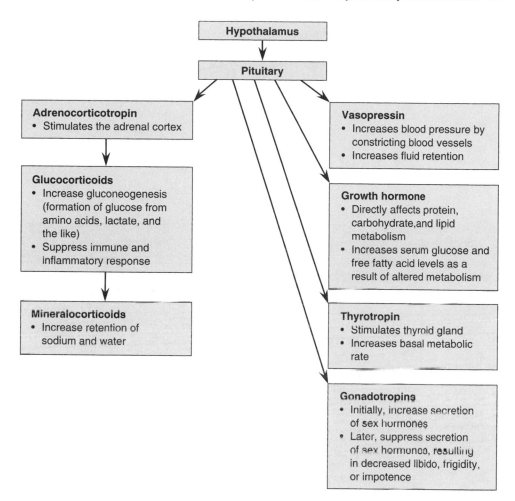

FIGURE 3-1
Components of sustained-stress response. When a continuing "fight or flight" response becomes a sustained-stress response, the whole body is affected. The hypothalamus stimulates the pituitary gland, which in turn directs the release of various hormones, including adreno-corticotropin, which stimulates the adrenal cortex: vasopressin, growth hormone, thyrotropin, and gonadotropins.

    b. **Serotonin** is a complex neurotransmitter associated with many aspects of brain functioning. Deficits or imbalance of serotonin in the amygdala are thought to be significant in anxiety and anxiety-related disorders.

    c. **Norepinephrine** is an excitatory neurotransmitter responsible for cardiovascular changes in stress and anxiety. The "noradrenergic dysregulation" theory implicates norepinephrine systems as either overactive or underactive in areas of the brain associated with anxiety (Glod, 1998).

  3. Kagan (1996) hypothesizes that biologic differences in some individuals can lead to an overly active stress response (ie, overproduction of hormones and neurotransmitters involved in the stress response).

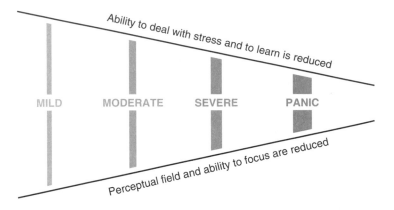

Anxiety Level	Effects	Nursing Interventions
Mild	Increased alertness; enhanced learning	Use cognitive strategies, stress-management education, and problem-solving approach
Moderate	Ability to focus on central concerns; difficulty staying attentive and being able to learn	Use relaxation techniques; assist in using problem solving approaches; teach about coping strategies; encourage verbalization of feelings
Severe	Inability to focus or problem solve; sympathetic nervous system activated	Encourage physical activity to stimulate large muscle groups and to release energy from "fight-flight" response: structured tasks or exercise useful
Panic	Complete inability to focus; disintegrated ability to cope; physiological symptoms from "fight-flight" response	Decrease environmental stimuli; stay with client; using quiet voice, assist client to perform relaxation breathing

FIGURE 3-2
Some effects of anxiety and descriptions of the four levels of anxiety.

4. **Genetic studies** have validated increased susceptibility to certain anxiety-related disorders in families.
D. **Psychological influences on stress response.** Four psychological variables are proposed as affecting the physiologic mechanisms of the stress response.
1. **Control:** the belief that one has some control over stressors can lessen the intensity of the stress response.
2. **Predictability:** stressors that can be predicted lessen the impact of the stress response as compared with the response to unpredictable stressors.
3. **Perception:** an individual's view of the world and perception of the current stressor either increases or decreases the intensity of the stress response.

DISPLAY 3-1. **Coping Strategies for Stress Reduction**

- Seek out a supportive person.
- Strive for self-discipline and perseverence.
- Vent strong emotions.
- Think through one's options and use problem-solving techniques.
- Perform physical activities and exercise to release energy.
- Use relaxation techniques, such as:
    Listening to music
    Taking warm showers or baths
    Meditating
    Performing imagery or visualization exercises
    Using progressive muscle relaxation techniques

---

4. **Coping responses:** the availability and effectiveness of anxiety-binding (ie, defense or coping) mechanisms may increase or decrease the stress response (Papero, 1997).

E. **Psychosocial theories of stress and anxiety**
   1. **Psychodynamic theory.** The unconscious conflicts resulting from repressed wishes and drives cause guilt and shame, which lead to anxiety. Anxiety threatens the ego, and protective defense mechanisms are used to respond to this threat.
   2. **Interpersonal theory.** Early interpersonal relationships directly affect development of self-concept and self-esteem. Individuals with poor self-concept and decreased self-esteem are more susceptible to anxiety and anxiety-related disorders.
   3. **Behavioral theory.** Anxiety is a conditioned response to internal and external stressors.
   4. **Cognitive theory.** The subjective feeling of anxiety is directly related to an individual's thoughts about oneself, one's future, and the world. Faulty cognitive patterns can lead to misperceptions about the meaning of events (and therefore cause anxiety).
   5. **Humanistic theory.** Anxiety is related to the loss of meaning in one's life.

II. **NURSING PROCESS OVERVIEW FOR Stress and Anxiety**

A. **Assessment**
   1. Review the client's **history** for precipitating stressors.
    2. **Note the physiologic symptoms of the client's anxiety (see Table 3-1).**
   3. **Determine the client's degree of anxiety (on a scale from mild to panic level; see Fig. 3-2). Ask the client to rate her subjective experience of anxiety on a scale of 1 to 10 (10 being the highest level of anxiety).**

    4. **Determine the client's cognitive responses,** including her belief about the degree of control she has, her perception of stressors, and her ability to concentrate and make decisions.

    5. **Observe the behaviors** typically noted in anxiety states, including irritability and anger, restlessness and pacing, crying and sighing, and complaints of tension and nervousness.

    6. **Determine the impact of the client's distress on her family,** including the family's involvement with the client, the quality of family relationships, and the level of support the family provides to the client.

    7. **Determine client's use of coping strategies** (see Display 3-1).

B. Nursing diagnoses

    1. Analyze the internal and external stressors affecting the client, and analyze the effectiveness of the client's coping strategies and defense mechanisms. (See Chapter 2, Table 2-1.)

    2. Establish an individualized nursing diagnosis for the client, the client's family, or both:

       a. Adjustment, impaired

       b. Anxiety

       c. Coping, ineffective individual

       d. Coping, ineffective family: compromised

       e. Decisional conflict (specify)

       f. Sleep pattern disturbance

       g. Violence, risk for: self-directed or directed at others

C. Planning and outcome identification

    1. Work with the client, the client's family, or both to set realistic goals.

    2. Establish desired outcome criteria, which are measures that can be used to evaluate the client's improvement as a result of nursing interventions and the client's independent change in thinking, feeling, or behaving.

       a. Acknowledge the presence of anxiety and stress.

       b. Identify the stressors causing the anxiety.

       c. Use coping strategies or learn new ones to reduce anxiety and stress.

       d. Modify thoughts and behaviors to enhance coping.

D. Implementation. The nurse assists the client in identifying precipitating stressors and teaches the client to monitor physical and psychological responses to stress (Client and Family Teaching 3-1).

    1. For a client with moderate anxiety level (see Fig. 3-2).

    2. **For a client with severe or panic anxiety level (see Fig. 3-2):**

       a. Stay with the client and provide support.

       b. Keep demands on the client to a minimum.

       c. Limit environmental stimuli (eg, turn off loud music; leave a room full of people).

       d. Encourage physical activity (eg, walking) to release energy.

       e. Administer prescribed anxiolytic medications in a timely manner.

       f. Assist the client in performing relaxation breathing techniques.

    3. **Other nursing implementations**

       a. Encourage the client to limit caffeine and nicotine intake.

CLIENT AND FAMILY TEACHING 3-1

Educating Families Who Have a Member With an Anxiety Disorder

- Anxiety-related disorders have both physical (brain chemical) and psychological causes (experience of stressful life events).
- The person with an anxiety disorder does not have control over symptoms. Part of the treatment is to learn how to control the anxiety.
- Remaining calm when the person with anxiety is upset, fearful, and panicky is very helpful. You cannot control anyone's response but your own.
- Treatment may take time, and providing encouragement for small changes in positive directions is helpful.
- Encouraging a person with an anxiety disorder to refrain from substances such as caffeine, nicotine, and alcohol can help reduce feelings of anxiety.
- Maintain your own normal life-style and functioning; giving up things you normally do in order to decrease the person's anxiety will create resentment.
- Learn about any medications used in treatment along with your family member.

b. Promote sleep with comfort measures (eg, warm bath, music, back rub).
c. **Protect the client from impulsive acts with one-to-one supervision.**
d. Facilitate the client's expression of her feelings through active listening and empathic responses.
e. Provide the client with information regarding community support systems, such as crisis hotline numbers, referral to a mental health center, self-help groups, and stress management clinics and programs.
f. Teach the client, the client's family, or both about prescribed medications, including the reason for use, dosage, times to take, measures to counteract minor side effects, side effects that require notification of health care provider, and what to do if dosage is missed.

E. Outcome evaluation. The client is evaluated to determine if established outcome criteria have been met as a result of nursing intervention.

1. The client recognizes and verbalizes her feelings of anxiety.
2. The client identifies the stressors causing anxiety.
3. The client reports a reduction in anxiety, an increased ability to cope, or both.
4. The client modifies his behaviors to enhance coping.

III. Anxiety-Related Disorders

A. Overview. Anxiety disorders are the most common of all psychiatric disorders. They cause an individual to feel frightened, distressed, and uneasy without a specific cause (ie, the specific stressor[s] may be out of the client's conscious awareness and therefore the client attributes uneasy feelings to "bad nerves").

1. More than 23 million people in the United States are afflicted with anxiety disorders yearly (approximately 1 out of every 4 persons). An individual with an anxiety disorder experiences the physiologic, cognitive, and behavioral symptoms of anxiety.

    2. The DSM-IV specifies the following types of anxiety disorders:

      a. Generalized anxiety disorder

      b. Panic disorders

      c. Obsessive-compulsive disorder

      d. Phobic disorder

      e. Post-traumatic stress disorder

B. Generalized anxiety disorder. The essential feature is excessive anxiety and worry occurring more days than not for at least 6 months. Other characteristics include restlessness, feeling keyed-up or on edge, being easily fatigued, difficulty concentrating, irritability and muscle tension, and sleep disturbances (DSM-IV, 1994).

    1. Etiology. The exact etiology is not established but associated factors include:

      a. **Biologic vulnerability.** This disorder is most likely associated with neurotransmitter abnormalities (ie, GABA, serotonin, or norepinephrine dysregulation) within the limbic system.

      b. **Gender.** Women are affected twice as often as men.

      c. **Other psychiatric disorders.** There is a high comorbidity rate with other psychiatric disorders, including major depression and panic disorder.

      d. **Psychosocial factors,** such as low self-esteem, decreased tolerance for stress, and tendency toward external locus of control beliefs.

    2. Management. Treatment for this disorder generally takes place in community settings, including the primary care physician's office.

      a. **Medication.** Antianxiety medications, especially benzodiazepines, are used on a short-term basis; long-term use is not recommended because these medications cause tolerance and dependence. Nonbenzodiazapine antianxiety medication, such as buspirone (BuSpar) and various antidepressants, are also used (Drug Chart 3-1).

      b. **Cognitive-behavioral therapy,** including relaxation training and biofeedback, is recommended. Other cognitive techniques (eg, questioning evidence, examining alternatives, reframing) are also useful (see Chapter 2).

C. Panic disorder is characterized by panic attacks that recur at unpredictable times, with intense apprehension, fear, and terror (Display 3-2).

    1. Types

      a. **Panic disorder without agoraphobia** is characterized by recurrent, unexpected panic attacks followed by at least 1 month of persistent concern about having another attack, worry about the possible implications or consequences of the attack, or a significant behavioral change related to the attack (DSM-IV, 1994).

      b. **Panic disorder with agoraphobia** is characterized by recurrent, unexpected panic attacks along with agoraphobia; that is, anxiety about being in places or situations from which escape might be difficult or embarrassing, or in which help may not be available in the event of having panic-like symptoms (DSM-IV, 1994).

    2. Etiology. The exact etiology is not established but associated factors include:

      a. **Biologic vulnerability,** resulting from irregularities in synthesis and release of norepinephrine, receptor hypersensitivity to serotonin or GABA, or both.

DRUG CHART 3-1. **Selected Medications Used for Clients with Anxiety Disorders**

Classification	Generic/ Trade Name	Adult Dosage* (mg/day)	Rationale for Use
Benzodiazapines	Alprazolam (Xanax) Clonazepam (Klonopin) Lorazepam (Ativan) Chlordiazepoxide (Librium)	0.25–1.5 0.5–6 0.5–2 5–25	Increases levels of GABA, which will decrease stimulation of limbic system, therefore decreasing anxiety. Used for *short-term* treatment of generalized anxiety disorder, panic disorder, social phobia.
Azapirones	Buspirone (BuSpar)	5–15	Acts on serotonin receptors, causing presynaptic neurons to release less serotonin. Decreased serotonin is thought to lead to decreased anxiety. Used for generalized anxiety disorder, panic disorder, social phobia.
Tricyclic antidepressants	Imipramine (Tofranil) Clomipramine (Anafranil)	75–300	Blocks reuptake of neurotransmitters (serotonin and norepinephrine), thus allowing increased levels at synapse. Deficits of serotonin in amygdala thought to be significant in anxiety disorders. Used for generalized anxiety disorder, panic disorder, social phobia, and for OCD.
Selective serotonin reuptake inhibitors	Paroxetine (Paxil) Fluoxetine (Prozac) Fluvoxamine (Luvox) Sertraline (Zoloft)	20–50 20–80 100–300 50–150	Selectively blocks serotonin reuptake at synapse, therefore increasing serotonin levels. Used for panic disorder (Paxil) and OCD.
Monoamine oxidase inhibitors	Phenelzine (Nardil)	45–90	Inhibits action of enzyme (monoamine oxidase) which breaks down serotonin, therefore increasing serotonin levels. Used for panic disorders, agoraphobia.
Beta blockers	Atenolol (Tenormin) Propranolol (Inderal)	50–100 80–240	Induces peripheral beta-adrenergic blockade, therefore reducing physiologic effects of anxiety. Used for social phobia, PTSD.

*These doses are usual adult dosage for a single dose of the drug. They are not usual daily dosage. The usual daily doses are included in Chapter 15
GABA = gamma-aminobutyric acid; OCD = obsessive-compulsive disorder; PTSD = post-traumatic stress disorder.

b. **Lactate sensitivity.** The chemical sodium lactate can produce physical symptoms associated with panic in about 4 out of 5 people with panic disorder, but only 1 out of 5 people in the general population; this sensitivity is often found in family members of people with panic disorder (Brown, 1996).

DISPLAY 3-2. **Characteristics of Panic Attacks**

- Physiologic symptoms of "fight-flight" response
    Racing heart
    Chest pains
    Dizziness and nausea
    Difficulty breathing
    Choking sensations
    Numbness and tingling sensations
    Trembling and diaphoresis
- Feeling that one is having a heart attack
- Feeling that one is "going crazy"
- Fear of loss of control
- Decreased perceptual ability
- Decreased cognitive abilities

---

    c. **Suffocation alarm theory** relates to rapid, heavy breathing (hyperventilation) that occurs during panic attacks. An individual with panic disorder may be receiving a false signal from the brain that there is a shortage of oxygen or an increase in carbon dioxide, triggering the panic attack (Brown, 1996).

    d. **Mitral valve prolapse.** Women with mitral valve prolapse have increased incidence of panic disorder. Both disorders appear to have a genetic basis (Brown, 1996).

    e. **Family history.** Individuals with a family history of panic disorders are 4 to 7 times more likely to develop this disorder.

    f. **Psychosocial factors,** including stressful life events and faulty thinking in such a way that normal bodily reactions are interpreted as catastrophic.

3. Management. The initial panic attack often is treated in the emergency department, because the individual may think she is having a heart attack. Other medical conditions must be ruled out before diagnosis of panic disorder is made.

    a. **Medication.** Antianxiety medications, such as benzodiazepines and buspirone, are used. Antidepressants, especially tricyclic antidepressants, have been validated as effective in treating panic disorder. The Food and Drug Administration (FDA) recently approved use of the selective serotonin reuptake inhibitors (SSRIs) paroxetine (Paxil) and sertraline (Zoloft) in treatment of panic disorder (see Drug Chart 3-1). Although monoamine oxidase inhibitors can be used, they require dietary restrictions (see Chapter 15).

    b. **Cognitive-behavioral therapy** targets the panic-generating thought process and behaviors that originate and maintain anxiety-laden symptoms. Specific techniques include client education and awareness, cognitive restructuring, and controlled relaxation breathing.

D. Obsessive compulsive disorder (OCD). The essential features are recurrent obsessions (persistent ideas) or compulsions (uncontrollable urge to perform an act repetitively) that are severe enough to be time consuming, cause marked distress, or lead to significant impairment in functioning (DSM-IV, 1994) (Display 3-3). The disorder often begins in childhood and adolescence.

1. **Etiology.** The exact etiology is not established but associated factors include:
   a. **Biologic vulnerability** associated with an increased serotonin responsiveness. This theory is validated by the success of antidepressant medications (both tricyclic antidepressants and the SSRIs) in treatment of OCD.
   b. **Striatum dysfunction theory.** The striatum is the part of the brain controlling voluntary movement. Repetitive motor acts, such as walking and chewing, stimulate release of serotonin, which in turn elevates mood. Individuals with OCD may be doing repetitive rituals to "self-medicate" for their serotonin deficiency.
   c. **Genetic vulnerability.** Risk is increased for an individual with family history of OCD.
2. **Management.** Once established, OCD tends to recur; many individuals experience increased symptoms associated with stressful events.
   a. **Medication.** Antidepressants, especially the tricyclic antidepressants (eg, clomipramine [Anafranil]) have been used for many years. Recently, the SSRIs fluvoxamine (Luvox), fluoxetine (Prozac), sertraline (Zoloft), and paroxetine (Paxil) have been recommended (see Drug Chart 3-1).
   b. **Cognitive-behavioral therapy** includes behavioral techniques, such as flooding and response prevention (ie, putting the individual in situations that usually trigger OCD behaviors and then preventing OCD response). Cognitive techniques also are used, in which cognitive distortions are identified and then restructured through psychoeducation.

DISPLAY 3-3. **Characteristics of Obsessive Compulsive Disorders**

- Obsessions and compulsions commonly occur together.
  The most common obsessions are repeated thoughts about contamination, repeated doubts, a need to have things in particular order, aggressive or horrific impulses, and sexual imagery.
  Most common compulsions involve washing and cleaning, counting, checking, requesting or demanding assurances, repeating actions, and ordering.
- The individual is aware of the unrealistic, intrusive, and inappropriate nature of obsessions and compulsions (described as ego-dystonic symptoms).
- Attempt to resist obsessive thought or compulsive behavior causes individual to experience increased anxiety.
- Indulgence in obsessive thoughts and performance of compulsive behaviors causes temporary anxiety relief (termed *primary gain*).

E. Phobic disorder. The essential feature is an irrational fear of a specific object, activity, or event (Display 3-4). Individuals may have panic attacks or severe anxiety when exposed to these situations or objects.

   1. Etiology. The exact etiology is not established but associated factors include:
      a. **Genetic susceptibility.** Twin studies suggest phobias have genetic factors.
      b. **Conditioned response.** Behavioral theory suggests that a phobia results from a conditioned response in which an individual learns to associate a phobic object with uncomfortable feelings; avoidance behaviors serve to reduce anxiety and reinforce the phobia.

   2. Management
      a. **In general, medications are not used to treat specific phobias.** Social phobia can be treated with benzodiazepines, certain antidepressants, and beta blockers (see Drug Chart 3-1).
      b. **Cognitive-behavioral techniques** are effective. Systematic desensitization is used; the individual learns the relaxation response, establishes a hierarchy of phobic situations, and then gradually is exposed to each situation while maintaining the relaxation response. Cognitive restructuring techniques are also useful to change the client's perception of phobic situations.

F. Post-traumatic stress disorder (PTSD). The essential feature is recurrent thoughts and feelings associated with severe, specific trauma (eg, combat experiences, rape, serious accident, severe deprivation or abuse) (Display 3-5).

   1. Etiology
      a. **There is a direct relationship between severe trauma and risk of PTSD.** The lifetime rate of this disorder in male veterans is 31%.
      b. **Psychosocial risk factors** can increase vulnerability to PTSD following severe trauma. These factors include separation from parents during childhood; family history of anxiety disorders; and pre-existing anxiety, or depression, or both.

   2. Management
      a. **Medication. Antianxiety medications, specifically benzodiazepines, are used cautiously because of risk for abuse or dependency. Antidepressants are used to treat coexisting depressive disorders. Beta blockers can be used to reduce the physiologic effects of anxiety (see Drug Chart 3-1).**

DISPLAY 3-4. **Characteristics of Phobic Disoder**

- Irrational fear of an object, person, or situation; the fear is accompanied by persistent avoidance of the object, person, or situation.
- Individual recognizes the fear as irrational and inappropriate (ego dystonic) but feels powerless to control it.
- *Simple phobia* is the fear of specific things (eg, elevators, airplanes, heights, insects).
- *Social phobia* is the fear of potentially embarrassing social situations (eg, the fear of eating or speaking in public or of using public rest rooms).

DISPLAY 3-5. **Characteristics of Post-traumatic Stress Disorder**

- Can be acute or delayed response; can also become chronic.
- Symptoms include an exaggerated startle response, sleep disorders, guilt (survivor's guilt), nightmares and flashbacks, anger with numbing of other emotions.
- Affected individuals often use drugs, alcohol, or both to self-medicate for distressful symptoms.

---

      b. **Cognitive-behavioral therapy** is used, especially cognitive restructuring to assist the individual to view self as survivor rather than victim.
      c. **Support group therapy,** especially with individuals who have experienced similar traumas (eg, combat veteran groups, rape trauma groups), is also used.

G. **Dissociative disorders.** The essential feature is an alteration in conscious awareness, which includes periods of forgetfulness, memory loss for past stressful events, feeling disconnected from daily events, or emergence of distinctly different personalities. Display 3-6 lists the subtypes of this disorder.

  1. Etiology
      a. **Trauma.** Dissociative disorders are generally associated with traumatic events. An individual reacts to trauma by "splitting off," or dissociating self, from the memory of the trauma.
      b. **Abuse.** Dissociative identity disorder is generally thought to result from severe, traumatic abuse in early childhood. There is a high comorbidity rate with substance abuse and depressive disorders.
      c. **Sexual and physical abuse in early childhood** has been found to affect neurodevelopment, especially in the left hemisphere and the limbic system. These alterations in normal brain development are associated with problems of mood, memory, and aggressive behavior.

DISPLAY 3-6. **DSM-IV Subtypes of Dissociative Disorder**

The DSM-IV identifies five separate disorders characterized by dissociation, or the feeling of being detached from usual experiences or in a dreamlike state.

1. *Dissociative amnesia* is the sudden inability to recall important personal information.
2. *Dissociative fugue* is the sudden, unexpected flight from home with an inability to recall events from one's past.
3. *Depersonalization disorder* is feeling detached from, and as if one is an outside observer of, one's thoughts or body.
4. *Dissociative identity disorder* is the presence of two or more distinct personalities, each with its own pattern of perceiving, relating to, and thinking about the environment.
5. *Dissociative disorder not otherwise specified* is a disorder that does not fit criteria for any of the other dissociative disorders.

    d. **Gender.** Diagnosis of dissociative identity disorder is 3 to 9 times more common in women than in men.

  2. **Management.** Dissociative disorders tend to be difficult to diagnose. An individual with this disorder often has had multiple psychiatric diagnoses; therefore, treatment is often lengthy.

    a. **Medications** are generally not used except for treatment of coexisting anxiety or depressive disorders.

    b. **Psychotherapy,** especially psychodynamic therapy with hypnosis, is used to bring a conscious awareness of traumatic events and to facilitate coping with them.

    d. **Support group therapy** has been useful in providing a supportive and psychoeducational approach.

IV. NURSING PROCESS OVERVIEW FOR Anxiety-Related Disorders

A. Assessment

 1. **Note the physiologic symptoms of anxiety (see Table 3-1).**

  2. Use key nursing assessment questions for clients with anxiety-related disorders (Table 3-2).

  3. Note the client's specific cognitive-behavioral responses that are congruent with established DSM-IV diagnostic criteria of an anxiety disorder.

  4. Use standardized assessment tools for detailed information regarding a particular anxiety-related disorder (eg, Yale-Brown Obsessive-Compulsive Scale, Dissociative Experiences Scale).

  5. Review client history for past experience of anxiety-related disorders.

  6. Discuss with the client his perception of current stressors or precipitating events, and determine the client's use of coping strategies (see Box 3-1).

  7. Determine the impact of the client's disorder on the family and its functioning, including specific role changes occurring in the family, degree of involvement of the family with the client, and the level of support provided to the client; determine if there is a family history of abuse.

B. Nursing diagnoses

  1. **Analysis.** Analyze the internal and external stressors affecting the client, the impact of symptoms on normal daily functioning, and the effectiveness of coping strategies and defense mechanisms (see Chapter 2, Table 2-1).

  2. **Nursing diagnosis.** Establish individualized nursing diagnoses for the client, the family, or both (see II.B.2).

    a. Denial, ineffective

    b. Personal identity disturbance

    c. Post-trauma response

    d. Role performance, altered

    e. Self-esteem disturbance

    f. Social isolation

C. Planning and outcome identification

  1. Work with the client, the family, or both in setting realistic goals.

TABLE 3-2
Key Nursing Assessment Questions

QUESTION	PROVIDES DATA ABOUT
• Have you noticed feelings of increased tension, worry, or unease?	• Subjective feelings of anxiety
• What kind of body sensations or symptoms do you experience when you are under stress?	• Client's awareness of unique experience of stress-related body sensations
• Do you have difficulty concentrating, feel restless, or have trouble making decisions?	• Symptoms related to generalized anxiety disorder
• Have you experienced severe distress in which your heart was racing, you had difficulty breathing, and you thought you may be having a heart attack?	• Symptoms related to panic disorder
• Do you find yourself constantly having recurrent thoughts that are difficult to control or stop?	• Symptoms of obsessive thoughts or compulsive behavior, related to obsessive-compulsive disorder
• Have you ever had to perform certain rituals or behaviors over and over again in order to feel calmer?	
• Do you have severe fears of persons, places, or things that prevent you from doing things you want?	• Symptoms related to phobic disorder
• Have you experienced a severe tragedy in your life that comes back to you in dreams or flashbacks?	• Symptoms related to post-traumatic stress disorder

 2. Establish desired outcome criteria.
  a. The client can identify specific anxiety responses.
  b. The client can identify stressors related to current experience of anxiety-related disorder.
  c. The client decreases or controls repetitive thoughts and behaviors.
  d. The client verbalizes relief or decrease in anxiety-related symptoms.
  e. The client performs normal daily activities without an increase in anxiety or distressful symptoms.
  f. The client uses a variety of coping strategies to reduce anxiety.
  g. The client verbalizes experiences of traumatic events.

D. Implementation
 1. For clients with generalized anxiety disorder or panic disorders, see II.D.
 2. Clients with OCD
  a. **Convey acceptance of the client, despite ritualistic behaviors.**
  b. Allow the client time to perform rituals; anxiety will increase if the client cannot perform compulsive behaviors.
  c. Encourage limit setting on ritualistic behaviors as part of the established treatment plan.
  d. Use active listening to encourage the client to verbalize his feelings; the best time for interaction is after the client completes a ritualistic behavior.

    e. Assist the client in listing all of the objects and places that trigger anxiety as part of exposure-response prevention program.

    f. Teach the client about coping measures and the medications used as part of the treatment plan.

    g. Encourage the client to use community support systems.

3. Clients with phobic disorder

    a. **Do not force the client to be in contact with a phobic object or situation.**

    b. Help the client describe his feelings prior to a response to a phobic object.

    c. Help the client identify alternative coping strategies to manage anxiety about encountering a phobic situation.

    d. Use cognitive strategies, such as reframing, to assist the client in placing thoughts and feelings in a different perspective.

    e. Practice relaxation techniques with the client.

    f. Participate as a member of the treatment team in the established program for systematic desensitization.

    g. Teach the client about prescribed medications used in treatment.

4. Clients with PTSD

    a. Use implementations related to anxiety (eg, relaxation techniques, encouraging expression of feelings, limiting caffeine and nicotine).

    b. **Validate for the client that the traumatic event he experienced was highly stressful.**

    c. Help the client verbalize all aspects of the traumatic event, including his thoughts and feelings.

    d. **Teach the client coping strategies to manage symptoms of anxiety that accompany memories of trauma.**

    e. Encourage the client to participate in self-help or support groups.

    f. Refer the client to Alcoholics Anonymous or Narcotics Anonymous if drug or alcohol abuse is a problem.

5. Clients with dissociative disorder

    a. **Establish a trusting relationship and provide support during times of depersonalization, amnesia, or emergence of new personalities.**

    b. Encourage the client to disclose and discuss her feelings in relation to painful memories becoming conscious.

    c. **Teach the client anxiety-binding techniques when reexperienced memories threaten to overwhelm the client.**

    d. Accurately record information on various personalities as part of an interdisciplinary team approach.

    e. Encourage the client's commitment to insight-oriented therapy with an experienced therapist.

E. Outcome evaluation

    1. Client identifies own anxiety responses.

    2. Client identifies stressors in past or current life situation contributing to anxiety response.

    3. Client utilizes coping strategies rather than symptomatic behaviors.

    4. Client identifies and actively participates in continued treatment plan.

STUDY QUESTIONS

1. Selye's general adaptation theory can be used to understand the relationship between stressful events and the body's response to stress. Which of the following statements best describes this relationship?
   - ✓(1) The body goes through predictable responses regardless of the type of stressor.
   - (2) The body's defenses become depleted from stressful events.
   - (3) The body reacts differently when the stress is psychological rather than physical.
   - (4) The body eventually adapts to any stress in a positive manner.

2. A client is pacing and complains of racing thoughts. The nurse asks the client if something upsetting happened, and the client's response is vague and not focused on nurse's question. The nurse assesses the client's level of anxiety as
   - (1) mild
   - (2) moderate
   - ✓(3) severe
   - (4) panic

3. A nurse is teaching a group of clients about antianxiety medications. She would explain that benzodiazapines affect a brain chemical called
   - (1) acetylcholine
   - ✓(2) gamma-aminobutyric acid (GABA)
   - (3) norepinephrine
   - (4) serotonin

4. A nurse is assessing a client for recent stressful life events. The nurse recognizes that stressful life events are both
   - (1) desirable and growth-promoting
   - ✓(2) positive and negative
   - (3) undesirable and harmful
   - (4) predictable and controllable

5. A nurse is teaching in a stress management program for clients. Which of the following beliefs will she advocate as a method for coping with stressful life events?
   - (1) Avoidance of stress is an important goal for living.
   - ✓(2) Control over one's response to stress is possible.
   - (3) Most people have no control over their level of stress.
   - (4) Significant others are important to provide care and concern.

6. A client limits her social events to only those in which a family member of hers is also present. The client is exhibiting behavior typical of which of the following anxiety disorders?
   - ✓(1) agoraphobia
   - (2) generalized anxiety disorder
   - (3) obsessive-compulsive disorder
   - (4) post-traumatic stress disorder

7. A nurse is teaching a client recently diagnosed with diabetes how to administer insulin injections. During the lesson, the client is having difficulty concentrating, has rapid respirations, and is fidgeting in the chair. The nurse recently performed a capillary blood glucose test, and the client's blood sugar range is normal. Which of the following is the next best step for the nurse to take?
   - (1) Instruct the client that it is vital to pay attention, because insulin injections will help provide a normal life.
   - (2) Leave the client alone at this time, instructing the client to review the literature before the next lesson.

(3) Stop the insulin lesson for a while and ask the client how things are going.

(4) Tell the client to relax and that if he does so, it will be easier to learn about injections.

8. A client is newly admitted to a psychiatric unit because of severe obsessive-compulsive behavior. Which of the following initial responses would be most therapeutic for the client?

(1) The nurse being accepting of the client's ritualistic behaviors

(2) The nurse challenging the client's need for rituals

(3) The nurse expressing concern about the harmfulness of the client's rituals

(4) The nurse limiting the client's rituals that are excessive

9. A client is scheduled for surgery and the nurse assesses a severe level of preoperative anxiety. Which of the following nursing actions is the priority?

(1) Asking the client about her perceptions and concerns about the surgery

(2) Informing the surgeon about the client's anxiety level

(3) Requesting family members to come and stay with the client

(4) Teaching the client facts about upcoming preoperative and postoperative care

10. A client is treated in a mental health clinic for a phobic disorder characterized by the client's fear of riding in an airplane. The treatment method used was systematic desensitization. The nurse would evaluate the treatment and deem it successful if

(1) the client plans a trip requiring airplane travel

(2) the client rides on an airplane for a short trip

(3) the client recognizes the unrealistic nature of the fear of riding on airplanes

(4) the client verbalizes a decreased fear about airplane trips

11. A client has been prescribed clomipramine (Anafranil) for treatment of obsessive compulsive behavior. The nurse understands the rational for this treatment is that the clomipramine

(1) decreases norepinephrine levels

(2) decreases levels of GABA

(3) increases dopamine levels

(4) increases serotonin levels

12. A nurse is planning care for a client with post-traumatic stress disorder. Which of the following would the nurse initially do?

(1) Avoid discussion of the traumatic event(s).

(2) Encourage the client to verbalize thoughts and feelings about the trauma

(3) Encourage the client to put the past in proper perspective.

(4) Instruct the client to use distraction techniques to cope with flashbacks.

13. A community nurse has a weekly caseload of many different types of clients and is involved in planning care for these clients. Which of the following clients would the nurse recognize as the most vulnerable to post-traumatic stress disorders?

(1) The child with asthma who has recently failed a grade in school

(2) The college student with diabetes who experienced date rape

(3) The man who has recently lost his wife to cancer

(4) The spouse of an individual with a severe substance abuse problem

14. Which of the following is the most appropriate outcome for a client with a dissociative disorder?

(1) The client will deal with uncomfortable emotions on a conscious level.

(2) The client will modify stress with the use of relaxation techniques.

(3) The client will identify his or her anxiety responses.

(4) The client will use problem-solving strategies when feeling stressed.

ANSWER KEY

1. The answer is (1). Selye's theory states that regardless of the stressor (ie, whether it is chemical, physical, or psychological), the body's physiologic response is the same (ie, an alarm reaction). If the stress continues and the body reaches the stage of exhaustion, then defenses are depleted. Adaptation may not occur if the stage of exhaustion is reached from continued stress.

2. The answer is (3). When the client has difficulty focusing and exhibits excessive motor activity, the level of anxiety is severe. Mild anxiety is characterized by increased alertness and problem-solving ability; the client described is unable to do this. Moderate anxiety is characterized by the ability to focus on central concerns, but the inability to problem solve without assistance; the client described is unable to do this. Panic level of anxiety is characterized by complete inability to focus and reduced perceptions; the client described is not at this point.

3. The answer is (2). Antianxiety medications stimulate the neurotransmitter GABA, which is a chemical associated with relaxation. The other neurotransmitters—acetylcholine, norepinephrine, and serotonin—are not affected by benzodiazapines.

4. The answer is (2). The concept of stressful life events is based on the research of Holmes and Rahe, who found that both positive and negative changes result in stress. Stressful life events are not always desirable and growth-promoting nor are they always undesirable and harmful. Some stressful life events can be predictable and controllable; however, many events are entirely unpredictable.

5. The answer is (2). When learning to manage stress, it is helpful to believe that that one has the ability to control one's response to stress. It is impossible to avoid stress, which is a normal life experience. Stress can be positive and growth-enhancing as well as harmful. The belief that one has *some* control is the significant factor in minimizing stress response. People who do not believe this is possible will experience increased stress. Significant others are important; however, reliance on the ability of oneself to cope is essential.

6. The answer is (1). Agoraphobia is a disorder characterized by avoidance of situations in which escape may not be possible or help may be unavailable. Generalized anxiety disorder, obsessive-compulsive disorder, and post-traumatic stress disorders are anxiety disorders, but they are not typically characterized by the behavior of the client described in the question.

7. The answer is (3). Because the client's anxiety is increased, the nurse should stop the insulin injection lesson and assess what is happening. Asking an open-ended question and conveying interest may reduce the client's anxiety and elicit information about the client's current concerns. Teaching is ineffective when a client is at a severe level of anxiety. The response in answer choice **(1)** assumes the client's concerns are about having a normal life. The response in answer choice

(2) ignores the client's anxiety. A client experiencing severe anxiety is unable to focus on relaxing, and the nurse is incorrectly responding to the client's anxiety level in answer choice **(4)**.

8. The answer is (1). It is important to accept the client's need to perform ritual-istic behaviors in this situation; admission to a psychiatric unit is stressful and this client will tend to increase rituals when anxious. Although the other answer choice responses may be appropriate as part of an ongoing treatment plan, they are not appropriate for a newly admitted client.

9. The answer is (1). The nurse should attempt to assess the specific client con-cerns regarding the surgical procedure. Following assessment, the nurse can address concerns and do appropriate teaching. If client anxiety remains elevated after further assessment by the nurse and appropriate teaching, the surgeon should be informed. Requesting family members to come and stay with the client may be part of the planned intervention following further assessment. Teaching the client about upcoming preoperative and postoperative care would be done following fur-ther assessment as specific concerns are elicited.

10. The answer is (2). Systematic desensitization is a behavioral technique in which a client with a specific phobia is gradually able to work through hierarchical fears until the most fearful situation is encountered. Success for this method would involve the client doing what is most fearful—riding in an airplane. The responses in answer choices **(1)** and **(4)** may occur earlier in treatment but are not indicative of success. In general, someone who is phobic recognizes that his or her fear is dis-proportionate to the thing feared.

11. The answer is (4). According to psychobiologic theory, dysregulation of the neurotransmitter serotonin is thought to contribute to obsessive compulsive behav-ior. Clomipramine (Anafranil) is used to increase serotonin levels and therefore decrease the need for obsessive-compulsive behaviors. The other answer choices do not describe the correct rationale for use of clomipramine (Anafranil) in treating obsessive-compulsive behaviors.

12. The answer is (2). Planning care for a client with post-traumatic stress disor-der would involve helping the client verbalize thoughts and feelings about the trauma. This strategy will help the client work through the strong emotions con-nected with the trauma and therefore assist in developing the belief that one is able to cope. The traumatic event needs to be dealt with in a conscious way, including recognizing strong emotions; therefore, answer choices **(1)** and **(4)** are inappropri-ate. Answer choice **c** may be an intervention that could occur after the client is able to verbalize strong emotions related to trauma; it is inappropriate as an initial inter-vention.

13. The answer is (2). Post-traumatic stress disorder is caused by the experience of severe, specific trauma. Rape is a severely traumatic event. Although the situa-tions in answer choices **(1), (3),** and **(4)** are certainly stressful, they are not at the level of severe trauma.

14. The answer is (1). Dissociative disorders occur when a traumatic event or events are beyond a person's recall, because these memories have been "blocked" from conscious awareness. Bringing the feelings associated with these events into conscious awareness and coping with these feelings will decrease the need for dissociation. The other answer choices would be general outcomes for other anxiety-related disorders and, although helpful, are not specific for a client with a dissociative disorder.

4 The Mind–Body Continuum: Common Disorders

Overview

Mind-body disorders are characterized by both psychological and physiologic symptoms and include somatoform disorders, sexual disorders, and eating disorders.

A. **Key definitions and concepts in mind-body disorders**
 1. **Holistic theory** is the belief that illness and wellness are the result of complex interactions among physiologic, cognitive, emotional, and sociocultural factors.
 2. **Systems theory** (ie, the whole is greater than the sum of its parts) provides useful perspective for conceptualizing relationships among physiologic, cognitive, emotional, and sociocultural factors in the individual, the family, and society.
  a. A systems model attempts to define all factors that interact to produce a particular clinical syndrome. Each factor affects the others, such that behavior or activity of any one factor cannot be understood out of context from its relationship to the others.
  b. Clinical disease develops through disturbance in balance of the relationship among all factors affecting the individual (Kerr, 1997).
 3. **Common components of mind-body disorders**
  a. Physiologic changes and symptoms may be real (as in diagnosable medical illnesses) or perceived by the individual to be actual (as in somatoform disorders).
  b. **Chronic physiologic or psychological stress.** The internal physiologic environment is altered as a result of the stress response and hyperfunctioning of the hypothalamic-pituitary-adrenal axis (see Chapter 3).
  c. **Psychological distress** either precedes, accompanies, or follows body changes and symptoms.
 4. **Psychoneuroimmunology** is the scientific discipline that attempts to explain how chronic physiologic or psychological stress alters the internal physiologic environment, including changes in hormonal levels and cellular responses.
 5. **Autoimmune disorders** are diseases resulting from the body's inappropriate reaction to a stressor, which stimulates an immune reaction to one's own cells and organ systems (Table 4-1).

TABLE 4-1
Medical Conditions Affected by Stress

IMMUNOLOGIC DISORDERS	GENERAL MEDICAL CONDITIONS
AIDS	Cardiovascular disorders
Addison's disease	Hypertension
Chronic hepatitis	Angina pectoris
Graves' disease	Respiratory disorders
Insulin-dependent diabetes mellitus	Asthma
Multiple sclerosis	Chronic obstructive pulmonary disease
Myasthenia gravis	Endocrine disorders
Pernicious anemia	Thyroid disease
Rheumatoid arthritis	Premenstrual syndrome
Rheumatoid disorders	Gastrointestinal disorders
Systemic lupus erythematosus	Peptic ulcer disease
	Irritable bowel syndrome
	Musculoskeletal disorders
	Acute/chronic back pain
	Osteoporosis
	Renal disorders
	Urinary tract infections
	Renal calculi
	Neoplastic disorders (cancers)

6. **Psychological, behavior, and sociocultural factors** play a potential role in the presentation or treatment of almost every general medical condition (see Table 4-1).

B. **Psychological factors affecting general medical conditions.** This diagnostic category in the *Diagnostic and Statistical Manual of Mental Disorders,* 4th edition, (DSM-IV) describes the presence of one or more specific psychological or behavioral factors that adversely affect a general medical condition.

1. Behavioral factors can contribute additional health risks for an individual (eg, failure to quit smoking despite significant hypertension).

2. Psychological factors can precipitate or exacerbate symptoms by eliciting the stress response (eg, chest pain precipitated by emotional upset in an individual with coronary artery disease).

3. Psychological factors can interfere with treatment (eg, an individual with insulin-dependent diabetes mellitus who refuses to take insulin because of fear of injections) (DSM-IV, 1994).

C. **Etiology.** Scientific research has identified multiple physiologic, cognitive, emotional, and sociocultural factors involved in the cause of mind-body disorders.

1. **Chronic stress,** whether from internal or external stressors, plays a major role.

a. The central nervous system and immune system work as an integrated whole to maintain homeostasis in response to stress. Communication between these systems occurs via chemical messengers, such as neuro-transmitters and immunohormones called interleukins.

b. Release of neurotransmitters and hormones is related to thoughts and feelings. When chronic stress is experienced, homeostasis is upset owing to the excessive stimulation of the neurotransmitters and hormones. Bodily defenses can become depleted if stress continues and the individual is at risk for physical or mental disease.

c. Cognitive, emotional, and sociocultural stimuli are among the most potent factors activating the biologic response to stress (Fontaine, 1999).

2. Increased reactivity or failure to respond to negative feedback mechanism in the hypothalamic-pituitary-adrenal axis leads to chronic elevations of glucocorticoids. This increased reactivity can be related to several factors:

a. Continuous real threat (as in chronic abuse) or continuous perceived or imagined threat (as in persistent cognitive distortions, chronic anxiety states)

b. Genetic predisposition

c. Learned responsiveness (Jones, 1994)

D. Management of mind-body disorders

1. **Holistic approach.** Treatment includes interventions directed toward both disease-specific management and stress reduction.

2. **Stress education interventions** are based on the concept that the individual can increase control over symptoms by learning how to anticipate situations that are upsetting and use measures to reduce the degree of anxiety experienced (eg, adequate sleep, good nutrition, relaxation techniques, and planning ahead).

3. **Education.** Management involves teaching an individual about his specific disorder, causative factors, reduction of risk, and medically prescribed treatments and medications.

4. **Specific mind-body therapies** include stress management training, relaxation techniques, biofeedback with relaxation training, support and self-help groups, guided imagery, art and movement therapies, meditation, and prayer.

5. **Alternative or complementary treatments** may also be used; these may rely on self-healing capabilities in which the role of the healer is more of a facilitator (Table 4-2).

a. These methods are becoming increasingly popular as consumers take a more active role in their health management.

b. People may seek alternative therapies if traditional therapies fail to relieve their illness or symptoms.

c. The U.S. Congress established the National Center for Complementary and Alternative Medicine at the National Institutes of Health.

d. Many cultures traditionally use alternative methods based on belief systems regarding the interrelationship between mind-body-spirit. Designated roles as healers are common to many different cultures.

TABLE 4-2
Examples of Alternative or Complementary Treatments

TREATMENT	DESCRIPTION
Acupuncture	Identifies patterns of energy flow and energy blockage among 12 principal meridians, which roughly correspond to points along peripheral nervous system. Balance is restored by inserting ultrathin needles at points along these meridians.
Ayurveda	Traditional Indian system involves understanding the body in its environment. Interventions include dietary modifications, cleansing procedures, herbal supplements, and spiritual healing.
Traditional Chinese medicine	Integrates use of herbs, diet therapy, acupuncture, massage, moxibustion (application of heat), and other techniques to restore balance and harmony to life energies.
Naturopathic medicine	Focuses on prevention of illness and use of nontoxic biologic therapies (homeopathic medicine).
Chiropractic	Based on premise that the spine is the most significant factor in health. Treating misalignments of the spine by manipulation, electrical stimulation, and heat can improve health.
Herbal therapy	Rapidly growing treatment approach involves using extracts of plant materials for a variety of physical and mental illnesses (see Chapter 15).
Therapeutic touch	Based on idea that illness is imbalance of energy field of human body. Practitioners use their hands to direct energy movement.

II.   Somatoform Disorders

A. General considerations. Somatoform disorders are characterized by complaints of physical symptoms that cannot be explained by known physical mechanisms.

   1. The affected individual experiences a loss or change in physical function, and the symptoms are not under the individual's voluntary control.
   2. Somatoform disorders are characterized by primary gain (anxiety relief) and secondary gains (special attention, relief from responsibilities). These disorders are usually ego syntonic (ie, they are congruent with the individual's view of self).
   3. Significant impairment occurs in social or occupational functioning.
      a. The individual becomes totally focused on the physical symptoms, which can severely restrict activities.
      b. Symptoms often contribute to relationship problems for the affected individual.
   4. The individual generally visits multiple health care providers and may undergo exploratory and unnecessary surgical procedures.
      a. The use of multiple prescribed and over-the-counter medication is common in these patients.

b. Dependence on pain relievers or antianxiety medications can lead to substance dependence.

c. Denial of psychological distress and resistance to psychiatric treatment is also common.

B. Types of somatoform disorders

1. **Somatization disorder** is characterized by a history of multiple physical complaints without organic basis, occurring before age 30 and persisting for several years. It is generally associated with the combination of pseudoneurologic, gastrointestinal, genitourinary and sexual symptoms, and pain.

2. **Hypochondriasis** is the unrealistic fear of having a serious illness; an individual's interpretation of body symptoms is without organic basis.

3. **Body dysmorphic disorder** is a preoccupation with an imagined defect in a normal-appearing person; if the individual actually has a defect, expressed concern is excessive.

4. **Pain disorder** is chronic pain in one or more anatomic sites; a medical condition, if present, plays a minor role in accounting for the pain.

5. **Conversion disorder** is a loss of or change in physical functioning that cannot be associated with any organic cause and seems to be associated with psychosocial stressors. These disorders generally are characterized by:

   a. **Sensory dysfunction,** such as blindness, deafness, or loss of tactile sense

   b. **Motor system dysfunction,** such as aphasia, impaired coordination, paralysis, or seizure

   c. *La belle indifference,* seeming unconcern with a fairly dramatic symptom, such as being unable to walk or move a limb

C. Etiology

1. **Psychobiologic theory**

   a. The individual experiences high levels of physiologic arousal (increased awareness of somatic sensations).

   b. **Alexithymia** is deficient communication between the brain hemispheres, resulting in difficulty expressing emotions directly; therefore, distress is expressed as physical sensations.

2. **Cognitive-behavioral theory**

   a. The child learns from her parents to express anxiety through somatization; secondary gains reinforce symptoms.

   b. The individual has cognitive distortions in which benign symptoms are magnified and interpreted as serious disease.

3. **Psychoanalytic theory.** The psychological source of ego conflict is denied and finds expression through displacement of anxiety onto physical symptoms.

4. **Sociocultural factors**

   a. Incidence of somatoform disorders is higher among individuals from lower socioeconomic groups, in rural areas, or with limited education.

   b. Somatic symptoms are common in cultures that view direct expression of emotions as unacceptable.

D. Management. The mainstay of treatment is a long-term relationship with a specific health care provider to prevent the client from seeking multiple providers with multiple recommendations for testing, treatment, and medications.

    1. Avoid treatment with medications that are characterized by tolerance and dependence (eg, antianxiety agents, analgesics).

    2. Encourage psychotherapy as part of the treatment plan.

        a. Assist the individual to express conflicts and emotions verbally.

        b. Focus on the individual's underlying psychosocial needs.

    3. Family education. Teach family members to avoid reinforcing secondary gains from symptoms.

    4. Encourage the client to participate in community-based self-help groups (eg, Recovery, Inc., encourages individuals to learn to control distressing symptoms through specific techniques and group support).

III. Sexual Disorders

A. General considerations

    1. Human sexuality includes gender identity (ie, the sense of maleness or femaleness) as well as desire for contact, warmth, tenderness, and love.

    2. Sexual health includes integration of somatic, intellectual, and social aspects of sexual being.

    3. Sexual expression is influenced by a variety of factors, including:

        a. Age, health status, and physical attributes

        b. Cultural, social, and religious views

        c. Environment and personal choice of sexual partner as result of personality development

    4. Normal sexual behavior is a sexual act between consenting adults, lacking force, performed in a private setting in the absence of unwilling observers. Sexual activity is legally unacceptable when it involves nonconsenting individuals, a child, or use of objects in such a way that bring physical or psychological harm to one of the partners.

    5. The **sexual response cycle** includes phases of desire, excitement, orgasm, and resolution.

B. Types of sexual disorders

    1. Sexual dysfunctions are characterized by a disturbance in the sexual response cycle or by pain associated with sexual intercourse.

        a. **Sexual desire disorders.** An individual has little or no sexual desire or an aversion to sexual contact.

        b. **Sexual arousal disorders.** An individual cannot maintain physiologic requirements for sexual intercourse (eg, in men, erectile dysfunction; in women, difficulty with lubrication response).

        c. **Orgasmic disorders.** An individual is unable to achieve orgasm.

        d. **Sexual pain disorders.** An individual experiences pain before, during, or after sexual intercourse.

e. **Sexual dysfunction due to general medical condition.** Evidence from history, physical examination, or laboratory and diagnostic study findings that the dysfunction is due to a direct physiologic effect from medical condition.

2. **Paraphilias.** Unusual or bizarre sexual acts or imagery are used to achieve sexual excitement. The individual with a paraphilia may prefer to use non-human objects.

   a. With a paraphilia, sexual activity with humans may involve real or simulated suffering (eg, sadism or masochism).

   b. The activity may involve children or other nonconsenting persons (eg, pedophilia).

   c. **Specific paraphilias** include fetishism, transvestism, zoophilia, pedophilia, exhibitionism, voyeurism, sexual masochism, sexual sadism.

3. **Gender identity disturbance.** An individual has a sense of discomfort and inappropriateness about his or her anatomic gender and wishes to be of the other sex.

C. **Etiology**

1. **Sexual dysfunctions**

   a. **Biologic factors** include altered levels of testosterone and serum prolactin; medical illness (eg, diabetes mellitus and vascular insufficiency can cause orgasmic dysfunction); and medication (eg, antihypertensive, antipsychotic, antidepressant, antianxiety, and anticonvulsant agents, or substance abuse).

   b. **Cognitive-behavioral theory.** Strongly negative emotions become associated with sexual activity.

2. **Paraphilias**

   a. **Biologic factors.** Possible destruction of parts of limbic system and temporal lobe disorders may be contributing factors to paraphilias, although evidence is inconclusive at this time.

   b. **System theory.** According to this theory, paraphilias are the result of multiple interrelated factors, including genetics, past learning, and stress, as well as physiologic, psychological, and sociocultural factors.

3. **Gender identity disorders**

   a. **Biologic factors.** Clients with gender identity disorders may have an abnormality in the temporal lobe, although studies are inconclusive.

   b. **Cognitive-behavioral theory.** According to this theory, the influence of social learning on gender development in childhood or parental dynamics that encourage identity with non–gender-based sex role may contribute.

D. **Management.** Treatment of gender identity disorders includes extensive evaluation of the specific problem and relationship dynamics coupled with education and supportive psychotherapy.

1. **Community-based treatment** that involves assessment and treatment of physiologic and psychosocial aspects is used.

2. **Cognitive-behavioral therapy** attempts to change an individual's thoughts and uses practice exercises to improve sexual activities.

3. Specialized training in **sex therapy** is advocated for professionals treating sexual disorders. The American Association of Sex Educators, Counselors, and Therapists (AASECT) provides training for certification.

IV. Eating Disorders

A. **General considerations.** Eating disorders are characterized by severe disturbances in eating behavior.

1. **Definitions**
   a. **Anorexia nervosa** is characterized by refusal to maintain minimally normal weight.
   b. **Bulimia nervosa** is characterized by repeated episodes of binge eating, followed by purging behaviors (DSM-IV, 1994).

2. Anorexia and bulimia are not diseases, but syndromes with multiple predisposing factors and a variety of characteristics (Fontaine, 1994).
   a. An individual can demonstrate symptoms of both disorders, or can revert from one to the other.
   b. Although eating disorders can exist in males, more than 90% of individuals with eating disorders are female.
   c. Onset generally is during adolescence (13 to 17 years of age).

3. **Cognitive distortions** are common among individuals with eating disorders.
   a. **Selective abstraction:** "I'm still too fat, see my big hands and my big feet."
   b. **Overgeneralization:** "Only thin people get ahead in life."
   c. **Magnification:** "If I gain 2 pounds I'll never get on the varsity team."
   d. **Superstitious thinking:** "If I gain weight, my boyfriend will leave me."
   e. **Dichotomous thinking:** "I'm not thin, I'm fat."

4. Eating disorders are a serious health problem that can cause death. The mortality rate in affected individuals is 10% to 15%, and the risk for suicide is increased (especially when the client also has a depressive disorder).

5. Eating disorders frequently coexist with other psychiatric disorders, including depression, social phobia, obsessive-compulsive disorder, panic disorder, and substance abuse.

6. Anorexia nervosa is an ego-syntonic disorder (ie, the individual views her behaviors as congruent with her self-image). Bulimia nervosa is an ego-dystonic disorder (ie, the individual views her behaviors as shameful or negative and incongruent with her self-image).

B. **Features and symptoms.** The characteristic features of anorexia nervosa and bulimia nervosa are listed in Table 4-3. Physical symptoms of both disorders are listed in Table 4-4.

C. **Etiology**

1. **Biologic theory**
   a. **Anorexia.** Changes in central nervous system pathways involving the neurotransmitters norepinephrine, dopamine, and serotonin may contribute.

TABLE 4-3
Features of Eating Disorders

Anorexia Nervosa
- Individual's weight is less than 85% of normal for age and height.
- Although underweight, individual has intense fear of becoming fat
- Body image disturbance (self-image related to weight)
- Strenuous exercising and peculiar food-handling patterns
- Lack of sense of control or competence in any area of life besides weight control
- Physical symptoms (see Table 4-4)

Bulimia Nervosa
- *Binge eating:* consuming enormous quantities of food in one continuous time period; anxiety often triggers binge
- *Purging:* compensatory behaviors to rid self of food and prevent weight gain. These behaviors include self-induced vomiting or misuse of laxatives, diuretics, enemas, or other medications or substances (eg, syrup of ipecac).
- Fasting or excessive exercise
- Binges commonly lead to feelings of loss of control, guilt, humiliation, and self-loathing
- Physical symptoms (see Table 4-4)

    b. **Bulimia.** Serotonin irregularities, especially in the hypothalamus where feelings of satiety are controlled, may contribute.

    c. **Research** about neurotransmitter irregularities is ongoing, although it is difficult to determine whether physiochemical changes precede, accompany, or follow behavior problems.

    d. **Genetics.** Relatives of individuals with eating disorders are 4 to 5 times more likely than the general population to have an eating disorder.

  2. Cognitive-behavioral theory. Cognitive distortions lead to abnormal eating behaviors, which become associated with anxiety relief and therefore are reinforced.

  3. Psychoanalytic theory. Disturbed relationships early in life lead to vulnerability in the child.

    a. **Separation-individuation conflicts,** which usually occur between the mother and daughter

    b. **Distorted body image** with misperception of internal needs

    c. **Control of anxiety is dependent on control of body and biologic needs.** The person who develops an eating disorder attributes or displaces anxiety to bodily function. Controlling the body and its functions relieves anxiety or becomes the defense against anxiety. The child or adolescent who has not successfully separated from the parent functions according to that parent's wishes or desires. The body is the only area in which the child can make decisions or exert any control.

  4. Sociocultural factors include a body image of thinness as promoted by popular culture and the media and peer pressure during adolescence (when self-perception is influenced by peer group ideals).

TABLE 4-4
Comparison of Physical Symptoms of Anorexia and Bulimia

BODY CHANGES	ANOREXIA NERVOSA	BULIMIA NERVOSA
Weight	Less than 85% of normal weight for age and height	Normal or near-normal weight for age and height
Cardiovascular changes	*Bradycardia, hypotension:* related to decreased cardiac muscle mass from starvation *Arrhythmias:* related to electrolyte imbalance	*Bradycardia, hypotension:* related to fluid deficit, possible heart muscle damage from overuse of syrup of ipecac to induce vomiting *Arrhythmias:* related to electrolyte imbalance
Fluid and electrolyte imbalances	*Hypokalemia:* related to laxative abuse or vomiting *Hypocalcemia:* related to lack of dietary intake *Dehydration:* related to lack of fluid intake, vomiting, and laxative abuse	*Hypokalemia, hyponatremia, and dehydration:* related to diuretic abuse, vomiting, and laxative abuse
Endocrine changes	*Amenorrhea:* starvation leads to loss of fat stores and estrogen loss, alteration in hypothalamic functioning *Hypoglycemia:* related to starvation	*Irregular menses, hypoglycemia:* alteration in hypothalamic functioning
Skin, hair, teeth, bone, voice changes	*Lanugo, dry skin, hypothermia, and hair loss:* starvation and loss of subcutaneous tissue *Osteoporosis:* related to loss of calcium stores	*Hoarseness:* irritation from vomiting *Dental caries:* loss of enamel from vomiting *Enlarged parotid glands:* inflammatory response from content irritation of vomiting
Gastrointestinal changes	*Constipation:* related to loss of bowel muscle tone and laxative abuse	*Constipation:* related to laxative abuse, fluid deficit, loss of bowel muscle tone *Esophagitis:* irritation from vomiting

5. **Family theory.** Symptoms of eating disorders allow a family to avoid dealing with conflict.
   a. Family members are enmeshed, lacking clear-cut boundaries among parents and children, leading to overinvolvement in the child's life.
   b. The family highly values perfection, and the child attempts to meet high standards.
   c. The eating disorder is a form of rebellion, in which the child gains a sense of control through the behavior.

D. Management. A multidisciplinary approach is important, with collaboration among medical, psychiatric, psychological, nutritional, and nursing team members.

1. **Acute care.** Hospitalization is recommended when the individual has persistent symptoms despite ongoing treatment, or when severe depression with suicidal impulses is present.

   a. **The priority is to maintain client safety and stabilize physiologic problems (eg, dehydration, electrolyte imbalance, arrhythmia).**

   b. A refeeding program is important to restore weight.

   c. Behavioral contracting is often used as part of treatment to reinforce appropriate eating and prevent harmful behaviors (eg, purging).

2. **Community-based treatment** is important because eating disorders are often persistent and require long-term management.

   a. Collaboration and communication between providers are important to ensure continuity of care.

   b. Support groups are often helpful for the client, the client's family, or both.

3. **Specific therapeutic approaches**

   a. **Psychotherapy** may be used, with an individual approach focusing on issues such as body image and self-esteem, self-control, and decision making, and relationships with peers and family.

   b. The **cognitive-behavioral approach** aims to reduce the client's symptoms by restructuring the faulty belief system that perpetuates the eating disorder.

   c. Family therapy assists family members to define appropriate boundaries, decrease controlling behaviors, and support the client in increasing self-responsibility (Client and Family Teaching 4-1).

4. **Pharmacological treatment** is aimed at treating accompanying depression, anxiety disorder symptoms, or both (Drug Chart 4-1).

DRUG CHART 4-1 Medications Used in Eating Disorders*

Classification	Generic/ Trade Name	Adult Dosage	Rationale for Use
Tricyclic antidepressant	Imipramine (Tofranil) Desipramine (Norpramine)	Used at low doses (10–25 mg/day)	More effective in treating bulimia than anorexia. Decreases frequency of binge eating and relieves anxiety and depression; affects serotonin levels.
Selective serotonin reuptake inhibitor (SSRI)	Fluoxetine (Prozac)	60 mg/day	Used to treat concurrent depression in eating disorders; restores serotonin levels

*See Chapter 15 for complete discussion.

CLIENT AND FAMILY TEACHING 4-1

Client With a Mind-Body Disorder

- Recognize that the person will experience worsening of symptoms when under stress.
- Expect person to function despite physical symptoms; doing things for them and making decisions will increase dependent behavior.
- A matter-of-fact attitude is helpful to decrease emphasis on dramatic symptoms.
- Expressions of concern should be directed toward real-life problems rather than bodily symptoms.
- Encourage family member to remain with one health care provider on long-term basis.
- Family therapy can be helpful to clarify roles, communication, and expectations.

 V.   **NURSING PROCESS OVERVIEW FOR Mind-Body Disorders**

A. Assessment

1. Note objective and subjective symptoms related to specific diagnosis established according to the DSM-IV.
2. Review client history and determine current internal and external stressors.
   a. Discuss the client's perception of the problem.
   b. Identify the client's self-concept and body image.
   c. Identify secondary gains from physical symptoms.
   d. Discuss significant relationship problems.
3. Ask key nursing assessment questions as appropriate for client problem or specific mind-body disorder (Table 4-5).

B. Nursing diagnoses

1. Determine the client's anxiety level, use of coping measures, and defense mechanisms. (See Chapter 3 for determination of anxiety level and coping measures.)
2. Determine what the physical symptoms mean to the individual client.
3. Analyze the client's insight into the relationship of physical symptoms and psychological distress.
4. Analyze the effect of the client's problem on family and relationship functioning.
5. Establish individualized nursing diagnoses for the client with a mind-body disorder, including but not limited to the following:
   a. Anxiety
   b. Body image disturbance
   c. Coping, defensive
   d. Coping, ineffective individual
   e. Decisional conflict (specify)
   f. Denial, ineffective
   g. Fatigue
   h. Health maintenance, altered
   i. Health-seeking behaviors (specify)
   j. Knowledge deficit (specify)

TABLE 4-5
Key Nursing Assessment Questions

QUESTION	PROVIDES DATA ABOUT
How would you rate your health: poor, fair, good, or excellent?	Self-reporting of health status reflects self-perception and can be used in comparing to objective symptoms
Who is your primary health care provider and how long have you been a client with this person?	A client with a somatoform disorder is likely to have frequent changes in health care providers
What prescription and nonprescription medications are you currently taking?	A client with somatoform disorder may be taking multiple prescribed and over-the-counter medications.
Are you using any alternative or nontraditional treatment measures?	A client with a sexual disorder may have medication-related symptoms.
	A client with an eating disorder may take a variety of medications for weight loss purposes.
	A client with psychological factors affecting general medical conditions may use nontraditional methods.
How has your illness affected your ability to function?	Significant impairment usually occurs in social and occupational functioning.
Are you experiencing any problems related to sexual activity or sexual relationship?	Affirmative response to this general question can be used to determine the need for more specific questions related to sexual health.
Are you satisfied with your eating patterns?	Direct questioning has been shown to be effective in screening for bulimia.
Are you on a strict diet?	Client with anorexia may admit to dieting behavior.

     k. Nutrition, altered, less than body requirement
     l. Pain
    m. Powerlessness
     n. Role performance, altered
     o. Self-esteem disturbance
     p. Sexual dysfunction
     q. Sexuality patterns, altered
     r. Social isolation
     s. Spiritual distress
     t. Violence, risk for self-directed

6. Establish a nursing diagnosis for the family of the client with a mind-body disorder, including, but not limited to the following:
     a. Coping, ineffective family: compromised
     b. Family processes, altered
     c. Management of therapeutic regimen: families; ineffective
     d. Knowledge deficit

C. **Planning and outcome identification.** Work with the client and family in setting realistic goals.

1. **Client who has psychological factors affecting a general medical condition.** Establish desired outcome criteria:
   a. Demonstrate the ability to cope with physical illness by using stress reduction measures.
   b. Use a combination of traditional and nontraditional modes of treatment.
   c. Identify specific stressors associated with physical illness.
   d. Adapt family coping to enhance health promotion (see Client and Family Teaching 4-1).

2. **Client or partner with a sexual disorder.** Establish desired outcome criteria:
   a. Identify relationship of stressors and decreased sexual functioning.
   b. Express desire to change variant or deviant sexual behavior.
   c. Communicate with partner about sexual issues without discomfort.
   d. Express satisfaction with one's own sexuality pattern.

3. **Client with a somatoform disorder.** Establish desired outcome criteria:
   a. Express anxiety and conflict verbally rather than with physical symptoms.
   b. Reduce or eliminate behavior that is demanding or manipulative in relationships with others.
   c. Reduce attention and other secondary gains for presence of symptomatic behaviors (see Client and Family Teaching 4-1).

4. **Client with an eating disorder.** Established desired outcome criteria:
   a. Achieve normal or near-normal weight for age and height.
   b. Replace maladaptive eating behaviors with stress-reduction measures.
   c. Identify positive self-concept and realistic body image.
   d. State feelings of control in areas of life other than eating.
   e. Establish open communication within the family and maintain boundaries (see Client and Family Teaching 4-1).

D. **Implementation**

1. **Clients with psychological factors affecting general medical condition**
   a. Assist the client in identifying and using positive coping measures to handle physical illness.
   b. Encourage the client to use specific support or self-help groups.
   c. Teach the client information related to the physical illness, effects of stress, and management of symptoms.
   d. Encourage client-selected alternative methods to enhance traditional treatments.

2. **Clients with a somatoform disorder**
   a. Report and assess new physical complaints, because organic disease is also a possibility for this client.
   b. Decrease reinforcement of secondary gains for physical symptoms (see Client and Family Teaching 4-1).
   c. Avoid fostering dependency, and encourage independent behaviors.
   d. Maintain therapeutic focus on feelings, emotional responses, and relationship problems rather than on somatic symptoms.
   e. Set limits on manipulative behaviors in matter-of-fact manner.

    f. Help the client identify and use positive means to meet emotional needs.

    g. Encourage maintenance of long-term relationship with primary health provider.

    h. Teach and encourage use of stress-reducing measures.

    i. Help identify relationship of stressful life events and somatic symptoms.

3. Clients with a sexual disorder

    a. Analyze one's own ability to be comfortable discussing sexual issues with a client.

    b. Educate the client about normal sexual behaviors and family planning issues.

    c. Correct misconceptions regarding sexuality and sexual functioning. Teach the client that sexuality is a normal human response and is not synonymous with any one sexual act. Complex relationships among self-concept, body image, family influence, and physical functioning all influence sexual expression.

    d. Review medications prescribed for client and identify side effects associated with sexual functioning.

    e. Identify physical illness and specific effects on sexual relationships.

    f. Refer client to qualified counselor for sex therapy.

4. Clients with an eating disorder

    a. Collaborate with other health team members.

    b. Reinforce dietician's prescription for healthy eating to accomplish realistic weight gain of 2 to 3 lb weekly, and reinforce treatment plan that establishes privileges and restrictions based on compliance.

    c. Decrease emphasis on specific "good" or "bad" foods.

    d. Weigh client twice weekly.

    e. In acute, hospital-based care, remain with client during meal and for first hour after meal.

    f. Discuss fears of weight gain and loss of control, and help client identify how feelings about self and problems are related to eating behaviors.

    g. Teach and encourage the client to use coping measures other than weight loss to maintain control and decrease anxiety.

    h. Encourage the client to verbalize role within family, identifying issues of dependence and independence. Assist the family to redefine roles and establish open communication.

    i. Promote the client's control by having her participate in treatment plan.

E. Outcome evaluation

    1. The client identifies relationship between specific stressors and physiologic symptoms.

    2. The client verbalizes anxiety about specific problems rather than expressing anxiety with physical symptoms.

    3. The client expresses satisfaction with self-concept, body image, and relationships with others.

    4. The client uses stress-management techniques and follows health-promoting lifestyle.

    5. The client assumes responsibility for self and expresses sense of internal locus of control.

    6. The client identifies and cooperates in continued treatment plan.

STUDY QUESTIONS

1. A client newly diagnosed with rheumatoid arthritis asks the community nurse how stress can affect his disease. The nurse would explain that
   (1) the psychological experience of stress will not affect symptoms of physical disease
   (2) psychological stress can cause painful emotions, which are harmful to a person with an illness
   (3) stress can overburden the body's immune system and therefore one can experience increased disease symptoms
   (4) the stress response of the body is only stimulated when there are major disruptions in one's life

2. A client with benign essential hypertension has been referred for biofeedback training. Which of the following criteria would the nurse use to evaluate the client's success with this method?
   (1) The client states that his stress level is under control.
   (2) The client's blood pressure is normal while on a decreased dose of antihypertensive medication.
   (3) The client uses relaxation methods on a regular basis.
   (4) The client follows recommended diet and medication plan without deviation.

3. A nurse is teaching a class on stress management. The nurse is questioned about the use of alternative treatments, such as herbal therapy and therapeutic touch. The nurse explains that the advantage of these methods would include all of the following *except*
   (1) that they can be congruent with many cultural belief systems

   (2) that they encourage the consumer to take an active role in health management
   (3) that they promote interrelationships between mind-body-spirit
   (4) that they usually work better than traditional medical practice

4. A client is preoccupied with numerous bodily complaints even after a careful diagnostic workup reveals no physiologic problems. Which of the following nursing interventions would be most therapeutic for this client?
   (1) Acknowledge that the complaints are real to the client and refocus the client on other concerns and problems.
   (2) Challenge the physical complaints by confronting the client with the normal diagnostic findings.
   (3) Ignore the client's complaints but request that the client keep a list of all symptoms.
   (4) Listen to the client's complaints carefully and question the client about specific symptoms.

5. A nurse is teaching a client about the medication sertraline (Zoloft), which has been prescribed for the client's depression. A significant side effect is interference with sexual arousal by inhibiting erectile function. How would the nurse approach this topic?
   (1) The nurse would not mention sexual side effects in order to prevent the client from having anxiety because of potential erectile problems.
   (2) The nurse would explain that the client should report any changes in sexual functioning, so medication adjustments can be considered.

(3) The nurse would explain that the client's sexual desire will likely decrease on this medication.

(4) The nurse would tell the client that sexual side effects are expected but will decrease when depression lifts.

6. A nurse is working with a client with a gender identity disorder. The client recently started living as a member of the opposite sex. Which of the following is an inappropriate outcome criterion for this nurse-client relationship?

(1) The client discusses feelings about reactions expected from family and friends.

(2) Feelings and issues regarding living in another gender role are discussed.

(3) A date is set for sex-change surgery as result of discussion.

(4) Support persons are identified who may be helpful during change from one gender to another.

7. The school nurse performing routine physical examinations would expect anorexia nervosa in an adolescent female after collecting which of the following data on her?

(1) bradycardia, hypotension, irregular menses for past 3 months

(2) complaints of constipation, excessive exercising, presence of dry, flaky skin

(3) hoarseness, multiple dental caries, near-normal weight

(4) weight less than 85% of normal, presence of lanugo, amenorrhea for past 3 months

8. A nurse is planning a psychoeducational discussion of topics for a group of adolescent clients with anorexia nervosa. Which of the following topics would the nurse select to increase understanding about central issues in this disorder?

(1) anger management

(2) parental expectations

(3) peer pressure and substance abuse

(4) self-control and self-esteem

9. A nurse understands that a client with bulimia nervosa feels shame and guilt over binge eating and purging. This disorder is therefore considered

(1) ego distorting

(2) ego dystonic

(3) ego enhancing

(4) ego syntonic

10. The psychoanalytic theory regarding etiology of anorexia nervosa includes which of the following concepts?

(1) achievement of secondary gain through control of eating

(2) conflict between mother and child over separation and individualization

(3) family dynamics that lead to enmeshment of members

(4) incorporation of body image ideal of thinness

11. A client hospitalized on an eating disorder unit is monitored by the nurse for one hour after eating. The rationale for this intervention is

(1) to develop a trusting relationship

(2) to maintain focus on importance of nutrition

(3) to prevent purging behaviors

(4) to reinforce behavioral contact

12. The initial treatment priority for a client hospitalized for anorexia nervosa on a special eating disorder unit is

   (1) to determine current body image

   (2) to identify family interaction patterns

   √**(3)** to initiate refeeding program

   (4) to promote client independence

13. The nurse evaluates the treatment of a client with somatoform disorder as successful if

   (1) the client practices self-medication rather than changing health care providers

   (2) the client recognizes that physical symptoms increase anxiety level

   (3) the client researches treatment protocols for various illnesses

   √**(4)** the client verbalizes anxiety directly rather than displacing it

14. Which of the following attitudes from a nurse would hinder a discussion with an adolescent client about sexuality?

   (1) accepting

   (2) matter-of-fact

   √**(3)** moralistic

   (4) nonjudgmental

ANSWER KEY

1. The answer is (3). The stress response causes stimulation of the hypothalamic-pituitary-adrenal axis and thus can further compromise an immune system that has been activated by the autoimmune disorder of rheumatoid arthritis. The individual can therefore expect an exacerbation of disease symptoms when under stress. The statement that stress will not affect symptoms of physical disease is false. Experiences of emotions that are painful are not necessarily harmful to someone with an illness. Learning to handle painful emotions can enhance coping. The stress response can be stimulated by major or minor disruptions in life, but the individual's perception of stress is more important than actual problem.

2. The answer is (2). Successful use of biofeedback enables the client to modify physiologic responses to stress, including blood pressure. A decreased need for an antihypertensive medication is an objective measurement of effectiveness. Although answer choices (1) and (3) are outcomes of stress management, they are not specific for biofeedback. Answer choice (4) would be a successful outcome of the medical treatment program.

3. The answer is (4). Alternative treatment methods are often used as adjuncts to medical treatment. Although an individual may choose a particular alternative treatment method, there is really no current scientific proof that these methods will work better than traditional medicine. This statement is quite global and therefore is not true. The other answer choice options are accurate regarding use of alternative treatment methods.

4. The answer is (1). After physical factors are ruled out, somatic complaints are thought to be expressions of anxiety. The complaints are real to the client, but the nurse should not focus on them. Prompting the client to talk about other concerns will encourage expression of anxiety and dependency needs. Confronting the client as demonstrated in answer choice (2) shows a lack of sensitivity to the unconscious nature of the problem and will increase client anxiety. Ignoring the client's complaints merely avoids the problem. Focusing on somatic symptoms will reinforce them (increases secondary gains).

5. The answer is (2). Clients often discontinue medications to avoid or correct sexual side effects and are less likely to do that if health professionals offer assistance with sexual issues. Clients generally will not raise sexual issues unless health professionals give permission by raising the issue first. Answer choice (1) does not promote discussion of this sensitive issue. More likely, it reflects the nurse's avoidance of uncomfortable feelings. Any impaired sexual desire most likely would be secondary to erectile dysfunction. Answer choice (4) reflects inaccurate information; not all clients will experience sexual side effects, and if experienced, will not necessarily decrease when depression lifts.

6. The answer is (3). Unless the nurse is a certified sex therapist, this would be an unexpected outcome from nursing care of this client. The other answer choices are important areas for the client to explore and are expected discussion topics in the nurse-client interactions.

7. The answer is (4). These assessments are most characteristic of a client who has anorexia nervosa. Severe restriction of eating leads to significant body weight loss. Subcutaneous tissue loss causes development of the fine, downy hair called lanugo. Loss of estrogen due to loss of fat stores causes amenorrhea. The symptoms in answer choice (1) could be associated with either anorexia or bulimia. Although the symptoms in answer choice (2) can occur in anorexia, the most significant and diagnostic symptoms for the disorder are those listed in answer choice (4). The symptoms in answer choice (3) are characteristic of bulimia.

8. The answer is (4). Self-control and self-esteem are central issues for the client with an eating disorder who maintains a sense of control only by controlling eating behaviors. A client with anorexia feels loss of control over other areas of life and experiences decreased self-esteem with severe doubts about self-worth. Anger management, parental expectations, peer pressure, and substance abuse are important issues for adolescent clients but are not necessarily specific for the client who has anorexia nervosa.

9. The answer is (2). An ego dystonic disorder is one in which the client views behaviors or symptoms as incongruent with self-image and therefore feels guilt, shame, and distress about the symptoms. Ego distorting and ego enhancing do not apply to the situation presented. An ego syntonic disorder is one in which the client views her behaviors as congruent with her self-image (eg, as in anorexia nervosa).

10. The answer is (2). According to psychoanalytic theory, early mother-child dynamics lead to difficulty with a child establishing a sense of separateness from the mother. Control of eating becomes one area in which the child establishes a sense of independence. Answer choice (1) is the behavioral view of anorexia nervosa. Answer choice (3) is the family theory view of anorexia nervosa, which deals with the issue of lack of generational boundaries. Answer choice (4) is the sociocultural view of anorexia nervosa, which identifies thinness as being a culturally determined ideal.

11. The answer is (3). The client may experience increased anxiety during treatment and therefore may resume behaviors designed to prevent weight gain, such as vomiting or excessive exercise. Although the other answer choices are important areas for nursing intervention, they do not provide the rationale for remaining with a client for one hour after eating.

12. The answer is (3). The physical need to reestablish near-normal weight takes priority because of the physiologic, life-threatening consequences of anorexia. The other answer choices are all important aspects of treatment, but they are not the highest priority in initial treatment.

13. The answer is (4). The client with somatoform disorder unconsciously displaces anxiety onto physical symptoms. The ability to recognize and verbalize anxious feelings directly rather than displacing them is a criterion of treatment success. The behaviors in answer choices **(1)** and **(3)** indicate continuation of a somatoform problem. Physical symptoms generally relieve anxiety by primary gain in a client with somatoform disorder. Some clients (eg, a client with hypochondriasis) may have increased anxiety over a particular symptom. The statement that the client recognizes a connection between physical symptoms and anxiety would not be the best indication that treatment is successful.

14. The answer is (3). Adolescents are not likely to feel free to ask questions and participate in a discussion if the nurse has a moralistic attitude toward sexual issues. Having an accepting, matter-of-fact, or nonjudgmental attitude will be helpful in allowing adolescents to feel comfortable discussing sexual issues.

5 Personality Disorders

Description

A. **Definition.** According to the *Diagnostic and Statistical Manual of Mental Disorders,* 4th edition, (DSM-IV), a personality disorder is an "enduring pattern of inner experience and behavior that deviates markedly from expectations of the individual's culture, is pervasive and inflexible, has an onset in adolescence or early adulthood, is stable over time, and leads to distress or impairment" (DSM-IV, 1994).

1. **Classification.** Personality disorders are coded on Axis II of the multiaxial diagnostic system used by the American Psychiatric Association. According to the DSM-IV, they are clustered into three broad groups:
   a. Odd, eccentric disorders (see I.B)
   b. Dramatic, emotional, erratic disorders (see I.C)
   c. Anxious, fearful disorders (see I.D)

2. **Characteristics.** Personality disorders are characterized by long-standing problems in behavior, mood, perception, and relationships. Behaviors are characterized by self-centeredness, rigidity and inflexibility, and poor ability to self-regulate (external locus of control).

3. **Self-perception.** Individuals with personality disorders generally do not perceive a problem with their behavior; they become distressed because of other people's reactions or behavior toward them.

4. **Treatment-seeking behavior.** Generally, individuals with personality disorders do not seek psychiatric treatment and usually are not hospitalized, unless they have a coexisting psychiatric disorder coded on Axis I.

5. **Functioning.** Although they experience problems in social and occupational functioning, individuals remain in the mainstream of society.

B. **Odd, eccentric disorders**

1. **Paranoid personality disorder.** Individuals with this disorder demonstrate a pattern of distrust and suspiciousness; the individual interprets other people's motives as threatening.

2. **Schizoid personality disorder.** Individuals with this disorder lack personal and social relationships. The individual is detached from others and withdraws from interactions.

3. **Schizotypal personality disorder.** Individuals with this disorder may have behaviors similar to those of someone with schizophrenia; however, psychotic episodes are infrequent. The individual may be acutely uncomfortable in relationships.

C. **Dramatic, emotional, erratic disorders**

1. **Antisocial personality disorder.** Individuals with this disorder have a pattern of disregard for and violation of the rights of others.
   a. **Diagnosis.** The individual must be at least 18 years of age and must have a history of some symptoms of conduct disorder before age 15.
   b. The individual usually exhibits behavior that is hostile to the well-being of society, and therefore frequently is found in the prison system. This individual is unable to follow rules, is grossly selfish and irresponsible, and generally is manipulative in relationships with others.

2. **Borderline personality disorder.** Individuals with this disorder are characterized by impulsive, unpredictable, and unstable moods; disturbed relationships with others; intolerance to being alone; and a chronic sense of boredom.
   a. The individual may use the defense mechanisms of **splitting** and **projecting** in relationships. In splitting, the individual views another person as either all good or all bad. Projection is seen when the individual is unable to recognize negative feelings or undesirable characteristics in the self and instead believes these feelings or characteristics belong to another person.
   b. Risk for self-mutilating behaviors and suicide is high with this individual.

3. **Histrionic personality disorder.** Individuals with this disorder are characterized by excessive emotionality and attention-seeking behaviors that are dramatic and egocentric.

4. **Narcissistic personality disorder.** Individuals with this disorder are characterized by grandiosity and the need for constant admiration of others. They will exaggerate their own importance and accomplishments.

D. **Anxious, fearful disorders**

1. **Avoidant personality disorder.** Individuals with this disorder are characterized by social inhibition, feelings of inadequacy, and sensitivity to potential rejection or criticism.

2. **Dependent personality disorder.** Individuals with this disorder are characterized by submissive and clinging behavior associated with an excessive need to be cared for by others.

3. **Obsessive-compulsive personality disorder.** Individuals with this disorder are characterized by a preoccupation with orderliness, perfectionism, and the need to be in control of situations, objects, and people.

II. Etiology

A. General considerations. Most theorists agree that a combination of factors, including negative childhood experiences, genetics, and environment, plays a role in the etiology of these disorders. Borderline and antisocial personality disorders have been researched more than the other disorders.

B. Psychoanalytic and developmental theories

1. These theories propose that the unsuccessful mastery of tasks in early developmental stages, along with **negative early childhood experiences,** lead to the development of personality disorders (ie, failure to establish trust in infancy owing to inconsistent or neglectful care can be correlated with later development of paranoid personality disorder).

2. Borderline personality disorder is believed to be associated with the failure to work through the separation-individuation process in early toddlerhood (around 2 years of age).
   a. The child may have been unable to separate from the mother without significant fear and anxiety (parent rewards clinging behavior and prevents autonomy).
   b. The mother may have been perceived by the child as both strongly nurturing at times and hateful and punishing at unpredictable times.

C. Sociocultural theory. A study by Zanarini (1997) of individuals with borderline personality disorder showed strong evidence of emotional and physical abuse in childhood by caretakers as well as sexual abuse by others who were not caretakers. Significant predictors of the development of this disorder include the following factors:

1. Female gender
2. Sexual abuse by a male
3. Emotional denial by male caretakers
4. Inconsistent treatment by female caretakers

D. Psychobiologic theory

1. **Antisocial personality disorder.** There is some evidence of genetic transmission and presence of specific neurologic deficits in individuals with this disorder. There may be a history of several individuals in the same family having this disorder, although no specific genes have been indicated.

2. **Borderline personality disorder.** There is some evidence of inadequate regulation of serotonin and dopamine in these individuals, which may be associated with impulsive behavior and mood instability (characteristics of this disorder).

E. Behavioral theory

1. **Antisocial personality disorder.** The child learns socially undesirable behavior from the parents, who reward acting-out behavior by giving in rather than setting limits.

2. **Borderline personality disorder.** The child is rewarded for clinging, dependent behaviors.

F. Family theory

1. **Antisocial personality disorder.** There is significant parental deprivation during the first 5 years of the child's life, with a chaotic home environment and inconsistent, impulsive parents.

2. **Borderline personality disorder.** According to family theory, an unstable family system leads to unstable personality development.

   a. The undifferentiation of the parents is played out in the relationship to the child. For example, the conflict and instability of the parental relationship may be handled by pulling the child into the parental conflict *(triangling)*.

   b. The life of the child is intensely connected and regulated by the chaotic emotional environment in the family.

III. Management

A. Acute care. An individual is not likely to present for help unless something has gone wrong in life (eg, relationship failures, job losses, legal problems).

1. Hospitalization is inappropriate unless the individual has an acute coexisting psychiatric disorder coded on Axis I.

2. An individual with borderline personality disorder may exhibit suicide risk and may also engage in self-mutilating behaviors. In this case, hospitalization may be recommended to reduce the risk for self-harm.

B. Community care. The treatment of choice for personality disorders is short-term psychotherapy focusing on solutions for specific life problems.

1. The individual with a personality disorder is not likely to be motivated for long-term treatment. The lack of motivation is related to the fact that the person does not think anything is wrong with him and would resent or resist treatment.

2. Group therapy may be appropriate if the client agrees to attend a sufficient number of sessions.

C. Medications are generally not recommended for personality disorders. If coexisting psychiatric disorders are present, then medications for the specific symptoms may be recommended.

IV. NURSING PROCESS OVERVIEW FOR Personality Disorders

A. Assessment

1. **General considerations**

   a. Note the objective and subjective symptoms related to the specific client diagnosis established and coded on Axis II.

   b. Identify specific current internal and external stressors (Table 5-1). Discuss the client's perception of the current or presenting problem, identify the client's significant relationships and level of family involvement, and determine the client's willingness to accept treatment and the expectations for therapy.

TABLE 5-1
Key Assessment Questions for Individual With a Personality Disorder

QUESTION	PROVIDES DATA ABOUT
What current problems in your life are causing you distress?	Client perspective regarding problem situations and degree of distress experienced
Who do you consider a support person(s) in your life?	Relationship system and degree of social isolation of client
What changes would you like to make in yourself or in your life?	Motivation for working on self-functioning; client reality perception
How do you handle anxious feelings?	Current use of defense or coping mechanisms
Have you ever done anything to hurt yourself?	Potential risk for self-harm (self-mutilating behavior common in individuals with borderline personality disorder)
Have you ever been in trouble with the legal system?	History of criminal behavior; individual with antisocial personality disorder often has conflict with rules and laws in society

2. **Paranoid personality disorder.** Assess the characteristics of an individual with this disorder:
   a. Is the client suspicious and mistrustful of others?
   b. Does the client use projection as a defense mechanism?
3. **Schizoid or schizotypal disorder.** Assess the characteristics of the individual with this disorder:
   a. Does the client withdraw socially and act emotionally aloof?
   b. Does the client display odd mannerisms, speech, and behaviors?
   c. Does the client show little interest in having sexual experiences with another person?
   d. Does the client respond with indifference to approval from or criticism by others?
4. **Borderline personality disorder.** Assess the characteristics of an individual with this disorder:
   a. Does the client have unstable moods and impulsive behavior?
   b. Does the client self-mutilate?
   c. Does the client have poor self-concept and an intense fear of being alone?
   d. Does the client express contradictory ideas or feelings about others? Does the client usually view others as all good or all bad (splitting)?
   e. Does the client manipulate others in relationships?
5. **Histrionic personality disorder.** Assess the characteristics of an individual with this disorder:
   a. Does the client have dramatic behavior with exaggerated emotions?
   b. Does the client have frequent temper tantrums?
   c. Does the client exhibit flamboyance with sexual overtones?
   d. Does the client lack commitment in relationships?

6. **Narcissistic personality disorder.** Assess the characteristics of an individual with this disorder:
   a. Does the client demonstrate grandiose thinking and an exaggerated sense of self-importance?
   b. Does the client display attention-seeking behaviors?
   c. Does the client rationalize failures?
7. **Antisocial personality disorder.** Assess the characteristics of an individual with this disorder:
   a. Does the client behave in a manipulative and controlling manner?
   b. Does the client act extroverted and have a superficial and charming manner?
   c. Does the client lack respect for the rights of others?
   d. Does the client have an impaired conscience, with lying, cheating, and possible criminal behaviors?
   e. Does the client lack commitment to and concern for a partner in a relationship?
   f. Does the client desire immediate pleasure and gratification?
8. **Avoidant personality disorder.** Assess the characteristics of an individual with this disorder:
   a. Does the client respond with hypersensitivity to others' reactions and criticisms?
   b. Does the client fear rejection and failure?
   c. Does the client desire attention but withdraw socially?
   d. Does the client fear being alone?
9. **Dependent personality disorder.** Assess the characteristics of an individual with this disorder:
   a. Does the client lack self-confidence and have poor self-esteem?
   b. Does the client display subordination in relationships?
   c. Does the client have difficulty making decisions?
   d. Does the client devalue any personal abilities?
10. **Obsessive-compulsive personality disorder.** Assess the characteristics of an individual with this disorder:
   a. Does the client strive for organization, order, and perfection?
   b. Does the client behave in a controlling and demanding manner in relationships?
   c. Does the client pay great attention to detail?
   d. Does the client form rigid, moralistic, and judgmental opinions of others?
   e. Does the client convey indirect expressions of anger, such as passive-aggressive behavior (eg, being consistently late for appointments)?

B. **Nursing diagnoses**
   1. **General consideration.** The nurse must analyze his own feelings and reactions to a client with a personality disorder. The nurse should seek direction from a peer or treatment team when his feelings interfere with therapeutic performance.

2. **Analyze the client's predominant manner of relating to others:**
   a. Withdrawn and suspicious (odd, eccentric personality disorders)
   b. Manipulative and controlling (dramatic, emotional, erratic disorders)
   c. Dependent (anxious, fearful disorders)
3. **Determine the client's level of self-esteem,** recognizing that poor self-esteem is present despite apparent egocentricity.
4. **Establish individualized nursing diagnoses for the client, family, or both** (Table 5-2).

C. **Planning and outcome identification.** Work with client and family in setting realistic goals.
   1. Establish desired outcome criteria for clients with an odd, eccentric personality disorder. The client will:
      a. Verbalize comfort in relating one-to-one with the nurse
      b. Participate in group situations with support
      c. Control or reduce unusual mannerisms
      d. Refrain from sharing bizarre or paranoid ideas with others
   2. Establish desired outcome criteria for clients with a dramatic, emotional, erratic personality disorder. The client will:
      a. Control impulsive behaviors, and refrain from self-destructive behaviors
      b. Verbalize anxiety and angry feelings rather than act out
      c. Decrease manipulative behavior and express needs in a direct manner
      d. Respect the rights and needs of others, and adhere to rules and regulations in structured environments and relationships with others

TABLE 5-2
Personality Disorders and Nursing Diagnoses

DIAGNOSTIC CATEGORY	SPECIFIC PERSONALITY DISORDERS	NURSING DIAGNOSES
Odd, eccentric	Paranoid	Social isolation
	Schizoid/Schizotypal	Social interaction, impaired
		Thought processes, altered
		Self-esteem, chronic low
Dramatic, emotional, erratic	Antisocial	Anxiety
	Borderline	Coping, ineffective individual
	Histrionic	Self-esteem disturbance
	Narcissistic	Self-mutilation, risk for violence, risk for: self-directed or directed at others
Anxious, fearful	Avoidant	Anxiety
	Dependent	Coping, ineffective individual
	Obsessive compulsive	Decisional conflict (specify)
		Self-esteem, chronic low
		Social interaction, impaired

3. Establish desired outcome criteria for client with an anxious, fearful personality disorder. The client will:
   a. Identify positive self-statements indicating improved sense of self-esteem
   b. Interact with peers in social situations
   c. Manage anxiety when daily living situations are not under individual control
   d. Make decisions in an independent manner
   e. Tolerate lack of perfection without undue anxiety
4. Establish desired outcome criteria for family with a member having a personality disorder. The family will:
   a. Maintain generational boundaries
   b. Identify areas of self-functioning
   c. Set consistent, appropriate limits
   d. Provide positive feedback for efforts to improve functioning

D. Implementation

1. Clients with an odd, eccentric personality disorder
   a. Adopt objective, matter-of-fact manner when interacting with the client, and maintain clear, consistent verbal and nonverbal communication.
   b. Provide daily structure for activities of daily living.
   c. Maintain focus on reality and reality-based topics.
   d. Help client identify feelings that are implied.
   e. Assist with problem solving for life issues identified as source of stress.
   f. Gradually involve client in group situations, providing support when necessary, and provide positive feedback for socially appropriate behavior.

2. Clients with a dramatic, emotional, erratic personality disorder
   a. **Prevent self-harm by observing the client frequently and developing a no-harm contract.**
   b. Give immediate feedback when confronting inappropriate or manipulative behavior, and help the client examine the consequences of appropriate and inappropriate behavior.
   c. Act as role model for appropriate expression of feelings and negative emotions.
   d. Work with treatment team in maintaining consistent feedback for client, reinforcing specific treatment objectives, and avoiding manipulations of staff by client.
   e. Avoid rescuing or rejecting client.
   f. Set limits; reinforce consequences of manipulative behavior or disregard for rights of others.
   g. Give positive feedback for goal achievement and independent behavior.
   h. Explore the client's feelings regarding rejection, being alone, and fear of abandonment.
   i. Use a problem-solving approach to help the client explore changes as necessary.
   j. Encourage follow-up treatment.

3. **Client with an anxious, fearful personality disorder**
   a. Establish a caring, consistent therapeutic relationship and clear expectations for responsible behavior.
   b. Expect the client to make decisions, and teach the client how to be assertive (or refer to training program for this behavior).
   c. Encourage the client to identify positive self-attributes.
   d. Provide positive feedback when the client interacts in social situations in appropriate manner.
   e. Teach the client to use stress-management and relaxation techniques to cope with anxiety.
4. Family of an individual with a personality disorder (Client and Family Teaching 5-1)
   a. Help the family members define and maintain generational boundaries.
   b. Provide positive feedback for efforts to define self-functioning.
   c. Encourage clear definitions of acceptable behavior for the client within family.
   d. Encourage parents to work on areas of conflict in their own relationship.
   e. Teach members to use stress-reduction measures to handle anxiety.
E. **Outcome evaluation.** The nurse will evaluate the effect on the client and family of nursing implementations and determine if outcomes have been achieved.
   1. The client maintains behavior that is appropriate in social situations.
   2. The client expresses satisfaction with self-concept and relationships with others.

CLIENT AND FAMILY TEACHING 5-1

Teaching Families Who Have a Member with a Personality Disorder

Teach information about the disorder and treatment:

- Personality disorder is a disorder that is persistent throughout life and that affects important areas of functioning, especially in relationships with others in social and occupational roles.
- Individual with a personality disorder may be suspicious and mistrustful of others, may form dependent relationships, or may take advantage of other person in a relationship.
- Individual with a personality disorder may lack motivation to change aspects of self-functioning, but may respond to problem-solving approach to specific issues.

Teach information about ways that family functioning can improve:

- It is useful for each member of the family to improve self-functioning rather than focus on changing another person.
- Maintaining clear expectations of each person's specific role in family is helpful in defining boundaries across the generations.
- Expectations about acceptable behavior for family members should be clearly specified and maintained.

3. The client avoids behaviors that are manipulative or exploitative of others.
4. The client expresses angry feelings verbally rather than acting out on self or others.
5. The client respects the rights and needs of others.
6. The client tolerates areas of imperfection in life without undue anxiety.
7. The client identifies the need for follow-up treatments and agrees to cooperate with appropriate referral.
8. The family members improve self-functioning.

STUDY QUESTIONS

1. A community nurse is following up on a client who was hospitalized with depressive disorder, not otherwise specified, following the death of a spouse. In reviewing the client's chart, the nurse notes that the client has an Axis II diagnosis of dependent personality disorder. Which of the following behaviors would the nurse anticipate in this client?
   (1) Difficulty making decisions, lack of self-confidence
   (2) Grandiose thinking, attention-seeking behaviors
   (3) Odd mannerisms, speech, and behaviors
   (4) Unstable moods and impulsive behaviors

2. A client with an Axis II diagnosis of histrionic personality disorder behaves in a dramatic fashion and displays intense emotions when having to wait in the health clinic for an appointment. Which of the following is the best way for a nurse to respond to this situation?
   (1) Call the health care provider and urge that the client be seen immediately because the behavior is disruptive to others.
   (2) Directly confront the client about the unreasonable nature of the behavior and point out that other people are also waiting.
   (3) Explain to the client the reason for the delay in a calm, non-threatening manner and offer to reschedule the appointment if the client wishes to do this.
   (4) Ignore the client's behavior and avoid confrontation, which can lead to escalation of problem.

3. A client is hospitalized following a suicide attempt. Chart history reveals a previous diagnosis of schizoid personality disorder. Which of the following behaviors would be atypical of a client with this disorder?
   (1) Actions designed to please the nurse
   (2) Limited expressions of feelings and emotions
   (3) Odd ideas and mannerisms
   (4) Reluctance to join group activities

4. A client has an anxious, fearful personality type, with difficulty accomplishing work assignments because of fear of failure. The client has been referred to the employee assistance program because of repeated absences from work and evidence of an alcohol problem. The most appropriate nursing diagnosis would be
   (1) Coping, ineffective individual
   (2) Decisional conflict
   (3) Thought processes, altered
   (4) Violence, risk for: self-directed

5. Which of the following statements about an individual with a personality disorder is true?
   (1) Psychotic behavior is common during acute episodes.
   (2) Prognosis for recovery is good with therapeutic intervention.
   (3) The individual remains in mainstream of society, although he or she has problems in social and occupational roles.
   (4) The individual usually seeks treatment willingly from symptoms that are personally distressful.

6. A client describes himself as "very religious" with strong opinions on "what is right and what is wrong." The client is quite judgmental about beliefs and life-styles that are "unacceptable." Which of the following statements support the analysis of the client's behavior as typical of someone with a personality disorder?
   (1) Inflexible behaviors, along with use of rigid defense mechanisms, are characteristic.
   (2) Judgmental behavior, including self-insight, is common.
   (3) Religious fanatics often have personality disorders.
   (4) Strong belief systems can be common and can help identify evidence of instability.

7. A client has a history of conflict-filled relationships. Despite an expressed desire for friends, the client acts in ways that alienate people. Which of the following would be an important nursing intervention for this client?
   (1) Establish a therapeutic relationship in which the nurse uses role modeling and role playing for appropriate behaviors.
   (2) Help the client select friends who are kind and extra caring.
   (3) Point out that the client acts in ways that alienate others.
   (4) Recognize that this client is unlikely to change and therefore intervention is inappropriate.

8. A hospitalized client with an antisocial personality disorder stole money from an elderly client on the unit. Which of the following is the most appropriate for a nurse to say to this client?
   (1) "Why did you take the money?"
   (2) "Let's talk about how you felt when you took the money."
   (3) "The consequences of stealing are loss of privileges."
   (4) "This client is defenseless against you."

9. A nurse is working with clients who have personality disorders. Which of the following techniques would the nurse use to deal with her own feelings that interfere with therapeutic performance?
   (1) Active listening techniques
   (2) Challenging client's assertions
   (3) Forming social relations
   (4) Seeking peer and/or supervisor direction

10. A client with borderline personality disorder is defensive, emotionally labile, and often becomes suddenly and explosively angry. When interacting with the client, the nurse would
    (1) point out how angry the client is becoming and confront the behavior
    (2) take a calm, quiet, and nonconfrontational approach and not argue
    (3) tell client to calm down and avoid becoming explosive or restraints will be used
    (4) use gentle touch and a caring approach to calm the client

11. A client with borderline personality disorder has a nursing diagnosis of *Violence, risk for: self-directed,* which is associated with the client's self-mutilation behavior (burning arms with cigarettes). Which client behavior would indicate a positive outcome of intervention?
    (1) The client denies feelings of wanting to harm anyone.
    (2) The client expresses feelings of anger toward others.
    (3) The client requests cigarettes at appropriate times.
    (4) The client tells the nurse about wanting to burn himself.

12. A nurse is working with the family of a client with a personality disorder. Which of the following would the nurse encourage the family members to work on?

    (1) Avoiding direct expression of problems within the family

    (2) Changing the client's problem behaviors

    (3) Improving self-functioning

    (4) Supporting the client's defenses

ANSWER KEY

1. The answer is (1). An individual who has a dependent personality disorder has anxious and fearful behavior and is reluctant to make decisions. Lack of self-confidence is reflective of chronic low self-esteem. The behavior in answer choice **(2)** is characteristic of someone with a dramatic, emotional, erratic personality disorder, such as narcissistic personality. The behavior in answer choice **(3)** is characteristic of someone with a schizoid or schizotypal personality disorder, in which odd, eccentric behavior is displayed. The behavior in answer choice **(4)** is characteristic of an individual with borderline personality disorder.

2. The answer is (3). The nurse is role modeling appropriate behavior to the client, using a calm and nonthreatening manner to avoid reinforcing the dramatic behavior. Offering to reschedule the client's appointment allows the client a choice, which respects the client's feelings in nonjudgmental way. Calling the health care provider and urging that he or she see the client immediately would serve to reinforce the inappropriate behavior being displayed by the client. Confrontation with this client would serve to increase anxiety and therefore the dramatic behavior would escalate. The nurse should attempt to decrease, not increase, a client's anxiety. Ignoring the client's behavior would be ignoring a problem that is disruptive not only to the client but also to other people in the clinic. Client behavior would likely become increasingly dramatic.

3. The answer is (1). A client with a schizoid personality disorder is detached, aloof, and socially isolated. This individual would have no interest in seeking the approval of another and would not behave in ways to please the nurse. The behaviors in the other answer choices are characteristic of an individual with a schizoid personality disorder and would be expected.

4. The answer is (1). This client is experiencing difficulty in occupational functioning as well as problems with alcohol. The client meets criteria for diagnosis of Ineffective coping. Answer choices **(2)** and **(3)** are incorrect because there is no evidence in this situation that the client has a conflict regarding a decision or any evidence of altered thinking. Answer choice **(4)** is incorrect, because the client has not expressed thoughts of self-harm or committed any acts designed to harm self; this diagnosis therefore does not apply to this situation.

5. The answer is (3). An individual with a personality disorder is usually not hospitalized unless a coexisting, Axis I psychiatric disorder is present. Generally, these people effect a marginal adjustment and remain in society although experiencing relationship and occupational problems related to rigid and inflexible behaviors. Personality disorders are chronic, life-long patterns of behavior. Acute episodes do not occur. Psychotic behavior is usually not common, although it can occur in either schizotypal personality disorder or borderline personality disorder. Because these disorders are enduring and evasive and the individual is inflexible, prognosis for recovery is not favorable. Generally, the individual does not seek treatment because he does not perceive problems with own behavior. Distress can occur based on other people's reaction to the individual's behavior.

6. The answer is (1). Individuals with a personality disorder have inflexible behavior patterns and rigid defense mechanisms. They are not likely to change over time. Individuals with a personality disorder generally lack self-insight and are more likely to have external locus of control thinking (ie, blaming others for problems). Religious fanatics may be motivated by other psychodynamics (eg, psychotic states). Strong belief systems do not necessarily mean mental instability. A mentally healthy person may have belief systems that are strong and that govern conduct.

7. The answer is (1). A therapeutic relationship will provide acceptance for client, and by using role modeling and role playing, the nurse can assist the client in learning appropriate behaviors. Answer choice **(2)** is an inappropriate and unrealistic solution to the client's problem behaviors. Answer choice **(3)** is an inappropriate intervention, because the client is not likely to accept direct criticism of the behavior. Individuals who have a personality disorder do not perceive a problem with their own behavior. Answer choice **(4)** negates an individual's potential for growth and improvement.

8. The answer is (3). The most appropriate response is to reinforce the consequences of behavior that disregard the rights of others. Answer choice **(1)** is incorrect because this client is likely to rationalize and excuse the behavior. Answer choice **(2)** is incorrect, because the nurse should not encourage the client to provide excuses or explanations of behaviors that are clearly against the rules. Answer choice **(4)** is incorrect, because the client with an antisocial personality disorder is not likely to have compassion for another and lacks respect for the rights of others.

9. The answer is (4). The nurse is likely to have strong reactions to a client with a personality disorder, especially those clients who display intense emotions and manipulative behaviors. Seeking the direction of peers and supervisors can help clarify issues and determine the best nursing responses to difficult behaviors. Active listening is for the benefit of the client. This question is asking about the nurse's performance. Challenging the client's assertions would be a nursing intervention that may be used with a client, but it does not answer this question. The nurse forming social relationships would not help in dealing with feelings that interfere with therapeutic performance.

10. The answer is (2). An important intervention with angry behavior is a calm, nonconfrontational, nonargumentative approach. This will avoid further escalating the client's behavior. Confronting the client's behavior could exacerbate anger and trigger explosive behavior. Telling the client to calm down minimizes client problems, and telling the client restraints may be used also may be perceived as threatening to the client. Touch may be perceived as threatening and is not recommended for a client who may become explosive.

11. The answer is (4). The fact that the client directly tells the nurse about feelings of wanting to self-mutilate, rather than *acting on* these feelings, is evidence of responding to nursing intervention. Answer choice **(1)** does not indicate that self-mutilating behavior is decreasing. Answer choice **(2)** does not indicate improvement with nursing diagnosis established. Answer choice **(3)** does not address the nursing diagnosis or positive outcomes.

12. The answer is (3). It is most useful for family members to work on improving self-functioning. This will facilitate ownership of problems among each individual involved in ongoing difficulties in relationships. The direct expression of problems is helpful and therefore should not be avoided. It is not possible to change another's behavior; the family would become quite frustrated if this were encouraged. The client's defenses are likely to be quite strong and this client is likely to blame others for problems; support for blaming others is not helpful.

6 Mood Disorders and Suicidal Behavior

I. Overview

A. Definitions. The mood disorders are characterized by disturbances in feelings, thinking, and behavior. Mood disorders may occur on a continuum ranging from severe depression to severe mania (hyperactivity) (Fig. 6-1).

1. **Depression** is an emotional state characterized by sadness, discouragement, guilt, decreased self-esteem, helplessness, and hopelessness.
2. **Mania** is an emotional state characterized by elation, high optimism, increased energy, and exaggerated sense of importance and invincibility.
3. **Unipolar depression** is a mood disturbance with only depression, but no occurrence of mania.
4. **Bipolar disorder** is a mood disturbance in which the symptoms of mania have occurred at least one time; an episode of depression may or may not have occurred.
5. **Grief** is a normal response to a loss (eg, death of a significant other, divorce, illness or hospitalization, job loss, or loss of personal possessions). Grief is differentiated from depression by the following factors:
   a. **Acute grieving** may occur up to 3 months after a significant loss.
   b. **Grief resolution** is characterized by the grieving person's ability to remember, comfortably and realistically, both the pleasures and disappointments associated with the loss. Grief resolution may take up to 3 years.
   d. **Maladaptive grief response** can lead to a mood disorder. The response may be delayed, inhibited, prolonged, or exaggerated.
   e. Loss of self-esteem in the grieving person is not characteristic of normal grieving, and may indicate a mood disorder.
6. **Suicidal behavior** involves thoughts of taking one's own life.
   a. **Suicidal threat.** A suicidal intent is usually accompanied by behavior changes; the threat includes a plan and the means to execute the plan.
   b. **Suicidal gesture.** This self-destructive act does not involve serious injury; however, it may be followed by a more serious attempt.
   c. **Suicidal attempt.** This self-destructive act has a potential outcome of death.

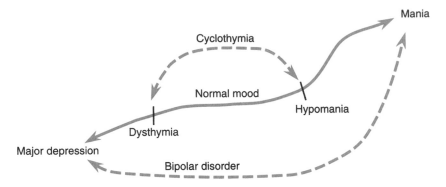

FIGURE 6-1
Relationships among mood disorders. Characterized by mood swings from elation to despair, mood disorders are related by their episodic and changing nature. Bipolar disorders consist of one or more manic episodes or one or more depressive episodes. Cyclothymia consists of both hypomanic (elevated or irritable) and dysthymic (chronically sad or depressed) mood swings. Situated between the extreme moods is a normal mood.

B. Impact of mood disorders

1. Mood disorders, especially depression, may become chronic and incapacitating without appropriate intervention.
2. A large number of clients who have a mood disorder are not diagnosed or are misdiagnosed.
   a. Clients may not seek treatment from a mental health care provider.
   b. Findings have indicated that only 16% to 23% of persons who meet DSM-IV criteria for mood disorders seek mental health care (Keltner, 1998).

C. Relevant statistics for mood disorders

1. **Prevalence.** The lifetime prevalence for major depressive disorder is 12.7% for men and 21.3% for women.
   a. No adequate explanation exists for the nearly twofold increase of depression in women.
   b. Some researchers think that social and cultural factors, such as role conflict, increased rate of victimization of women, tendency toward negative self-evaluation, and the tendency to internalize stress, may account for the increased rate in women.
2. **Incidence**
   a. Adolescents between 14 and 16 years of age have a 4.7% incidence of major depression.
   b. Individuals who are 65 years and older have a 10% to 15% incidence of major depression, with a 30% incidence of dysthymia. These statistics indicate that depression is a significant problem for elderly individuals.
   c. Estimates suggest that 10 to 14 million Americans are afflicted with some form of mood disorder.

3. **Episodes of major depressive disorder**
   a. Of persons with major depressive disorder, 50% to 85% will experience more than one episode of depression. The average is four episodes across a lifetime.
   b. The **age of onset** of a depressive episode is most frequently between ages 25 and 44. However, individuals born after World War II typically have an earlier age of onset.
4. **Bipolar disorder** affects 1% of the U.S. population.
   a. Persons with this disorder typically will experience 10 episodes across a lifetime; 30% of individuals with bipolar disorder will begin to show symptoms before 25 years of age.
   b. Bipolar disorder affects men and women equally, although women may have depression as their first experience of this disorder.
D. **Effect on family.** Family members of individuals with a mood disorder are severely impacted.
   1. Changes in energy levels, role functioning, and socialization that occur in an individual with a mood disorder affect every aspect of family life.
   2. Children of depressed mothers have increased vulnerability for emotional problems.
E. **Cultural considerations**
   1. African Americans have a lower rate of mood disorders than Whites and Hispanic Americans
   2. People of Asian background manifest more somatic symptoms, whereas people from Western cultures have mood and cognitive symptoms. For example, somatic symptoms such as general fatigue and unexplained body aches or pains would be more common in people of Asian background, whereas people in Western cultures would have symptoms such as depressed mood and decreased ability to concentrate.

 Types of Mood Disorders

A. **Major depressive disorder**
   1. Major depressive disorder is characterized by at least 2 weeks of a depressed mood or loss of interest in pleasure and activities. In addition, at least four of the following symptoms of depression must be present:
      a. Increase or decrease in appetite
      b. Increase or decrease in sleep
      c. Psychomotor agitation or retardation
      d. Fatigue and loss of energy
      e. Decreased ability to think and concentrate
      f. Recurrent thoughts of suicide
   2. **DSM-IV specifiers of major depressive disorder**
      a. **Melancholic features.** The individual experiences either anhedonia in relation to all activities or lack of mood reactivity to usually pleasurable

stimuli. This specifier is also characterized by early morning awakening, feeling worse in the morning, and excessive guilt.

b. **Atypical features.** The individual exhibits mood reactivity (ie, ability to respond to positive environmental stimuli), increased levels of anxiety, changes in appetite and sleep, and increased sensitivity to interpersonal rejection.

c. **Psychotic features.** The individual's depression is accompanied by delusions and hallucinations. The theme of the psychotic symptoms is usually mood congruent with depression.

d. **Postpartum onset.** The onset of symptoms occurs within 4 weeks of delivery. The symptoms are similar to that of a typical major depressive disorder; however, psychotic features may also be present. Postpartum depression affects 1 in 10 new mothers.

e. **Seasonal pattern specifier.** Although seasonal affective disorder (SAD) is currently not classified as a diagnostic category in DSM-IV, it is included as a specifier. This disorder commonly occurs in the fall and winter and is associated with the decrease in sunlight. Common symptoms include hypersomnia, overeating and carbohydrate craving, and weight gain.

B. Dysthymia

1. Dysthymia is characterized by a chronically depressed mood occurring most of the day, for more days than not, for at least a 2-year period. During the periods of depressed mood, at least two or more of the other symptoms of depression must be present (see II.A.1.a–f).

2. This disorder usually does not affect social or occupational functioning.

C. Bipolar disorder

1. **Bipolar I disorder** is characterized by one or more manic or mixed episodes, usually accompanied by a major depressive episode. Symptoms of a manic episode include the following:
   a. Inflated self-esteem or grandiosity
   b. Decreased need for sleep
   c. Increased or pressured speech
   d. Flight of ideas
   e. Distractibility
   f. Increased involvement in goal-directed activities
   g. Excessive involvement in pleasurable activities that have a high potential for painful consequences (eg, charging expensive items on a credit card that is already at maximum limit; sleeping with multiple partners without regard to safe sex practices)

2. **Bipolar II disorder** is characterized by one or more major depressive episodes accompanied by at least one hypomanic episode. A hypomanic episode is one in which at least three or more of the symptoms of mania are present (see II.C.1.a–g).

D. Cyclothymia is characterized by at least 2 years of several periods of hypomanic symptoms not as severe as those in a manic episode (Table 6-1).

TABLE 6-1
Common Risk Factors Associated With Mood Disorder and Suicidal Behaviors

RISK FACTOR	MOOD DISORDERS	SUICIDAL BEHAVIORS
Sex	Depression twice as likely in women as men (2:1) Bipolar more likely in women than men (1.2:1)	Increased risk in men
Age	Higher in young women and older men	Risk increases with age (but adolescents make more attempts)
Marital status	Higher in married women and single men Lower in married men	Risk lower among married men and women
Family history	Higher risk among first-degree relatives	Higher risk among family members of suicide victims
Precipitators (recent life events)	Birth in family within 6 months Loss of significant other Job problems Separation or divorce Physical illness	Increases with Solitariness (eg, living alone) Unemployment Recent loss Recent surgery or childbirth Social disgrace
Other	Seasonal pattern: depression higher in fall and winter	High risk with alcohol and drug abuse Increased risk in those with mood or thought disorders

E. Pseudodementia is a disorder associated with depression in the elderly.

1. The clinical presentation of depression is similar to symptoms associated with a cognitive impairment disorder

2. Treatment of depression that is successful in eliminating the symptoms of dementia will establish this diagnosis.

III. Etiology

A. General considerations

1. **The exact causes for mood disorders have not been established.** The current general consensus is that these disorders result from complex interactions among a variety of factors.

2. **Implicating factors** that have been studied include genetic predisposition, neurochemical imbalances (affecting neurotransmission and neuroendocrine regulation), certain medications, medical conditions, and psychosocial and environmental processes.

B. Genetic predisposition

1. **Mood disorders**

   a. The risk of developing a mood disorder is 1.5 to 3 times greater in individuals with a first-degree relative with a mood disorder.

   b. Twin studies reveal a higher rate of concordance in monozygotic twins than dizygotic twins, indicating genetic component.
   c. Researchers are currently investigating a defective gene on chromosome 4. People with this defective gene are 26 times more likely to be hospitalized for severe depression and suicide attempt. Research also is focused on genes on chromosomes 11, 18, and 21.
2. **Bipolar disorders**
   a. The risk for developing bipolar disorder is 4% to 24% increased in first-degree relatives of people with bipolar disorder.
   b. Twin studies of monozygotic twins indicate a 65% concordance rate.
   c. Research indicates that defective genes located somewhere within chromosomes 18 and 21 are important in the causation of bipolar disorder (Keltner, 1998).

C. **Neurotransmission dysregulation**
   1. **Biogenic amine theory.** This theory postulates that there is a norepinephrine and serotonin deficiency in individuals with a depressive disorder, and increases in these neurotransmitters in individuals with a bipolar disorder. Changes in quantity and sensitivity of receptor sites are also important.
   2. **Kindling theory.** First described by Post (1992), this theory states that external environmental stressors activate internal physiologic stress responses, which trigger the first episode of a mood disorder. The first episode then creates electrophysiologic sensitivity to future episodes so that less stress is required to evoke another episode.

D. **Neuroendocrine dysregulation**
   1. **Hypothalamic-pituitary-adrenal (HPA) axis.** Laboratory findings indicate that some individuals with depressive disorders exhibit increased cortisol levels, resistance of cortisol to suppression by dexamethasone (dexamethasone suppression test), and blunted adrenocorticotropin hormone response to corticotropin-releasing factor challenge as compared to normal controls. Elevated corticotropin-releasing factor has also been found in cerebrospinal fluid.
   2. **Subclinical hypothyroidism** has been found in some individuals with depressive disorders, especially women. Blunting of response of thyroid-stimulating hormone to thyrotropic-releasing factor has been found in approximately 25% of euthyroid individuals with depressive disorders.
   3. **Circadian rhythm changes.** Studies indicate abnormal sleep electroencephalograms in many individuals with mood disorders. This has led to the theory that mood disorders reflect abnormal regulation of circadian rhythms (Keltner, 1998).

E. **Medications.** Some medications have side effects that include depression. These medications include:
   1. **Hormones:** eg, oral contraceptives, glucocorticoids
   2. **Cardiovascular drugs:** eg, beta-blockers, calcium channel blockers, thiazide diuretics, and digitalis preparations
   3. **Psychotropics:** eg, benzodiazepines, neuroleptics

4. **Anti-inflammatory and anti-infective drugs:** eg, nonsteroidal anti-inflammatory drugs, antituberculosis drugs, and sulfonamides
5. **Anti-ulcer medications:** eg, cimetidine, ranitidine

F. **Medical conditions.** Clinically significant depressive symptoms are detected in approximately 12% to 36% of individuals with a nonpsychiatric general medical condition (Agency for Health Care Policy and Research, 1993). Some examples include:

1. CVA
2. Cognitive impairment disorders (dementia)
3. Diabetes
4. Coronary artery disease
5. Cancer
6. Chronic fatigue syndrome
7. Acquired immunodeficiency syndrome (AIDS)

G. **Psychosocial and environmental theories**

1. **Psychoanalytic (psychodynamic) theory.** Freud's theory describes the occurrence of a significant loss (object loss) that is associated with anger and aggression, which is turned inward and leads to negative feelings about self associated with depression.

2. **Cognitive-behavioral theory.** Beck's theory proposes that depression is a problem of cognitive patterns that have developed in an individual over time. The individual holds negative views of self, the world, and the future; views self as unattractive and incompetent; and views the outward environment as demanding and unyielding and the future as hopeless. Table 6-2 lists and defines the most common negative cognitions.

3. **Environmental stressors.** Experiences such as recent loss of family member through death, divorce, or separation; lack of social support system, or significant health problem have all been associated with the onset of a mood disorder. Sleep deprivation has been associated with the occurrence of another manic episode in an individual with a history of bipolar disorder.

IV. Management

A. **General considerations.** Clients may receive treatment in various settings, including acute psychiatric hospitals, community-based treatment in outpatient program, or private psychotherapy with a primary practitioner.

B. **Acute, psychiatric, hospital-based care.** This setting may be recommended when a client's mood disorder is severe or danger for self-harm exists.

1. Clients with suicidal behavior require hospitalization for protection, so they can receive:
   a. Supportive psychotherapy and milieu management
   b. Cognitive-behavioral therapy
   c. Medication with antidepressants, neuroleptics (if psychotic level symptoms occur), or mood-stabilizing agents (Drug Chart 6-1)

TABLE 6-2
Common Negative Cognitions

NEGATIVE COGNITION	DESCRIPTION	EXAMPLE
Overgeneralization	Believing that everything will go wrong because of a single negative occurrence: the act of blowing things out of proportion. Key words include "never" and "always."	After scoring a low grade in algebra, a student says, "I will never learn this stuff."
All-or-nothing thinking	Viewing everything in extremes— either "black or white," with no middle ground	John takes pictures of his friend's wedding. All but three of the pictures are perfect. John is dissatisfied because all the pictures are not perfect and considers himself to be a failure at photography.
Should statements	Using "should," "shouldn't," "must," and "ought to" statements to establish standards for self and others. "Should" statements in general lead to frustration. Those directed toward oneself lead to guilt; those directed at others lead to anger and resentment.	John (from previous example) says to himself, "I should have taken all of the pictures right."
Labeling	Applying negatively loaded labels to oneself or others	After the student was unable to comprehend the 300 pages of her nursing text, she says, "I'm an idiot."
Mind reading	Jumping to conclusions regarding another person's reactions without checking those reactions with the other person	Pat is having an enjoyable lunch with a friend, but the friend looks dejected. Pat asks what the problem is. After coaxing, the friend says, "I know you think that I'm a bad person."
Fortune telling	Being absolutely convinced that things will not turn out right, no matter what the evidence to the contrary	Ellen has received several letters of commendation from her boss, but when it's time to apply for a promotion, she states, "I'd better not apply; my boss will never give me a promotion; I only perform mediocre work."

DRUG CHART 6-1. Selected Medications Used in Treatment of Mood Disorders

Classification	Generic/ Trade Name	Adult Dosage (mg/day)	Rationale for Use
Antidepressants			
Tricyclic antidepressants (TCAs)	Amitriptyline (Elavil) Clomipramine (Anafranil) Desipramine (Norpramin) Nortriptyline (Pamelor)	75–300 mg 75–250 mg 75–300 mg 50–150 mg	Act by blocking reuptake of neurotransmitters at presynaptic neuron. The TCAs act on both serotonin and norepinephrine; therefore, they are nonselective in action. Provides elevation of mood, increased activity level, and appetite stimulation.
Monoamine oxidase inhibitors (MAOIs)	Phenelzine (Nardil) Isocarboxazid (Marplan) Tranylcypromine (Parnate)	45–90 mg 30–50 mg 20–60 mg	Act by inhibiting enzyme monoamine oxidase, which is responsible for metabolizing norepinephrine and serotonin. When the enzyme is inhibited, increased amounts of neurotransmitters remain at the synapse and act to elevate mood and increase activity level.
Selective serotonin reuptake inhibitors	Fluvoxamine (Luvox) Fluoxetine (Prozac) Paroxetine (Paxil) Sertraline (Zoloft)	100–300 mg 40–80 mg 20–50 mg 50–150 mg	Act specifically on serotonin, preventing its reuptake. Because it is selective, it does not have side effects of the TCAs and MAOIs (related to increasing norepinephrine at synapse).
Atypical antidepressants	Bupropion (Wellbutrin) Mitrazapine (Remeron) Nefazodone (Serzone) Venlafaxine (Effexor) Trazadone (Desyrel)	150–300 mg 15–45 mg 200–400 mg 75–300 mg 150–300 mg	Act similar to the TCAs. Antidepressant effects are not yet well understood; however, have fewer side effects than TCAs.
Herbal remedy	Hypericum perforatum (St. John's Wort)	No standard dose yet recommended	May relieve mild-to-moderate depression. Study currently ongoing.
Mood Stabilizers			
Antimanic	Lithium carbonate (Eskalith, Lithobid, Lithonite)	600–2100 mg/day (blood level of 0.8 to 1.5 mEq/L.)	Lithium acts by interfering with a neuropathway called the phosphoinositide (PI) second messenger system in the limbic system. This helps to stabilize neurochemical regulation in the brain and therefore stabilize mood.
Anticonvulsants	Carbamazepine (Tegretol) Valproic acid (Depakote)	800–1200 mg/day 800–1200 mg/day	Acts by affecting sodium and calcium channels and thereby decreasing release of neurotransmitters. Thought to inhibit process of kindling from occurring.

2. Electroconvulsive therapy may be recommended for severe depression that is unresponsive to antidepressant therapy (see Chapter 15).

C. Community-based treatment

    1. Primary prevention may be accomplished through identification of at-risk populations and teaching self-care measures to decrease occurrence of mood disorders. Self-care measures may include:

        a. Adequate exercise and rest

        b. Good nutrition

        c. Stress management

        d. Use of support systems

        e. Verbalizing rather than internalizing feelings

        f. Assertiveness training programs

    2. Case finding occurs when health care practitioners identify individuals in the community who have symptoms of a mood disorder but are not in treatment. Case finding can promote early intervention and decrease chronicity. The client, family, or both can be educated about:

        a. The nature and course of the disorder

        b. Recognizing individual symptom patterns

        c. Self-monitoring for symptom return and seeking prompt treatment

        d. Self-care measures (see IV.C.1.a–f)

    3. Crisis intervention services should be used for those individuals with suicidal behavior.

    4. Medication management (see Drug Chart 6-1) and use of ultraviolet light therapy for seasonal affective disorder.

    5. Cognitive-behavior therapy is the recommended type of psychotherapeutic approach for a client with a mood disorder.

        a. In some studies, it has been found to be as effective as antidepressant therapy (Glod, 1998).

        b. This approach includes identifying and challenging the accuracy of the client's negative cognitions, reinforcing more accurate perceptions, and encouraging behaviors that are designed to counteract the depressive symptoms.

D. Resources for client and family

    1. Community support groups (eg, Depressives Anonymous; Recovery, Inc.)

    2. National Depressive and Manic Depressive Association, which provides information and assistance

    3. National Alliance for the Mentally Ill, which provides information, support groups, and political action for legislative efforts on behalf of individuals with mental illness and their families

V.   **NURSING PROCESS OVERVIEW FOR**
Stress and Anxiety

A. Assessment (Table 6-3)

    1. Review the client's history for precipitating stressors and significant data about:

        a. Genetic-biologic vulnerability (eg, family history)

TABLE 6-3
Comparison of Assessment Data in Mood Disorders

CHARACTERISTICS	DEPRESSIVE DISORDERS	BIPOLAR (MANIC) DISORDERS
Physiologic responses	Altered appetite (increased or decreased) Altered sleep patterns (hypersomnia or insomnia) Constipation due to dietary factors	Reduced appetite due to hyperactivity Little sleep due to excess energy (insomnia) Constipation possible Boundless energy leading to physical exhaustion Physiologic responses ignored
Cognitive responses	Indecisiveness Reduced concentration and attention span Rumination (constant preoccupation with same thoughts), somatic delusions, poverty of thought	Impaired judgement Reduced concentration and attention span, distractible, flight of ideas Grandiose beliefs and delusions, tangential thinking
Emotional responses	Sadness and despondency Anger, agitation, resentfulness Guilt and worthlessness Hopelessness and helplessness Apathy	Euphoria, elation Anger, irritability, rage Lack of guilt, narcissism Exaggerated sense of ability Emotional lability
Behavioral responses	Poor personal hygiene Psychomotor retardation Decreased motivation Anhedonia Frequent complaints and demands Lack of spontaneity Lack of exercise Fatigue Somatic complaints Restless and undirected activity	Poor personal hygiene Psychomotor agitation Impulsiveness, lack of inhibition Hypersexuality, increase in high-risk sexual behavior Manipulative, domineering Inappropriate singing, dancing, joking Undirected hyperactivity

    b. Stressful life events and recent losses

    c. Results of standardized assessment tools for depression (eg, Beck Depression Inventory, Hamilton Rating Scale of Depression, Geriatric Depression Scale, and Self-Rating Depression Scale).

    d. Past episodes of mood disorder or suicidal behaviors

    e. Medication history

    f. Drug and alcohol use

    g. Education and employment history

  2. Note characteristic physiologic, cognitive, emotional, and behavioral responses of individual with a history of a mood disorder (see Tables 6-3 and 6-4).

  3. **Assess suicidal risk factors and lethality of client's suicidal behavior (Display 6-1; see also Table 6-1)**

    a. The **client's intent** (eg, for relief from stress, solution to difficult problems)

    b. The **suicidal plan,** including whether the client has an organized plan and means to carry out the plan

TABLE 6-4
Key Nursing Assessment Questions for Clients With a Mood Disorder

CLIENT	QUESTIONS	PROVIDES DATA ABOUT
Client with depression	What is the feeling of depression like for you? How long have you felt this way? How would you rate your feeling of depression on a scale from 1–10? What are the activities or things in your life that give you pleasure? Do you sleep excessively or have difficulty sleeping? Have you lost weight recently or have a poor appetite? Have you experienced any losses or changes in your life? Are you experiencing thoughts of suicide? Do you have a specific suicide plan?	Individual experience of depression Severity of depressive symptoms Presence of anhedonia Disturbance of sleep patterns Presence of altered appetite Recent losses Suicide intent
Client with mania	Have you experienced racing thoughts or find that you can't speak your thoughts quickly enough? What projects or activities have you recently been doing? Have you completed things you have started? Have you become impatient or easily angered with others? How many hours a night do you sleep? How would you describe your mood?	Presence of flight of ideas or pressured speech Hyperactivity Inability to complete tasks Irritability, impulsiveness Inadequate sleep patterns Presence of elation, euphoria

    c. The client's **mental state** (eg, presence of thought disorder, level of anxiety, severity of mood disorder)

    d. **Support systems** available

    e. **Current stressors** affecting the client, including other illnesses (both psychiatric and medical), recent losses, and history of substance abuse

  4. Assess the family support system and assess the client or family's knowledge base about specific mood disorder symptoms, medications and treatment recommendations, signs of relapse, and self-care measures.

B. Analysis and nursing diagnosis

  1. Analyze the client's predominant mood, anxiety level, degree of self-esteem, and severity of symptoms.

    a. **Determine the client's risk for suicide, understanding that a client with a mood disorder is at increased risk. (Suicide is most likely when going into or coming out of a depression.)**

    b. Determine the level of family support available.

DISPLAY 6-1. **Quick Assessment of Suicide Risk Factors**

- Sex (males more than females)
- Age (adolescent or older than 50 years of age)
- Previous attempt (increases risk)
- Alcohol/substance abuse
- Presence of thought disorder
- Lack of support system
- Unmarried, divorced, widowed
- Presence of physical illness (especially chronic)
- Organized plan

---

2. Establish individualized nursing diagnoses for the client or family with a depressive disorder, bipolar disorder, or suicidal behaviors and prioritize these:

a. Anxiety
b. Coping, ineffective family; compromised
c. Coping, ineffective individual
d. Family processes, altered
e. Grieving, dysfunctional
f. Hopelessness
g. Knowledge deficit (specify)
h. Nutrition, altered: risk for less than body requirement
i. Powerlessness
j. Self-esteem disturbance
k. Sexuality patterns, altered
l. Sleep pattern disturbance
m. Social isolation
n. Spiritual distress
o. Thought processes, altered
p. Violence, risk for: self-directed or directed at others

C. Planning and outcome identification. Work with the client in setting realistic goals.

1. Establish desired outcome criteria for a client with a mood disorder.

a. The client will demonstrate decreased anxiety.
b. The client will identify aspects of self-control over current life situation.
c. The client will proceed through the grieving process, verbalizing feelings to supportive persons.
d. The client will reestablish sleep patterns, including at least 6 to 7 hours of uninterrupted sleep nightly.
e. The client will eat nutritious meals, either three meals or six smaller meals a day.
f. The client will verbalize positive, realistic self-statements.
g. The client will report increased hope for the future.

    h. The client will identify thoughts that are not reality based.
    i. The client will interact in social situations, reporting satisfaction and feelings of belonging.
    j. The client will agree to report feelings of wanting to harm self to treatment staff in timely manner.
    k. The client will refrain from any acts of harm to self or others.
    l. The client will reestablish normal sexual patterns.
  2. Establish desired outcome criteria for families with a member having a mood disorder.
    a. The family will express feelings about individual concerns.
    b. The family will verbalize knowledge about mood disorders, treatment plans, relapse signs, and symptom management (Client and Family Teaching 6-1).

D. Implementation

  1. For the client with a depressive disorder
    a. Accept the client, avoiding any action that could be interpreted as criticism.
    b. Facilitate adequate nutrition, considering the client's food preferences.

CLIENT AND FAMILY TEACHING 6-1

Educating Families Who Have a Member With a Mood Disorder

1. Educate the family about the specific disorder:
   Depression is a disorder characterized by sadness, hopelessness, and decreased self-esteem. No single cause has been established, but research indicates genetics, chemical imbalance in the brain, and life changes (eg, losses).
   Mania is a disorder characterized by elation, feelings of boundless energy, and belief that one is superior and gifted. An individual with mania may be too busy to sleep or eat and may spend money wildly or engage in risk-taking behaviors. No single cause has been established, but research indicates genetics, chemical imbalance in the brain, and life changes.
   An individual with a mood disorder generally experiences thoughts of suicide. Times of increased risk would be going into or coming out of a depression.
2. Educate the family about treatment:
   Medications are used—antidepressants for depression and mood-stabilizing agents for mania.
   It is important to take medication as prescribed.
   Antidepressants may not have an effect immediately; it may take 2 to 4 weeks for mood improvement.
   Blood levels will be important if the individual is taking a mood-stabilizing agents.
   Talk therapy can also be an effective treatment, along with medication.
3. Educate the family about handling symptoms:
   Attempts to either cheer up a person with depression or to bring down a person with mania are not helpful.
   Matter-of-fact acceptance of individual's current mood is helpful.
   Reassurance that mood will improve with treatment is supportive.
   Encourage regular routine of activity and rest (balance of both).
   Talk about suicide should be taken seriously; contact health care provider.

    c. **Implement suicide precautions according to assessments about the client's intent.**
    d. Avoid excessive cheerfulness, sympathy, or superficiality.
    e. Assist the client in developing a daily schedule that includes activities and rest.
    f. Promote sleep with bedtime relaxation interventions (eg, quiet time, back rubs, music or relaxation tapes, or guided imagery).
    g. Encourage participation and social interaction, offering support as needed.
    h. Assist the client to identify feelings and reduce negative cognitions (see Table 6-2).
    i. Encourage success in achieving goals by helping the client structure simple, manageable tasks.
    j. Question or express doubt about the client's negative self-statements.
    k. Facilitate movement through the grieving process by accepting feelings expressed.
    l. When a client expresses delusional beliefs, use reality reinforcement techniques (see Chapter 7).
    m. **Administer medications as prescribed, monitoring laboratory study findings indicating appropriate blood levels (for mood-stabilizing medications). (See Chapter 15.)**
    n. Monitor the client for expected effects as well as untoward side effects of medications.
    o. Teach the client about the disorder, including the etiology, symptom identification and management, treatment recommendations, medications, and long-term self-management.
    p. Collaborate with other health team members, especially activity therapists, in providing activities (eg, art, music, dance therapy) that allow client to express feelings.
    q. Encourage the client to participate in self-help or other support groups in the community.

2. For the client with a bipolar disorder (manic behaviors), use the implementations described for the client with a depressive disorder in addition to the following:
    a. Promote adequate nutrition by providing high-calorie foods that can be eaten on the run.
    b. Remove the client from excessively stimulating environment when hyperactivity escalates.
    c. Promote rest periods and encourage use of quiet activities if client is unable to rest.
    d. Take a matter-of-fact, consistent approach in describing acceptable behavior and realistic limits.
    e. Assist the client to think through the consequences of impulsive behaviors.
    f. Refrain from laughing or otherwise encouraging inappropriate behaviors.
    g. **Provide a safe environment and monitor the client to prevent accidents and injury.**

  h. Provide the client with simple tasks that focus attention and yield successful completion.
  i. Assist the client in identifying realistic goals and future plans.

3. For the client with suicidal behavior

  a. Establish a supportive relationship, aligning oneself with the part of the client that wishes to live.
  b. Monitor the client closely, using suicidal precautions according to agency protocol.
  c. Question the client directly about suicide, including asking about a specific plan and a means to accomplish the plan. (Note: Asking the client does not increase the risk.)
  d. Remove dangerous and potentially lethal materials or objects, according to agency protocol.
  e. Encourage the client to discuss stressors, feelings of pain, anger, and anguish.
  f. Encourage the client to agree to a no-suicide contract as part of behavioral agreement.
  g. Assist the client with the problem-solving process when specific problems are identified.

E. Outcome evaluation. The nurse uses the following criteria to evaluate client outcomes and the effectiveness of nursing implementations.

  1. The client verbalizes decreased anxiety and normal mood.
  2. The client does not harm self, and reports wanting to live.
  3. The client eats nutritious meals each day, maintaining a normal weight.
  4. The client exhibits normal sleep patterns, allowing for adequate energy during the day.
  5. The client verbalizes feeling able to cope with current life changes and is able to identify specific ways for coping.
  6. The client voices positive self-statements.
  7. The client expresses hope for the future.
  8. The client expresses satisfaction with improved social interaction and identifies support systems available.
  9. The client demonstrates clear thinking patterns, with no evidence of delusions, excessive guilt, or flight of ideas.
  10. The client and family use knowledge about the disorder, treatment program, medications, and symptoms to manage the disorder on an ongoing basis.

STUDY QUESTIONS

1. Using cognitive-behavioral therapy, which of the following would be involved in the treatment of a client with depression?
   (1) challenging negative thinking
   (2) encouraging analysis of dreams
   (3) prescribing antidepressant medications
   (4) using ultraviolet light therapy

2. The nurse assessing a client diagnosed with bipolar disorder would expect to find a history of which of the following?
   (1) a depressive episode followed by prolonged sadness
   (2) a series of depressive episodes that reoccur periodically
   (3) symptoms of mania that may or may not be followed by depression
   (4) symptoms of mania that include delusional thoughts

3. A client completing requirements for student teaching reports to the nurse an incident in which a student was rude and disrespectful. The client states, "None of the students respect my teaching ability." The nurse identifies this as an example of which of the following common negative cognitions?
   (1) labeling
   (2) fortune telling
   (3) overgeneralization
   (4) "should" statement

4. Which of the following behaviors in a client with the DSM-IV diagnosis of bipolar disorder, single manic episode, would be assessed by a nurse?
   (1) apathy, poor insight, poverty of ideas
   (2) anxiety, somatic complaints, insomnia
   (3) elation, hyperactivity, impaired judgment
   (4) social isolation, delusional thinking, clang associations

5. A client with manic behavior is creating considerable chaos in a day treatment program with dominating and manipulative behavior. Which of the following nursing interventions is most appropriate?
   (1) Allow the peer group to intervene.
   (2) Describe acceptable behavior and set realistic limits with the client.
   (3) Recommend the client to be hospitalized for treatment.
   (4) Tell client that his behavior is not appropriate.

6. According to the biogenic amine theory, an individual with depression has a deficiency in which of the following neurotransmitters?
   (1) dopamine and thyroxin
   (2) GABA and acetylcholine
   (3) cortisone and epinephrine
   (4) serotonin and norepinephrine

7. An elderly client has a chronic illness. She has increased risk for depression if she is taking
   (1) an antacid preparation
   (2) a benzodiazapine
   (3) a bronchodilator
   (4) a laxative

8. A nurse is teaching a client and her family about the most significant factor in the causation of depression. Which of the following causative factors would the nurse emphasize?
   (1) brain structure abnormalities
   (2) chemical imbalance in the brain
   (3) social environment
   (4) recessive gene transmission

9. When evaluating an imminent suicide risk, which of the following
information given by the client
would be *most* significant?
   (1) at least a 2-year history of feeling depressed more days than
   not
   (2) divorced from spouse 6 months
   ago
   (3) feeling loss of energy and
   appetite
   (4) reference to suicide as best
   solution to identified problems

10. A client in an acute psychiatric hospital unit tells a nurse about his
plans for suicide. The priority nursing intervention is to
   (1) allow the client time alone for
   reflection
   (2) encourage client to use problem solving
   (3) follow agency protocol for suicide precautions
   (4) stimulate the client's interest in
   activities

11. Which of the following mood disorders has a defining characteristic of
feeling depressed most of the day
for a 2-year period?
   (1) cyclothymia
   (2) dysthymia
   (3) melancholic depressive disorder
   (4) seasonal affective disorder

12. The community nurse is speaking
to a group of new mothers as part
of a primary prevention program.
Which of the following self-care
measures would be *most* helpful as
a strategy to decrease occurrence of
mood disorders?
   (1) keeping busy, so as not to confront problem areas

   (2) medication with antidepressants
   (3) use of crisis intervention services
   (4) verbalizing rather than internalizing feelings

13. The husband of a client who has
recently lost her job tells the clinic
nurse that the client's moods are
constantly changing from extremely
happy and elated to sadness and
crying. As part of an immediate
assessment of the family situation,
the nurse should question the husband and wife about which of the
following?
   (1) the client's academic and work
   history
   (2) the specific history of psy-
   chopathology in client's family
   (3) the client's specific symptoms,
   the duration of the symptoms,
   and the impact of the symptoms
   on the family
   (4) the quality of couple's marital
   relationship

14. During a daily community meeting,
a client with bipolar disorder, manic
type, begins pacing around the
room and talking in a loud voice
with rapid speech. Which of the following is the most appropriate
nursing intervention?
   (1) asking the client to accompany
   you and moving to a quieter
   room
   (2) allowing the community group
   to handle the client's behavior
   (3) ending the community meeting
   at this time
   (4) offering antianxiety medication
   to the client

ANSWER KEY

1. The answer is (1). Cognitive-behavioral therapy includes identifying and challenging a client's negative cognitions. The belief is that these negative thoughts influence the feelings and behaviors in depression. Dream analysis would be used in psychoanalytic psychotherapy. Antidepressant medication could be part of a treatment program for an individual with depression; however, this would not be considered cognitive-behavioral therapy. Ultraviolet light therapy would be a somatic approach to treatment for seasonal affective disorder.

2. The answer is (3). The definition of bipolar disorder is a mood disturbance in which the symptoms of mania have occurred at least one time. Depression may or may not occur as a separate episode in bipolar disorder. None of the other answer choices indicate a correct understanding of bipolar disorder.

3. The answer is (3). The client in this situation is overgeneralizing the response of one particular student, such that the notion is that the entire class has this attitude. The client is blowing one incident out of proportion to reality. Labeling is the applying of negative labels to oneself or others. Fortune telling is the conviction that things will not turn out right, despite contrary evidence. "Should" statements refer to statements establishing standards for self and others.

4. The answer is (3). A client with bipolar disorder, manic episode, would demonstrate symptoms, such as flight of ideas and hyperactivity, as part of the increased psychomotor activity. The mood is one of elation and the feeling is that one is invincible; therefore, judgment may be quite impaired. The symptoms in answer choice (1) would be more characteristic of an individual with long-term schizophrenia. The symptoms in answer choice (2) would be more characteristic of an individual with an anxiety disorder, although the person who has mania may not sleep because of excessive energy. The symptoms in answer choice (4) would be more characteristic of an individual with a problem of schizophrenia.

5. The answer is (2). The nurse's response is an alternative behavior for the unacceptable ones in order to assist the client in self-control. It is not the responsibility of the peer group to monitor the client's behavior. The client's behavior does not warrant hospitalization. The intervention in answer choice (4) is inappropriate because the client is told only what is unacceptable and is not given any alternatives.

6. The answer is (4). The biogenic amine theory of depression describes deficiencies in the neurotransmitters serotonin and norepinephrine. Antidepressant medications increase the levels of these neurotransmitters and therefore help to relieve depressive symptoms. According to current research, dopamine, thyroxin, GABA, acetylcholine, cortisone, and epinephrine are not directly related to depression.

7. The answer is (2). Certain categories of medications are known to cause depression as a side effect. In an elderly individual with a chronic illness, this side effect can increase the risk for a depressive episode. The benzodiazepine group of medications is one of these categories. Other drug groups include hormones, certain cardiovascular drugs, anti-inflammatory medications, and anti-ulcer medication. Antacids are used for clients with ulcer disease because they have a buffering effect on excess gastric acid. They do not have any side effects of depression. The medications that are histamine-2 blockers, cimetidine and ranitidine, have depressive side effects. Bronchodilators and laxatives do not produce depression as a side effect.

8. The answer is (2). Chemical imbalance of neurotransmitters in the brain is a major factor in depression. Exact causation has not been established, so that other factors may also play a role in causation. Although genetic transmission certainly may be a factor, there is no definite pattern of transmission. Social environment in terms of lack of support systems can increase risk for depression, but the most significant factor would be chemical imbalance in the brain.

9. The answer is (4). An individual who talks about suicide as a solution to problems is at high risk. Suicidal threats need to be taken seriously, because this individual does not see any other viable solutions to problems in living. All of the factors in the other answer choices would increase the client's risk for depression; however, actual statements about intent for suicide are red flags for the nurse of imminent danger.

10. The answer is (3). The nurse must act to safeguard the client from danger, including self-harm. Implementation of specific agency protocol for suicidal precautions would be protective for client. A client with suicidal intent should not be left alone. One-to-one observations are generally part of suicide precautions. Encouraging the client to use problem solving and stimulating the client's interest in activities would be helpful for a client with depression; however, the priority intervention is to protect the client, and therefore the appropriate intervention is suicide precautions.

11. The answer is (2). Dysthymia is characterized by at least a 2-year history of depression, occurring most of the day for more days than not. Cyclothymia is characterized by at least 2 years of several periods of hypomanic symptoms. Melancholic depressive disorder is characterized by either anhedonia in relation to all activities or lack of mood reactivity to usually pleasurable stimuli. Seasonal affective disorder is characterized by its occurrence in fall and winter, associated with loss of sunlight.

12. The answer is (4). Individuals who develop mood disorders often have difficulty expressing feelings, especially feelings of anger toward significant others. Internalizing those feelings can contribute to loss of self-esteem and guilt, and therefore negative cognitions and depression. Ignoring problems is not a helpful strategy. Recognizing problems and using problem-solving methods will contribute to mental health. Antidepressants are certainly necessary in the treatment of the mood disorder of depression; however, they are not used in primary prevention. Crisis intervention would be a strategy useful in the immediate treatment of a crisis of a mood disorder. It is not a tool of primary prevention.

13. The answer is (3). Assessment of the current family situation would include identifying the client's symptoms, duration of symptoms, and the unique impact on this particular family. The assessment data related to answer choices **(1)** and **(2)** would be important, but the immediate assessment would be more specific to the current family crisis. The quality of the marital relationship would be one aspect of the entire family situation.

14. The answer is (1). The most appropriate intervention when a client with mania begins to escalate is to remove the client from an overstimulating environment. The community meeting is not an appropriate place for a client who is becoming agitated. The community group may be intimidated by client behavior and reluctant to intervene. The nurse is responsible for limit setting and intervention when client behavior is inappropriate. The community meeting is an important forum for client participation and should not be terminated because one client is upset. Removing the client from an overstimulating environment may be sufficient in helping a client regain self-control. The least restrictive means should be offered prior to use of chemical restraints.

7

Schizophrenic Disorders

I. Description

A. Definition. Schizophrenic disorders are a group of psychotic reactions that affect multiple areas of an individual's functioning, including thinking and communicating, perceiving and interpreting reality, feeling and demonstrating emotion, and behaving in a socially acceptable manner.

B. DSM-IV criteria

1. The disturbance lasts for at least 6 months and includes at least 1 month of active-phase symptoms involving two or more of the following: delusions, hallucinations, disorganized speech, grossly disorganized or catatonic behavior, negative symptoms (ie, affective flattening, alogia, or avolition).
2. Other criteria
   a. Social and occupational dysfunction are present.
   b. Schizoaffective disorders and mood disorder with psychotic features have been ruled out.
   c. The disturbance is not due to physiologic effect of a substance or a general medical condition.

C. Common symptoms of schizophrenia

1. **Delusions:** fixed false beliefs that cannot be discounted by use of logic (Display 7-1)
2. **Loose associations:** lack of logical relationships between thoughts and ideas, which may be reflected in a variety of symptoms (Table 7-1)
3. **Hallucinations:** false sensory perceptions involving any of the five senses; in schizophrenia, auditory hallucinations are most common
4. **Illusions:** misinterpretations of environmental stimuli
5. **Depersonalization/derealization:** feeling of the individual that the "self" has been fundamentally changed or altered
6. **Affective flattening:** absence of emotional response; affect can also be described as **blunted** (dulled response) or **inappropriate** (opposite to what is expected of a situation)
7. **Ambivalence:** presence of conflicting or opposite emotions leading to difficulty making a choice or a decision
8. **Avolition:** lack of motivation to persist in goal-directed activity
9. **Alogia:** decreased speech patterns or poverty of speech

---

DISPLAY 7-1. **Common Delusions in Schizophrenia**

Delusions of reference—everything occurring in environment has direct significance to oneself
Delusions of persecution—people or institutions are plotting against or attacking oneself
Delusions of external influences—one is controlled by others or outside forces
Somatic delusions—appearance or functioning of one's body is altered
Grandiose delusions—inflated self-worth, power, knowledge, or identity

---

10. **Echopraxia:** senseless copying of another's actions
11. **Anhedonia:** lack of pleasure in activities and things that the individual would normally perceive as pleasurable or enjoyable
12. **Concrete thinking:** difficulty on the part of the affected individual with abstract thought, who instead interprets another's communication in a literal manner. Concrete thinking can be tested by asking person to interpret a common proverb.

D. **Classification.** Schizophrenia can be classified as positive or negative type. Most clients with this disorder have a mixture of both types of symptoms.
   1. **Positive symptoms** include hallucinations, delusions, loose associations, and bizarre or disorganized behavior.
   2. **Negative symptoms** include restricted emotion (flat affect), anhedonia, avolition, alogia, and social withdrawal.
E. **Types**
   1. **Paranoid schizophrenia**
      a. Essential features are systematized delusions or auditory hallucinations.
      b. The individual may be suspicious, argumentative, hostile, and aggressive.
      c. Behavior is less regressive, there is less social impairment, and the prognosis is better than that of other types.

TABLE 7-1
Symptoms of Loose Associations

SYMPTOM	DESCRIPTION
Neologism	Making up new words (eg, *potlomp, lemopty*)
Word salad	Words in a sentence that may seem connected but do not compose coherent thought (eg, *The blue isn't silly eating upwards time.*)
Illogical or paralogical thinking	Syllogistic thinking that defies logic (eg, *Blessed Mary is a virgin. I am a virgin. Therefore, I am Blessed Mary.*)
Echolalia	Senseless repetition of the words of another person
Echopraxia	Senseless copying of another person's behavior or actions
Clang association	Words that rhyme are put together without coherent thought (eg, *The sky and pie, for my and dye.*)

2. Disorganized schizophrenia

   a. Essential features are disorganized speech and behaviors, as well as flat or inappropriate affect; associative disturbances are common.

   b. The individual may have odd mannerisms, exhibit extreme social withdrawal, and neglect hygiene and appearance.

   c. Onset usually occurs before 25 years of age, and the course may be chronic.

   d. Behavior is regressive, with poor social interaction and poor reality contact.

3. Catatonic schizophrenia

   a. Essential features are marked psychomotor disturbances, which may involve immobility or excessive activity.

   b. **Catatonic stupor.** The individual may exhibit inactivity, negativism, and waxy flexibility (abnormal posturing).

   c. **Catatonic excitement** involves extreme agitation and may be accompanied by echolalia and echopraxia.

4. Undifferentiated schizophrenia

   a. Essential features are delusions, hallucinations, incoherent speech, and disorganized behaviors.

   b. This classification is used when criteria for other types are not met.

5. Residual schizophrenia

   a. The essential feature is the current absence of acute symptoms but history of past episodes.

   b. Negative symptoms, such as marked social isolation, withdrawal, and impaired role functioning, may be present.

F. Onset and course

1. **Onset** of symptoms usually occurs in late adolescence or early adulthood. The onset can be gradual or sudden.

2. **Course** of schizophrenia is variable, and remissions may occur. Some clients recover completely; some have a chronic, unremitting disorder.

G. Relevant statistics

1. It is known that approximately 1% of the population will experience schizophrenia in their lifetime.

2. For 95% of people with schizophrenia, the disease lasts a lifetime.

3. People with schizophrenia occupy 25% of inpatient hospital beds.

4. An estimated 33% to 50% of homeless people in the United States suffer from schizophrenia.

5. More than 50% of people with schizophrenia have alcohol or drug problems, which may represent an attempt to self-medicate the distressing symptoms.

H. Perception of reality and communicative patterns

1. The psychotic thinking and communicative patterns in clients with a schizophrenic disorder indicate severe impairment in perception of reality or a disturbance in ego function.

2. Individuals affected may not perceive any abnormality and may have difficulty developing any insight into problems. An individual who has insight would question his perceptions of reality, acknowledge the illness, and

understand the necessity for medications and the periodic assistance of others.

3. Individuals affected have poor sense of identity as well as lowered self-esteem.
4. Individuals affected may have difficulty filtering out extraneous environmental stimuli, resulting in an inability to focus on tasks and conversations.

I. **Interpersonal relationships** of an individual with a schizophrenic disorder are characterized by the following:

1. Withdrawal from interactions (ego protection)
2. Fear of interactions (reflects a poor sense of identity)
3. Basic feeling of rejection and lack of trust

J. **Family considerations**

1. Family members of individuals with schizophrenia are also severely impacted by this disorder, and living with a person who suffers from schizophrenia can be very difficult. These families experience stress and are required to cope with a variety of problems.
2. The National Alliance for the Mentally Ill (NAMI) provides support for the family and advocacy for the severely mentally ill.

II. Etiology

A. **General considerations**

1. The exact cause of schizophrenia remains unclear. The current general consensus is that these disorders result from complex interactions among a variety of factors.
2. Factors that have been studied and implicated include genetic predisposition, neurodevelopmental abnormalities, brain structural abnormalities, neurochemical imbalances, and psychosocial and environmental processes.

B. **Genetic predisposition**

1. Although genetics provide a significant risk factor, a single genetic marker has not been identified. It is likely that multiple genes may be involved.
2. Research has focused on chromosomes 6, 13, 18, and 22. Risk of developing schizophrenia if the disorder exists in the family is as follows:
   a. One affected parent: 12% to 15% risk
   b. Both parents affected: 35% to 39% risk
   c. Sibling affected: 8% to 10% risk
   d. Dizygotic twin affected: 15% risk
   e. Monozygotic twin affected: 50% risk

C. **Neurodevelopmental abnormalities**

1. Research indicates that minor fetal malformations developed during early gestation may play a role in later manifestation of schizophrenia.
2. Factors that can affect neurodevelopment and that are identified as increasing risk include:
   a. Individuals whose mothers had influenza during the second trimester

b. Individuals who experienced trauma or injury at birth

c. Infant or early childhood abuse or trauma

D. Brain structural abnormalities. In some subgroups of people with schizophrenia, brain imaging techniques (CT, MRI, and PET) have shown abnormalities in the structure of the brain, including:

1. Enlarged ventricles
2. Decreased cortical blood flow, especially in prefrontal cortex
3. Decreased metabolic activity in certain brain areas
4. Cerebral atrophy

E. Neurochemical (neurotransmitter) imbalances

1. Early research focused on the **dopamine hypothesis,** which stated that excessive dopamine activity in cortical areas of the brain was related to the positive symptoms of schizophrenia.
2. Current research indicates the importance of other **neurotransmitters,** including serotonin, norepinephrine, glutamate, and GABA.
3. **Homeostasis,** or the relationship between neurotransmitters, may be more important than relative amounts of specific neurotransmitters.
4. **Receptor sites** for specific neurotransmitters are also important. Changes in numbers and types of receptors can affect level of neurotransmitters. Psychotropic medications can affect neurotransmitter receptor sites (see Chapter 15) as well as the neurotransmitters.

F. Psychosocial and environmental process

1. **Developmental theories.** Theorists such as Freud, Sullivan, and Erikson proposed that the lack of warm, nurturing attention in the earliest years of life contributes to the lack of self-identity, reality misinterpretation, and relationship withdrawal in the individual with schizophrenia.
2. **Family theories.** Theories related to the role of the family in causation of schizophrenia have not been validated by research. An area of family functioning that has been implicated in increased relapse rates of individuals with schizophrenia is high expressed emotion (HEE). Families with this characteristic are described as emotionally overinvolved, hostile, and critical.
3. **Socioeconomic status.** A consistent research finding is the strong association between schizophrenia and low socioeconomic status.
4. **Stress-vulnerability model.** An interactional model that has been proposed suggests that people with schizophrenia have a genetic, biologically based vulnerability for schizophrenia. This vulnerability, when accompanied by exposure to life stressors, can then produce symptoms in the individual.

III. Management

A. General considerations

1. **Continuity of care is important.** Clients may receive treatment in various settings, including acute psychiatric hospitals, long-term psychiatric hospitals, and community-based programs.

2. Level of care depends on severity of symptoms as well as availability of family and social supports. Treatment is generally provided in least restrictive setting possible.
3. **Case management approach** is important because client care is generally long term, requiring collaboration with multiple care providers to ensure services are provided in coordinated manner.

B. **Brief psychiatric hospitalization** is used for management of acute symptoms and provides safe, structured environment and a variety of treatments, including:
1. Pharmacologic treatment with antipsychotic medications (Drug Chart 7-1)
2. Milieu management
3. Supportive therapy, which is generally reality oriented, with use of cognitive-behavioral approach
4. Psychoeducation for client and family
5. Discharge planning to ensure continuity of care

C. **Long-term psychiatric hospitalization**
1. Long-term hospitalization is used for clients with persistent symptoms who may pose a danger to self or others.
2. The goal is to stabilize and transfer the client as soon as possible to a less-restrictive setting.

D. **Community-based treatment** provides the following comprehensive client and family services.
1. **Supportive housing** includes transitional living halfway houses; cooperative living arrangements; crisis community residences; foster care; and board and care homes.

DRUG CHART 7-1. Selected Antipsychotic Medications Used for Schizophrenia*

Classification	Generic/ Trade Name	Adult Dosage (mg/day)	Rationale for Use
Typical antipsychotics	Chlorpromazine (Thorazine)	30–800	Acts by blocking selected dopamine receptors in both striatal and limbic areas of brain. Also affects other receptors including those for histamine, acetylcholine, serotonin. Provides antipsychotic effect, decreasing positive symptoms of schizophrenia.
	Thioridazine (Mellaril)	150–800	
	Trifluoperazine (Stelazine)	2–40	
	Fluphenazine (Prolixin)	0.5–40	
	Haloperidol (Haldol)	1–50	
	Thiothixene (Navane)	6–120	
	Molindone (Moban)	15–225	
Atypical antipsychotics	Clozapine (Clozaril)	300–900	Produces selective dopamine and serotonin receptor blocking in limbic system. Provides antipsychotic effect (positive symptoms) and will also decrease negative symptoms. Advantage—fewer side effects than typical antipsychotics.
	Olanzapine (Zyprexa)	5–20	
	Quetiapine (Seroquel)	150–750	
	Risperidone (Risperdal)	4–16	
	Serindole (Serlect)	12–24	
	Ziprasidone (Zeldox)	80–160	

*See Chapter 15 for complete discussion.

2. **Day treatment programs** offer group therapy, social skills training, medication management, and socialization and recreation.
3. **Supportive therapy** involves a case manager and therapists for the client and family.
4. **Psychoeducation programs** exist for the client, family, and community groups.
5. **Outreach services** exist for case finding and preventive treatment programs for individuals and families at increased risk.

E. **Psychosocial rehabilitation**
   1. Psychosocial rehabilitation emphasizes development of skills and supports necessary for successful living, learning, and working in the community.
   2. This approach can be part of the treatment program in any of the settings where service is provided. Use of a clubhouse where clients can gather to work together and socialize while learning necessary skills may be part of community services in some areas.

 IV. NURSING PROCESS OVERVIEW FOR
Schizophrenic Disorders

A. **Assessment** (Table 7-2)
   1. **History.** Review client history for precipitating stressors and significant data.
      a. Genetic-biologic vulnerability (family history)
      b. Stressful life events

TABLE 7-2
Key Nursing Assessment Questions

QUESTIONS	PROVIDES DATA ABOUT
Do you believe you have an illness? What is your explanation of your illness?	Reality perception Level of insight
Have you been in treatment before? What was helpful for you at that time?	Past history
What do you think are your strengths? What do you think are your problem areas?	Level of self-esteem Stressful life events Knowledge base regarding illness
Do you hear voices that others do not hear or see things that others do not see?	Hallucinations Delusions
Do you believe that someone or some group is plotting against you or trying to harm you?	
What medications do you take? Do you have any problems with your medications?	Compliance with medication regimen Knowledge of and problems with medications
Whom do you consider a support person in your life?	Level of supportive relationships
What are your activities during a typical day? What activities and events do you enjoy?	Thought process in terms of description Anhedonia Self-care ability

    c. Results of mental status examination
    d. Past psychiatric history and treatment compliance
    e. Medication history
    f. Drug and alcohol use
    g. Education and employment history
  2. Assess client for characteristic symptoms (see Tables 7-2 and 7-3)
  3. Assess family and community support systems, including:
    a. Current living arrangements and degree of supervision
    b. Family involvement and support
    c. Case manager or therapist
    d. Participation in community treatment programs
  4. Assess client and family knowledge base. Assess whether the client and family are knowledgeable about:
    a. Disorder of schizophrenia
    b. Medications and treatment recommendations
    c. Relapse signs
    d. Stress-reducing measures
  5. Assess client for side effects of antipsychotic medications (see Chapter 15)
    a. **Extrapyramidal system effects (EPS).** Use specific tools, such as the AIMS scale or Simpson neurologic scale, to make assessment.
    b. Anticholinergic effects
    c. Cardiovascular effects
    d. Other (see Table 15-2)
B. Nursing diagnoses
  1. Analyze positive and negative symptoms.
  2. Analyze client strengths and weaknesses, including:
    a. Self-care ability
    b. Socialization
    c. Communication

TABLE 7-3
Common Symptoms of Schizophrenia

THINKING AND COMMUNICATING	PERCEIVING AND INTERPRETING	FEELING AND AFFECT	BEHAVING AND INTERACTING
Loose associations	Delusions	Flat*	Relationship withdrawal*
Alogia*	Hallucinations	Blunted	Motor hyperactivity or hypoactivity
Concrete thinking	Illusions	Inappropriate	Ambivalence
Lack of insight	Depersonalization		Anhedonia*
	Attending to irrelevant stimuli		Avolition*
	Poor reality testing		Poor personal hygiene

*Indicates negative symptoms.

      d. Reality testing

      e. Job skills

      f. Support systems

  3. Analyze factors increasing risk for acting-out behavior, including:

      a. Agitation

      b. Anger

      c. Suspiciousness

      d. Presence of threatening hallucinations

  4. Establish and prioritize individualized nursing diagnoses for client and family.

      a. Self-esteem, chronic low

      b. Family coping: ineffective: compromised

      c. Home maintenance management, impaired

      d. Coping, individual, ineffective

      e. Knowledge deficit (specify)

      f. Therapeutic regimen: families, ineffective management

      g. Therapeutic regimen: individual, ineffective management

      h. Noncompliance

      i. Role performance, altered

      j. Self care deficit (specify)

      k. Sensory/perceptual alterations: visual, auditory, kinesthetic, gustatory, tactile, olfactory (specify)

      l. Thought processes, altered

      m. Violence, risk for: directed at self/others

C. Planning and outcome identification

  1. Work with the client in **setting realistic goals.** Initially, one may have to establish goals that are limited, depending on the client's assessed degree of impairment.

  2. Establish desired outcome criteria for client with schizophrenic disorder. The client will:

      a. Demonstrate decreased anxiety level.

      b. Interact on one-to-one basis with nurse or treatment team member.

      c. Maintain personal hygiene and activities of daily living.

      d. Decrease or refrain from behaviors that are considered bizarre or inappropriate.

      e. Differentiate between thoughts and feelings that are from inside self and those that are from external environment.

      f. Increase appropriate social interaction.

      g. Identify positive self statements.

      h. Cooperate with established treatment plan and agree to follow up with community care recommendations.

      i. Verbalize knowledge about the disorder, treatment plans, medications, relapse signs, and stress management techniques.

  3. Establish desired outcome criteria for families with a member having a schizophrenic disorder. The families will:

      a. Express feelings about individual concerns.

    b. Verbalize knowledge about the disorder, treatment plans, medications, relapse signs, handling crises, and symptom management.

D. Implementation

1. Withdrawn and isolated client
    a. Use self in therapeutic manner.
    b. **Initiate planned, short, frequent, and undemanding interactions.**
    c. Plan simple one-on-one activities.
    d. **Maintain consistency and honesty in interactions.**
    e. Gradually encourage the client to interact with peers in nonthreatening situations.
    f. Provide social skills training.
    g. Use measures to enhance self-esteem.

2. Clients exhibiting regressive or unusual behaviors
    a. **Assume a matter-of-fact approach to bizarre behaviors (do not reinforce these behaviors).**
    b. Treat the client as an adult, despite regression.
    c. Monitor the client's eating patterns; encourage and assist when necessary.
    d. **Assist with hygiene and grooming, performing these tasks only when the client is unable to.**
    e. Be cautious with touch because it may be perceived as threatening.
    f. Establish a routine schedule of activities of daily living.
    g. Give simple choices of two items for the ambivalent client.

3. Clients with unclear communication patterns
    a. **Maintain own communication in clear, unambiguous manner.**
    b. Maintain own communication as verbally and nonverbally congruent.
    c. **Clarify any ambiguous or unclear meanings related to the client's communication (Display 7-2).**
    d. Use therapeutic communication techniques (see Chapter 2).

4. Highly suspicious and hostile clients
    a. Establish a professional relationship; overfriendliness may be threatening.
    b. **Be cautious with touch because it may be perceived as threatening.**

DISPLAY 7-2. **Implementation: Clarifying Communication**

Client: "The skirts in the sky are flying high and I'm not going with them."
Nurse: "You are trying to tell me something, but I don't understand what it is. Can you tell me in a different way?"
Client *(pointing to a nurse walking briskly down the hall):* "They are all in a hurry. . . ."
Nurse: "You're telling me that the nurses are very busy and that you feel left out?"
Client: "Yes, I need help with my bath . . ."
Interpretation. In this example, the client is using highly symbolic language to try to communicate. The nurse indicates that she does not understand what is being said. When the client tries again, the nurse thinks she understands and repeats, directly to the client, the message she thinks the client is trying to communicate. The client then confirms the message.

   c. Allow client as much control and autonomy as possible within the limits of the therapeutic setting.

   d. Work on establishing trust through short interactions that communicate interest and respect.

   e. Explain any treatments, medications, and laboratory tests before initiating.

   f. Avoid focusing on or reinforcing suspicious thoughts or delusions.

   g. Identify and respond to emotional needs underlying suspicious thoughts or delusions (Display 7-3).

   h. Intervene when the client shows signs of increased anxiety and of potential acting-out behavior.

   i. Be careful not to behave in a manner that can be misinterpreted by the client.

5. Client with hallucinations or delusions

   a. Do not focus attention on hallucination or delusions. Interrupt hallucinatory experience of client by initiating one-to-one interaction that is reality based.

   b. Point out that you do not share client's perception (eg, "I do not hear the voices you say you hear."), but validate that you believe the hallucination is real to the client.

   c. Do not argue with the client about hallucinations or delusions.

   d. Respond to the feelings communicated during hallucinatory or delusional experiences (eg, "You seem frightened.").

   e. Redirect and focus the client on a structured activity or reality-based task.

   f. Move the client to quieter, less stimulating environment.

   g. Wait until the client is not experiencing hallucinations or delusions before initiating a teaching session about them.

   h. Explain that hallucinations or delusions are symptoms of psychiatric disorders.

DISPLAY 7-3. **Implementation: Responding to Suspicious Thoughts or Delusions**

Client *(furtively standing by the nurse's station, looking at the tape recorder on the desk):* "That tape recorder is used to record my thoughts. People here are against me."

Nurse: "It doesn't seem to me that this is so. The night nurse uses this tape recorder to make the evening report. I believe that you are safe here."

Client: "I don't feel safe here. Can I stay by the desk while you are here?"

Nurse: "Yes. I'll be here for 5 more minutes, until the lunch trays come. Here's a newspaper for you to read."

Client: "I'll stay here and read the paper."

Interpretation: In this example, the client misinterprets the environment by drawing an unwarranted conclusion about the tape recorder kept at the nurses' station. The nurse responds by presenting reality to the patient in a matter-of-fact manner. Similarly, the nurse responds to the underlying meaning of the client's communication by saying that the client is safe and can remain close by. Then, the nurse refocuses the client on another environmental object, the newspaper.

    i. Point out that anxiety or increased stimuli from environment may stimulate hallucinations.

    j. Help the client control hallucinations by focusing on reality and by taking prescribed medications.

    k. If hallucinations persist, help the client learn to ignore them and act in appropriate manner despite hallucinations.

    l. Teach cognitive strategies and tell client to use **self-talk** ("The voices are not reasonable") and **thought stopping** ("I won't think about this").

  6. Client with agitated behavior and potential for violence

    a. Observe for early cues of agitation; intervene before the client begins acting out.

    b. Provide a safe, quiet environment; decrease stimuli when the client becomes agitated.

    c. Avoid retaliating when the client is verbally hostile; use a quiet, calm tone of voice. Provide personal space and avoid physical contact.

    d. Encourage the client to talk about, rather than act out, feelings.

    e. Offer medications as needed (prn) to the agitated client.

    f. Isolate the client from general milieu if agitation increases.

    g. Set limits on unacceptable behavior and consistently follow institutional protocol for intervention.

    h. Follow institutional protocol for responding to the client with acting-out behavior.

    i. Ensure that staff members are available when attempting to subdue a violent client. If restraints are necessary, apply them in a safe and nonpunitive manner, follow protocol, and provide safe care.

  7. The family of the client with a schizophrenic disorder

    a. Encourage each member to discuss feelings and needs.

    b. Assist family members to define basic rules about respecting one another's privacy and living together.

    c. Encourage interaction for each family member with a wider social environment.

    d. Encourage family members to become involved in support groups.

    e. Assist members to identify anxiety-producing situations and plan specific coping strategies.

    f. Teach the family about schizophrenia and its management (Client and Family Teaching 7-1).

E. Outcome evaluation

  1. The client identifies internal feelings of anxiety and uses learned coping measures to decrease anxiety.

  2. The client independently maintains personal hygiene.

  3. The client follows routine schedule for activities of daily living (ADLs).

  4. The client demonstrates appropriate behavior in social situations.

  5. The client communicates without evidence of loose, dissociated thinking.

  6. The client differentiates between thoughts and feelings that are stimulated from within self and those that are stimulated from the external environment.

CLIENT AND FAMILY TEACHING 7-1

Educating Families Who Have a Member With Schizophrenia

1. Educate the family about schizophrenia:
   Schizophrenia is a brain disorder that affects all aspects of functioning.
   No single cause is established, but research indicates genetics, changes in brain structure and chemicals, and stress-related factors.
   Symptoms can include hearing voices (hallucinations), beliefs that are false (delusions), communicating in ways that are difficult to understand, and poor occupational and social functioning.
   Symptoms may improve and can also recur throughout life.
2. Educate the family about treatment:
   Antipsychotic medications are used; it is important for the client to take as prescribed.
   Side effects are common and can be managed if reported promptly to health care provider. (*Provide specific information regarding individual client's medications.*)
   Follow-up treatment with therapist or care manager is vital.
3. Educate the family about handling the client's symptoms:
   Identify events that are typically upsetting to client and provide extra support as needed.
   Note when client is becoming upset and encourage measures to reduce anxiety.
   Anxiety-reducing measures include time outs, relaxation techniques, balanced rest and activity, and proper diet.
   Note the symptoms that client exhibits when ill, and when these recur encourage client to contact health provider (if resistant, contact health provider on your own).
   Do not agree with hallucinations or delusions; point out reality but do not argue with client.
4. Additional information:
   Educate the family members about self-care.
   Encourage family members to talk about feelings and concerns with health care provider.
   Encourage family to consider joining community support group such as National Alliance for Mentally Ill (NAMI).

7. The client exhibits decreased or controlled magical thinking, delusions, hallucinations, and illusions.
8. The client demonstrates improved social interaction with others.
9. The client displays affect that is appropriate to a given feeling, thought, or situation.
10. The client exhibits decreased suspiciousness, negativity, and anger.
11. The client identifies positive aspects of self.
12. Family members use effective coping strategies to handle anxiety-producing situations.
13. The client participates in the treatment plan and agrees to follow up in community treatment.
14. The client and family use knowledge regarding the disorder, treatment program, medications, symptoms, and crisis management on an ongoing basis.

STUDY QUESTIONS

1. Which of the following behaviors would a nurse assess in a client with the DSM-IV psychiatric diagnosis of schizophrenia, disorganized type?
   (1) absence of acute symptoms, impaired role function
   ✓ (2) extreme social withdrawal, odd mannerisms and behaviors
   (3) psychomotor immobility, presence of waxy flexibility
   (4) suspiciousness toward others, increased hostility

2. In planning care for a client with schizophrenia who has negative symptoms, the nurse would anticipate a problem with
   (1) auditory hallucinations
   (2) bizarre behaviors
   (3) ideas of reference
   ✓ (4) motivation for activities

3. The family of a client with schizophrenia asks the nurse if there is a genetic cause of this disorder. To answer the family, which of the following facts would the nurse cite?
   (1) Conclusive evidence indicates a specific gene transmits the disorder.
   (2) Incidence of this disorder is variable in all families.
   (3) There is little evidence that genes play a role in transmission.
   ✓ (4) Genetic factors can increase the vulnerability for this disorder.

4. Which of the following nursing interventions would be most appropriate for a client with schizophrenia, paranoid type?
   ✓ (1) establishing a nondemanding relationship

   (2) encouraging involvement in group activities
   (3) spending more time with the client
   (4) waiting until client initiates interaction

5. A client tells the nurse that psychotropic medicines are dangerous and refuses to take them. Which of the following interventions should the nurse use first?
   (1) Ask client why medicines are dangerous.
   (2) Ask client if an injection is preferable.
   ✓ (3) Hand client medicine with instruction to take it.
   (4) Withhold medicine until client is less suspicious.

6. A client is admitted for acute psychiatric hospitalization. Nursing assessment includes the following: client refuses to bathe or dress, remains in room most of the day, speaks infrequently to peers or staff. The priority nursing diagnosis is
   (1) Anxiety
   (2) Decisional conflict
   (3) Self-care deficit
   ✓ (4) Social isolation

7. In a 20-year-old client newly diagnosed with schizophrenia, which of the following statements is correct?
   ✓ (1) Age of onset is typical for schizophrenia.
   (2) Age of onset is later than usual for schizophrenia.
   (3) Age of onset is earlier than usual for schizophrenia.
   (4) Age of onset follows no predictable pattern in schizophrenia.

8. Which of the following factors are associated with increased risk for schizophrenia?
(1) alcoholism
(2) adolescent pregnancy
(3) overcrowded schools
✓**(4)** poverty

9. An appropriate nursing strategy to deal with a client's withdrawal would be
(1) to not attempt to establish a relationship
(2) to make group interactions the main focus of therapy
(3) to hold in-depth, one-on-one counseling sessions
✓**(4)** to keep interactions short, frequent, and nondemanding

10. When evaluating care for a client with schizophrenia, the nurse should keep in mind which of the following points?
✓**(1)** Frequent reassessment is needed and is based on the client's response to treatment.
(2) The family does not need to be included in the care because the client is an adult.
(3) The client is too ill to learn about his illness.
(4) Relapse is not an issue for a client with schizophrenia.

11. A male client tells the nurse that the FBI is monitoring and recording his every movement and that microphones have been planted in the unit walls. Which of the following actions would be the most therapeutic response?
(1) Confront the delusional material directly by telling the client that this simply is not so.
✓**(2)** Tell the client that this must seem frightening to him but that you believe he is safe here.

(3) Tell the client to wait and talk about these beliefs in his one-on-one counseling sessions.
(4) Isolate the client when he begins to talk about these beliefs.

12. Which of the following client behaviors documented in the chart would validate the nursing diagnosis of risk for violence directed at others?
(1) The client describes being endowed with super powers.
✓**(2)** Frequent angry outbursts noted toward peers and staff
(3) Refusal to eat cafeteria food
(4) Refusal to join in group activities

13. The nurse educates the family about symptom management when the individual with schizophrenia becomes upset or anxious. Which of the following would the nurse state is helpful?
(1) Call the therapist to request medication change.
✓**(2)** Encourage use of learned relaxation measures.
(3) Request hospitalization until crisis is over.
(4) Wait until anxiety becomes worse before intervening.

14. A client who has had auditory hallucinations for many years tells the nurse that the voices prevent participation in the social skills training program of the community mental health center. Which of the following would the nurse teach the client to do?
(1) Analyze the content of the voices.
(2) Participate when the voices cease.
(3) Take medication as prescribed.
✓**(4)** Use thought stopping techniques.

ANSWER KEY

1. The answer is (2). Disorganized type of schizophrenia is characterized by regressive behavior with extreme social withdrawal and frequently odd mannerisms. The absence of acute symptoms and impaired role function are more characteristic of schizophrenia, residual type. Psychomotor immobility and presence of waxy flexibility are more indicative of schizophrenia, catatonic type. Suspiciousness toward others and increased hostility is more characteristic of schizophrenia, paranoid type.

2. The answer is (4). In a client demonstrating negative symptoms of schizophrenia, avolition or the lack of motivation for activities is a common problem. All the other symptoms listed are the positive symptoms of schizophrenia.

3. The answer is (4). Research shows that family history statistically increases the risk for development of schizophrenia. However, no single gene has yet been identified. Answer choices **(2)** and **(3)** are both incorrect because genetics play a role in the etiology of schizophrenia.

4. The answer is (1). A nonthreatening, nondemanding relationship helps decrease the mistrust that is common in a client with schizophrenia, paranoid type. Encouraging involvement in group activities and spending more time with the client would be threatening for a client who is suspicious of other people's motives. This client is unlikely to initiate interaction, and the nurse is responsible for initiating a relationship.

5. The answer is (3). A matter-of-fact attitude is best when trying to get a client who has delusional beliefs to take medications. A nurse's apparent uncertainty will add to client's mistrust and fear. The nurse already knows the client believes medicine is dangerous, and asking the client why the medicine is dangerous would reinforce these beliefs. Asking the client if an injection is preferable may add to the client feeling threatened. Withholding medication prescribed to relieve delusional beliefs will likely intensify paranoid thoughts and feelings.

6. The answer is (4). These behaviors indicate the client's withdrawal from others and possible fear or mistrust of relationships. There is no indication of anxiety or decisional conflict given the information in the question. Although the client refuses to bathe or dress, self-care deficit would not be the priority nursing diagnosis.

7. The answer is (1). The primary age of onset for schizophrenia is late adolescence through young adulthood (17 to 27 years of age). Paranoid schizophrenia may sometimes have a later onset. All of the other answer choices are incorrect.

8. The answer is (4). Low socioeconomic status or poverty is an identified environmental factor associated with increased incidence of schizophrenia. Although alcoholism, adolescent pregnancy, and overcrowded schools may be stressful, research does not show they increase the risk for schizophrenia.

9. The answer is (4). The nurse must proceed slowly, building trust gradually with a client who is withdrawn and initiating contact by showing interest in the client's daily activities, hygiene, and so forth. Not making any attempt to establish a relationship suggests ignoring the client, which is inappropriate. Making group interactions the main focus of therapy or having in-depth, one-on-one counseling sessions may be potentially overwhelming to a withdrawn client.

10. The answer is (1). Because clients respond to treatment in different ways, the nurse must constantly evaluate the client and the client's potential. Premorbid adjustment must also be considered. Most clients with schizophrenia go home, and the family should be involved and supported. The client can learn about the illness if information is provided gradually and in easy-to-understand terms. Relapse is common in schizophrenia.

11. The answer is (2). The nurse must realize that these perceptions are very real to the client. Acknowledging the client's feelings provides support; explaining how the nurse sees the situation in a different way provides reality orientation. Confronting the delusional material directly will not work with this client and may decrease trust. Telling the client to wait and talk about these beliefs in his one-on-one counseling session will reinforce the delusion. Isolation will increase anxiety. Distraction with a radio or activities would be a better approach.

12. The answer is (2). Anger is an important factor that indicates potential for acting out. The client is also angry with both peers and staff, indicating that the acting out, if it occurs, would be toward others. The client describing being endowed with super powers and refusing to eat cafeteria food indicate that the client may have delusional beliefs but not necessarily a risk for violence. Refusal to join in group activities indicates discomfort with a group, but no threat of violence is apparent.

13. The answer is (2). The client with schizophrenia can learn relaxation techniques, which help reduce anxiety. The family can be supportive and helpful by encouraging the client to use these techniques. Anxiety is a common experience for everyone, and is no reason to change medication. Handling anxiety is a learned skill that is important to reinforce. There is no indication that the client is in crisis. It is much easier to intervene early in anxiety rather than waiting until escalation occurs.

14. The answer is (4). Clients with long-lasting auditory hallucinations can learn to use thought-stopping measures to accomplish tasks. Analyzing the content of the voices may be indicated when hallucinations first occur to establish whether the voices are threatening to the individual or instructing the client to harm others. Focusing on content at this point would reinforce this symptom. The voices have lasted many years; the client should participate despite the voices. There is no indication that the client is not taking medication as prescribed.

8 Substance-Related Disorders

Overview

A. **Definitions**
   1. **Psychoactive substances** are drugs or chemicals that alter one or several of the following: perception, awareness, consciousness, thinking, judgment, decision making, insight, mood, or behavior. Commonly abused substances include alcohol, amphetamines, caffeine, cannabis, cocaine, hallucinogens, inhalants, nicotine, opioids, phencyclidine, barbiturates, nonbarbiturate sedative-hypnotics, and anxiolytics.
   2. **Substance abuse** is the misuse of a substance with significant and recurrent adverse consequences related to repeated use.
   3. **Substance dependence** is a cluster of cognitive, behavioral, and physiologic symptoms indicating continued use of substance despite significant life problems related to that use. The diagnosis of substance dependence requires at least three of the following symptoms occurring over 12 months (DSM-IV, 1994).
      a. **Tolerance:** the need for greatly increased amounts of a substance to obtain the desired effect; or diminished effect with continued use of the same amount of the substance
      b. **Withdrawal:** the behavioral, physiologic, and cognitive symptoms that occur when blood or tissue concentrations of a substance abruptly decline
      c. Compulsive drug-taking behavior
      d. Inability to reduce substance use
      e. Excess time spent obtaining drugs
      f. Impairment in social or occupational functioning or recreational activities
      g. Continued substance use despite negative consequences
   4. **Polysubstance abuse** is the use of more than one abusive substance.
   5. **Substance intoxication** is the development of a reversible substance-specific syndrome induced by ingestion or exposure to substance, which produces physiologic effects on the central nervous system (CNS).
   6. **Dual diagnosis** is the presence of another psychiatric diagnosis in an individual with a substance-specific disorder. Studies have identified associations between alcohol use and anxiety disorder, depression, schizophrenia, eating disorder, and antisocial personality disorder.

7. **Cross-tolerance** (addiction) is demonstrated when a person dependent on one substance requires higher doses of another substance in the same general category. For example, an individual who develops tolerance to alcohol—a CNS depressant—will require higher-than-normal doses of another CNS depressant (eg, benzodiazepine) to achieve the desired effect.

8. **Detoxification** is controlled withdrawal from an abusive substance in a medically prescribed program using gradually tapered sedation, a controlled environment, and nutritional supplements.

9. **Codependence** is the enabling behaviors of individuals in the family or social system of a person who is substance dependent; these behaviors inadvertently promote continued use by protecting the individual from the consequences of his actions.

B. **Classification.** Commonly abused substances are classified in the following categories (Table 8-1):

1. **CNS depressants** produce their effects by stimulating inhibitory neurotransmitters (gamma-aminobutyric acid; GABA) or altering excitatory neurotransmitters (dopamine and norepinephrine) (see Table 8-1).
   a. Chronic use of CNS depressants may reduce the production and supply of inhibitory neurotransmitters.
   b. Neuroexcitation occurs when CNS depressants are abruptly withdrawn. Rebound norepinephrine and dopamine stimulation accounts for the withdrawal symptoms.

2. **CNS stimulants** produce their effects by increasing the release of dopamine and norepinephrine from presynaptic neurons and preventing their reuptake (see Table 8-1).
   a. This presynaptic blockade eventually causes catecholamine depletion, and therefore increased need for the stimulating substance.
   b. When CNS stimulants are abruptly withdrawn, excitatory neurotransmitters are profoundly depleted and severe dysphoria and depression occur.

3. **Opioids** are both CNS depressants and powerful analgesics (see Table 8-1).
   a. Opioids are thought to block release of substance P and attach to endorphin receptors to relieve pain. They stimulate the opioid receptors in the nucleus ceruleus and suppress noradrenergic neurotransmitters.
   b. When opioids are abruptly withdrawn, rebound release of large amounts of norepinephrine occurs.

4. **Hallucinogens** excite presynaptic receptors in the pontine nuclei and produce visual, proprioceptive, and perceptual disturbances (see Table 8-1).
   a. The hallucinogen phencyclidine (PCP) acts at several neurotransmitter sites, thereby releasing dopamine, norepinephrine, and serotonin as well as inhibiting GABA.
   b. Withdrawal of hallucinogens produces unpleasant effects (eg, anxiety, insomnia, panic) related to neurotransmitter imbalances.

5. **Cannabinoids** are difficult to categorize. They are related to hallucinogens (ie, effects include alteration in perceptions) and to CNS depressants (ie, depressing higher brain centers).
   a. Other effects include euphoria, short-term memory loss, and decreased concentration.

TABLE 8-1
Classification of Common Abusive Substances

CNS DEPRESSANTS	CNS STIMULANTS	HALLUCINOGENS	CANNABINOIDS
Alcohol Beer Wine Liquor **Barbiturates** Pentobarbital (Nembutal) Secobarbital (Seconal) Amobarbital (Amytal) **Nonbarbiturate Sedative/Hypnotics** Methaqualone (Quaalude) Ethchlorvynol (Placidyl) Glutethimide (Doriden) Chloral hydrate (Noctec) **Anxiolytics** Diazepam (Valium) Chlordiazepoxide (Librium) Oxazepam (Serax) Alprazolam (Xanax) Lorazepam (Ativan) **Inhalants** Hydrocarbon solvents, (eg, in gasoline, glue, paint thinners, cleaning fluids) Aerosol propellants (eg, in spray cans) Anesthetic gases (eg, chloroform, nitrous oxide) **Opioids (Narcotic Analgesics)** Heroin, opium Morphine and derivatives (MS Contin, Roxanol) Codeine Oxycodone (eg, in Percodan) **Synthetics** Meperidine (Demerol) Methadone (Dolophine) Propoxyphene (Darvon) Pentazocine (Talwin)	**Amphetamines** Dextroamphetamine (Dexedrine) Methamphetamine (Desoxyn) Amphetamine sulfate (Benzedrine) **Nonamphetamine Stimulants** Methylphenidate (Ritalin) Pemoline (Cylert) Phenmetrazine (Preludin) Cocaine (crack, coke) **Nicotine** Cigarettes Chewing and pipe tobacco Snuff **Caffeine** Coffee Cola Tea	Mescaline (in peyote cactus) Psilocybin (in psilocybe mushrooms) Lysergic acid (LSD) Phencyclidine (PCP) **Others** STP, MOMA (variants of amphetamines)	Cannabis (marijuana) Hashish (hash) Dronabinol (Marinol)

    b. Withdrawal of cannabinoids can produce effects of excess stimulation because the depressant action of the substance is stopped.

  6. Inhalants act as CNS depressants and rapidly cross the blood-brain barrier (see Table 8-1).

    a. They are particularly dangerous because the dosage of an inhalant cannot be controlled.

    b. Inhalants do not produce withdrawal symptoms when abruptly stopped.

C. Selected statistics

  1. Alcohol is the most commonly abused substance in the United States, with a 13.8% incidence, out of a lifetime prevalence of 10% to 16%. Alcohol is ranked as the third major health problem in the United States when morbidity is considered.

  2. Gender. Substance abuse is 2 to 3 times more common in men than women. However, women who are substance abusers suffer a more virulent course with more severe physiologic and psychological consequences (Bradley, et al, 1998).

  3. High-risk groups. Groups who experience high rates of substance abuse include the unemployed, those who are 18 to 25 years of age, and members of the medical profession (30 to 100 times higher than the general population).

  4. Suicide risk. Individuals who are substance abusers are at increased risk for suicide, 20 times higher than the rate for nonabusers.

  5. Crack cocaine continues to dominate the illicit drug problem in the United States (NIDA, 1999).

  6. Heroin use has been increasing since 1992, with a large proportion of recent new users under age 26 (NIDA, 1999).

  7. The resurgence of **marijuana** use continues, especially among adolescents (NIDA, 1999).

D. Cultural differences in alcohol use. Because alcohol has religious, social, and cultural significance, different cultural groups use alcohol in markedly different ways, thus affecting the abuse rate in various groups.

  1. Asian cultures have an overall low prevalence of alcohol-related disorders. This may be related to genetic inheritance factors that regulate alcohol metabolism in this cultural group.

  2. Black and white Americans have nearly identical rates of alcohol abuse and dependence.

  3. Hispanics have a somewhat higher rate of alcohol-related disorders.

  4. Native Americans have a high incidence of alcohol-related disorders.

E. Women and substance abuse. Research indicates that certain risk factors are common in women who become substance abusers (Mynatt, 1996), including:

  1. Growing up in a chaotic family

  2. Suffering from victimization (eg, abuse) in childhood

  3. Having decreased level of self-esteem

F. Nursing profession and substance abuse

  1. A study by Mynatt (1996) found that 80% of chemically dependent nurses surveyed reported occurrence of a traumatic event prior to the development of chemical dependence.

2. Practicing nurses must identify and report nurses who may be suffering from chemical dependency. Some state nurse practice acts include provisions for mandatory reporting of impaired nurses.
3. Many state nursing associations, supported by national nursing organizations, have established peer support systems to help nurses who abuse substances to recover (Fontaine and Fletcher, 1999).

G. **Defense mechanisms** are common in individuals who abuse substances.
   1. **Denial** is manifested when the individual is unable to acknowledge how destructive substance use has become and the effect of use on the individual's problems.
   2. Other common defense mechanisms used by substance abusers include **rationalization** and **projection.** (See Chapter 2.)

H. **Common personality traits** are identified as being associated with substance abusers. Controversy exists about whether the traits or the abuse occurs first.
   1. **Dominant and critical behavior** toward others (which masks self-doubt and passivity)
   2. **Personal insecurity** and **decreased self-esteem**
   3. **Rebellious attitude** toward authority
   4. **Difficulty with intimate relationships** and tendency toward narcissism

I. **Laboratory testing** for abusive substances
   1. Blood levels are used to detect recent use of substances.
   2. For most psychoactive drugs (eg, opioids, CNS depressants and stimulants) urinalysis will detect evidence 2 to 4 days after use; it will detect hallucinogens up to 1 month after use.

J. **Substance abuse and the family.** About 50% of all families in the United States have problems related to the abuse of substances.
   1. The family system can become chaotic and disorganized, especially when a parent is a substance abuser.
   2. Children of a substance abuser exhibit stress, guilt, and difficulties in relationships with others. They may attempt to compensate for the parent by adopting various roles (eg, caretaker, scapegoat).
   3. Adolescents in families where a parent is a substance abuser have been found to have low levels of warmth, increased anger and rebelliousness, and difficulty with trust and intimacy (Frisch & Frisch, 1998).
   4. Codependent (enabling) behaviors may permit the abuser to avoid the consequences of addiction.
      a. The family members who are codependent develop behavioral patterns that present problems in many areas of life. For example, codependent family members tend to become caretakers in friend or work relationships, ignoring their own needs to fulfill the needs of others, which can result in bitterness, anger, resentment, and depletion of emotional and physical energy.
      b. Incidence of depression is high in these family members.

II. Types of Substances

A. **Alcohol**
1. **Immediate effects.** Acute intoxication causes slurred speech, lack of coordination, unsteady gait, and impaired attention and memory. High doses can cause stupor and coma.
2. **Chronic use** causes multisystem dysfunction.
   a. **Gastrointestinal effects** include gastritis, pancreatitis, and cirrhosis of the liver.
   b. **CNS effects** are related to the effect of thiamin (vitamin B_1) deficiency.
      (1) **Wernicke's syndrome** is an acute confusional state characterized by ataxia, delirium, and peripheral neuropathy. Treatment with thiamin can reverse this disorder.
      (2) **Korsakoff's syndrome** is a chronic cognitive impairment (dementia) characterized by cerebral atrophy and memory loss. This disorder is treated in a supportive manner as with other disorders of dementia (see Chapter 11).
   c. **Cardiovascular problems** include anemia, cardiomyopathy, and clotting disorders.
   d. **Blackouts** (antegrade amnesia) occur with chronic alcohol use and are characterized by loss of short-term memory. The individual functions during a blackout in social situations but later will have no memory of what occurred during this time.
   e. **Reproductive problems** include fetal alcohol syndrome (FAS) in infants of impaired mothers. FAS is characterized by low birth weight, abnormal facial features, microcephaly, mental retardation, cardiac and genital abnormalities, and vision and hearing problems.
3. **Blood alcohol level** (BAL) is important in the legal definition of intoxication. BAL is the determining criteria for legal action related to driving under the influence (DUI).
   a. BAL peaks within 50 minutes to 3 hours after heavy drinking ends.
   b. The legal definition of intoxication varies by state, ranging from a BAL of 80 to 100 mg/dL (0.08 to 0.1 g/dL).
   c. Coma generally occurs with a BAL of 0.4 g/dL and severe respiratory depression with a BAL of 0.5 g/dL.
   d. An individual who has developed tolerance can have increased BAL with minimal behavioral changes and therefore can be at risk for severe withdrawal (Antai-Otong, 1996).
4. **Withdrawal symptoms**
   a. **Mild tremulousness ("the shakes")** can occur 3 to 36 hours after the last drink and is characterized by anxiety, agitation, tremors, anorexia, nausea, sweating, and increased pulse and blood pressure.
   b. **Severe alcohol withdrawal syndrome (delirium tremens)** can occur 24 to 72 hours after the last drink and is characterized by increased temperature, pulse, and blood pressure; severe diaphoresis; auditory, visual, and tactile hallucinations; agitation; confusion; and seizures.

B. Other CNS depressants, including barbiturates, nonbarbiturate sedative-hypnotics, and anxiolytics

1. The **method of use** is oral.
2. **Immediate effects** include euphoria, impaired attention and memory, sedation, psychomotor retardation, flushed face, bradycardia, and hypotension. High doses can cause respiratory depression, coma, and death.
3. **Chronic use.** Psychological effects (eg, depression, paranoia) caused by chronic use depend on the specific substance used and its effects on body systems.
4. **Synergistic properties.** The effects of CNS depressants are additive with one another and also with alcohol. Therefore, the depressant effects are compounded when more than one substance in this group is taken; results are unpredictable and often may be fatal.
5. **Overdose**
   a. There is no antidote to an overdose of CNS depressants.
   b. CNS stimulants may temporarily arouse the individual with an overdose, but no drug currently is available to displace the depressants from brain receptors and reverse their effects.
6. **Withdrawal symptoms** are similar to those of alcohol withdrawal.
   a. Withdrawal occurs 24 to 72 hours after the last dose. In substances with long half-life (eg, diazepam), withdrawal symptoms may not occur for up to 1 week.
   b. Withdrawal is characterized by anxiety, tremors, insomnia, anorexia, nausea, and vomiting. More severe symptoms, such as hypertension, tachycardia, delirium, and hallucinations, can also occur.
   c. For treatment of withdrawal, see Table 8-2.

C. Opioids (CNS depressants and analgesics)

1. The **method of use** may be oral, smoking, inhaling or injection.
2. **Immediate effects** include euphoria, agitation, apathy, decreased sensation of pain, impaired attention and memory, sedation ("nodding out"), psychomotor retardation, pinpoint pupils, nausea, and vomiting. More severe effects include decreased blood pressure, hypothermia, respiratory depression, and death.
3. **Chronic use** can cause physical problems and greatly impair social and occupational functioning.
   a. A heroin abuser's **lifestyle** is characterized by drug-seeking behaviors to the exclusion of other activities of living.
      (1) Heroin abusers seldom maintain a steady job that will support their habit.
      (2) Obtaining funds illegally (eg, stealing, prostitution) is common.
   b. **Physical effects**
      (1) **Gastrointestinal effects** include a slowing of peristalsis and chronic constipation.
      (2) Individuals who abuse heroin intravenously may develop **multiple skin abscesses** on their extremities as well as darkened, hardened, and scarred veins ("tracks") (Fontaine & Fletcher, 1999).

TABLE 8-2
Treatment of Withdrawal from Abusive Substances

SUBSTANCE	TREATMENT	RATIONALE
CNA Depressants Alcohol Barbiturates Nonbarbiturate sedative/ hypnotic	Benzodiazepines (eg, diazepam, chlordiazepoxide, lorazepam, oxazepam) administered in scheduled doses with gradual tapering of frequency and amount over 5–10-day period. Anticonvulsants (eg, phenytoin, carbamazepine)	Restores depleted GABA levels and prevents neuroexcitation response to withdrawal of CNS depressants.
Anxiolytics	Nutritional supplements (multi-vitamins, folic acid, and thiamin) Nonsteroidal anti-inflammatories (eg, Ascriptin)	Prevents seizures that can occur with excessive neuroexcitation during severe withdrawal. Restores depleted nutrients (eg, thiamin is important for alcohol abusers, who generally develop thiamin deficiency). Analgesia for common complaints of headache, muscle soreness.
Opioids	Central-acting adrenergic stimulant (eg, clonidine) Synthetic opioid (eg, methadone) Narcotic antagonist (eg, buprenorphine)	Stimulates alpha-adrenergic receptors in CNS, which reduces norepinephrine rebound when opioid is stopped. Decreases opiate dependence when administered in scheduled doses with gradual tapering over 14–28-day period; can also be administered as long-term maintenance therapy to replace dependence on illegal narcotics. Suppresses acute opioid withdrawal symptoms.
CNS Stimulants Amphetamines Cocaine	Dopamine agonist (eg, bromo-criptine, amantadine) Antidepressant (eg, desipramine) Antipsychotic (eg, haloperidol)	Restores dopamine, which is depleted by chronic use of CNS stimulant. Restores serotonin, which is depleted by chronic use of CNS stimulant, and counteracts severe depression occurring from withdrawal. Treats psychotic symptoms, which may occur.
Hallucinogens LSD PCP	Benzodiazapines (eg, diazepam, lorazepam) Antipsychotic (eg, haloperidol)	Treats panic response, which can occur during withdrawal. Treats psychotic symptoms by counteracting excessive dopamine release caused by hallucinogenic substance.
Cannabis	Calm environment, supportive care	Physiologic withdrawal symptoms do not occur.

(3) Use of contaminated needles may lead to **multiple infectious diseases,** including hepatitis B, C, and D and acquired immunodeficiency syndrome (AIDS).

4. Overdose

a. Opioid overdose is a medical emergency that places an individual in danger of respiratory arrest.

b. Naloxone (Narcan), an opioid antagonist, is given intravenously to reverse the overdose. It is short acting and must be given in repeat doses, and the client must be closely observed for hypotension.

c. Volume replacement is used to treat hypotension.

5. Fetal exposure

a. Fetal exposure to opioids has been associated with an increased rate of prematurity and a 5 to 10 times higher risk of sudden infant death syndrome (SIDS).

b. Newborns of addicted mothers suffer withdrawal symptoms, including noise sensitivity, sweating, irritability, tremors, nasal congestion, and feeding difficulties (Fontaine and Fletcher, 1999).

6. Withdrawal symptoms

a. Symptoms may occur 6 to 24 hours after last dose.

b. Symptoms are distressing, but medically benign, and include nausea, vomiting, muscle aches, cramping, lacrimation, rhinorrhea, piloerection, sweating, fever, and insomnia. Tachycardia and hypertension can also occur from norepinephrine rebound.

c. For treatment of withdrawal, see Table 8-2.

D. Inhalants

1. The **method of use** is to inhale the fumes of the substance through the nose and mouth.

2. Immediate effects include euphoria, dizziness, ataxia, uninhibited behavior, the sensation of floating, and perceptual changes (including hallucinations). Inhalants can cause respiratory and cardiac depression, leading to sudden death.

3. Chronic use may lead to kidney, liver, and brain damage.

4. Epidemiology

a. Adolescents most often use inhalants, frequently as part of peer group activity and pressure.

b. Although inhalant use is widespread and dangerous, only a small percentage of users become dependent.

5. Withdrawal symptoms

a. Although a withdrawal syndrome has not been well established, symptoms have been documented 24 to 48 hours after last dose.

b. Symptoms include sleep disturbances, tremor, irritability, diaphoresis, nausea, and fleeting illusions (DSM-IV, 1994).

E. Amphetamines and related drugs (CNS stimulants)

1. The **method of use** includes oral, smoking, or injection.

2. **Immediate effects** include increased energy, euphoria, extreme vigilance, hostility, impaired judgment, increased blood pressure, tachycardia, dilated pupils, insomnia, decreased appetite, nausea, and vomiting.
3. **Chronic use of amphetamines**
   a. Chronic use may cause paranoia and malnutrition.
   b. Intravenous (IV) use can lead to infectious diseases, such as hepatitis B, C, and D and AIDS.
   c. Individuals who are chronic users are at increased risk for cerebrovascular and cardiovascular accidents.
4. **Pattern of use.** Individuals who are amphetamine abusers may have binges followed by a period of exhaustion, depression, and withdrawal ("crash").
5. **Caffeine and nicotine** are currently the most widely used stimulants in the United States (Townsend, 1999).
   a. **Caffeine.** An intake of 500 to 600 mg/day (equivalent to 4 cups of coffee) can cause anxiety, insomnia, and depression.
      (1) Tachycardia and arrhythmias may also occur.
      (2) Withdrawal from caffeine has not been included in the *Diagnostic and Statistical Manual of Mental Disorders,* 4th edition (DSM-IV); however, symptoms documented include headache, fatigue, anxiety or depression, nausea, and vomiting.
   b. **Nicotine** continues to affect 30% of the population.
      (1) Besides the well-documented overall health risks (eg, lung cancer, emphysema), nicotine causes tachycardia and increased blood pressure.
      (2) Nicotine withdrawal causes depression, insomnia, irritability, anxiety, bradycardia, and increased appetite.
      (3) Treatment of nicotine withdrawal includes use of nicotine gum (Nicorette) or nicotine patch (Nicotrol) in gradually decreasing doses over a period lasting from 3 weeks to 3 months) (Fiume, 1997).
6. **Withdrawal symptoms** from amphetamines and related substances
   a. Withdrawal symptoms occur within a few hours to several days after cessation of the drug.
   b. Withdrawal is characterized by depression, fatigue, vivid and unpleasant dreams, insomnia or hypersomnia, paranoia, and psychomotor retardation or agitation.
   c. For treatment of withdrawal, see Table 8-2.
F. **Cocaine** (CNS stimulant)
   1. The method of use may be snorting, smoking, or injection.
   2. **Immediate effects** include euphoria, anxiety, anger, impaired thinking and judgment, and hypervigilance.
      a. More severe physical effects include tachycardia, cardiac arrhythmias, pupil dilation, elevated blood pressure, confusion, and seizures.
      b. Death can occur as result of cardiac dysrhythmias or intracranial hemorrhage caused by severe hypertension.
   3. **Chronic effects** include perforated nasal septum (from snorting the drug), lung damage, and chronic infectious diseases (hepatitis B, C, D, and AIDS)

caused by IV transmission. Cocaine produces extreme euphoria and there-fore can cause psychological dependence after initial use.

4. Fetal exposure

  a. Fetal exposure to cocaine during the first trimester is associated with neu-rologic damage, leading to learning and behavior problems.

  b. After birth, these infants experience abnormal sleep patterns, tremors, seizures (occasionally), irritability, and feeding difficulties (Fontaine & Fletcher, 1999).

6. Withdrawal symptoms are similar to withdrawal from other stimulants (see II.E.6). Treatment of withdrawal is covered in Table 8-2.

G. Hallucinogens

  1. The **method of use** may be oral, injection, smoking, or sniffing.

  2. Immediate effects include intensified perceptions, including heightened response to color, textures, and sounds.

  a. Illusions and hallucinations, anxiety, and depression may also occur. Some drugs in this group (eg, LSD, PCP) can cause dilated pupils and tachycardia.

  b. Effects produced by these drugs are unpredictable and may be related to the specific drug and dosage as well as the individual's mental state.

  c. A **panic reaction ("bad trip")** is characterized by an intense level of anxiety, fear, and paranoia.

  3. Chronic use

  a. Flashbacks (ie, transient spontaneous repetition of previous hallucinogenic experience occurring in absence of substance), psychotic disorders with delusions, and mood and anxiety disorders may occur with chronic use.

  b. PCP use and dependence can lead to symptoms such as belligerence, assaultiveness, impulsive behaviors, psychomotor agitation, and impaired judgment. Physical responses include hypertension, tachycardia, and decreased pain responsiveness.

  4. Withdrawal symptoms include lethargy, depression, and possible panic attacks. Treatment of withdrawal is covered in Table 8-2.

H. Cannabis (CNS depressant and hallucinogen)

  1. The **method of use** is oral or smoking.

  2. Immediate effects include altered sensory perceptions, euphoria, impaired coordination, social withdrawal, conjunctival irritation, increased appetite, dry mouth, and tachycardia.

  3. Chronic use may lead to lethargy and mild depression; paranoid reactions are possible.

  a. Chronic use may lead to a chronic cough and an increased risk for chronic lung diseases, such as emphysema and cancer.

  b. Decreased testosterone levels also occur.

  c. Cannabis crosses the placenta and is associated with low birth weight and small head circumference.

  4. The **major psychoactive ingredient** in cannabinoids is **tetrahydrocanna-binol (THC)**. The most beneficial reported use for this drug is to counteract chemotherapy-induced nausea and vomiting (Townsend, 1999).

5. Withdrawal symptoms include restlessness, irritability, insomnia, tremors, and nausea. Treatment of withdrawal is usually supportive (see Table 8-2).

III. Etiology

A. **General considerations.** The exact cause of substance abuse remains unclear. Genetic factors, biochemical mechanisms, environment, and interpersonal factors, as well as cultural attitudes about substances and their use, all may be implicated.

B. **Genetic theory.** Evidence exists for a genetic component to substance abuse; however, most of this research has been done on alcohol abuse.
   1. **Alcohol metabolism** has a genetic component, which helps to explain differing rates of alcoholism in various cultural groups.
   2. **Statistics**
      a. The risk of becoming an alcoholic for first-degree relatives of alcoholics is as high as 50%.
      b. The concordance rate for monozygotic twins when one twin has an alcohol problem is 70%, while the rate for dizygotic twins is 30%.
      c. Chromosomes 1, 3, and 7 are implicated in vulnerability to alcohol abuse.

C. **Psychobiologic theory.** Research indicates that addictive substances activate neurotransmitters in the mesolimbic dopaminergic reward pathways in the brain.
   1. Stimulation of these pathways leads to the reinforcing properties of "highs."
   2. When neurotransmitter balance is altered in the brain, the need exists to continue the addictive substance.

D. **Psychosocial and environmental theories**
   1. **Developmental (psychodynamic) theories**
      a. The individual has an ego impairment and a disturbance in sense of self; reliance on a substance enhances self-esteem and improves the person's ability to interact with others.
      b. Feelings of guilt and shame are allayed by continued use of substance.
   2. **Family theory** implicates a dysfunctional family system, particularly characterized by enmeshed families in which children feel increased dependency and turn to substances for pseudoseparation (rebellion).
   3. **Sociocultural theory**
      a. Substances are used to relieve the hopelessness experienced with poverty and chronic unemployment.
      b. Societal ambivalence about substance use is seen when the predominant message from advertising is that taking medicine (ie, drugs) solves problems. For example, popular magazines and newspapers carry advertising for antianxiety agents and antidepressants; the advertisements indicate that people who experience anxiety in daily life and social situations should take medicine.
   4. **Cognitive-behavioral theory.** Substance abuse is a learned response to stressful stimuli; the response is reinforced because substance use temporarily decreases anxiety and increases feeling of well-being.

IV. Management

A. General considerations. Treatment decisions, including the recommended care, depend on factors affecting the individual client, including:

1. Type of substance abused and severity of dependence
2. Risk for withdrawal symptoms
3. Current social and occupational functioning
4. Number of previous relapses
5. Willingness of client to accept help

B. Hospital or residential programs

1. These programs are usually recommended for clients with severe substance dependence or failure to achieve success in community-based programs. Follow-up care is recommended after treatment in an inpatient setting.
2. **Types of programs**
   a. **Medical detoxification units** located in community hospitals provide detoxification for several days to a week. Referral is then made for either another residential program or a community-based follow-up program.
   b. **Chemical dependency** units located in psychiatric hospitals or special residential treatment centers. Short-term (3 to 6 weeks) programs provide treatment, usually based on 12-step programs (eg, as recommended by Alcoholics Anonymous [AA] and Narcotics Anonymous [NA] models).
   c. **Long-term residential programs** (3 to 6 months) may be recommended for individuals with a long history of substance abuse and multiple problems as a result of that abuse. These programs provide a therapeutic community setting for treatment of abuse as well as training in life skills.

C. Community-based programs are more common in today's managed care environment, which emphasizes cost containment and treatment in the least restrictive setting.

1. **Partial hospitalization programs** may provide treatment for up to 20 hours weekly, with therapeutic group support and education regarding substance abuse, coping skills, and self-esteem building.
2. **Outpatient counseling** may be provided by either an individual therapist, a group therapy program, or a specific drug and alcohol counselor employed by local drug and alcohol clinics or mental health centers.
3. **Self-help groups,** such as AA and NA, provide support and a specific program designed to establish and maintain sobriety and drug-free lifestyles (Table 8-3).

D. Prevention

1. **Description.** Community educational programs target vulnerable groups as well as the general population. For example, members of the health care team, including community nurses, serve as speakers and use written materials for education.
2. Elements of prevention programs include:
   a. Teaching the concept of substance abuse and dependence, including symptoms and warning signs

TABLE 8-3
Self-Help Treatment Programs

Examples
Alcoholics Anonymous (AA)
Narcotics Anonymous (NA)
Alanon (for spouse or significant others of alcoholics and substance users)
Alateen (for adolescent children of alcoholics)
Adult Children of Alcoholics (ACOA)

Characteristics of These Programs
Use the original 12-Step Model from AA; reinforce the disease concept of substance abuse; and emphasize recovery occurring one day at a time. AA and NA groups rely on help from members who are also substance abusers but who have been successful in the recovery process. A special one-to-one relationship with a sponsor who has been successful in recovery is recommended.

b. Teaching about the consequences of substance abuse and the effect of substances on the body and general life functioning
c. Teaching about the options available for assistance and treatment
d. Teaching about alternative coping mechanisms to avoid substance abuse

E. Pharmacologic management
   1. **Heroin.** Methadone maintenance programs attempt to replace a person's reliance on heroin with the use of a medically controlled dose of methadone (or other synthetic narcotic).
      a. Methadone provides a noneuphoric state that frees the addicted person from the physiologic craving for heroin (Drug Chart 8-1).
      b. Methadone programs have been controversial owing to failure to bring about drug-free states in heroin-dependent individuals.
   2. **Alcohol.** Several pharmacologic alternatives are currently available for alcoholics (see Drug Chart 8-1).

F. Family support
   1. **Family therapy.** Family members of a substance abuser are encouraged to define and maintain responsible self-functioning, thus decreasing codependent behaviors.
   2. **Support groups,** such as Alanon, Alateen, and Adult Children of Alcoholics (ACOA), provide support to families using the 12-step program. These programs focus on family members changing their own behavior rather than trying to change the behavior of the individual with the substance abuse problem.

 NURSING PROCESS OVERVIEW
V. Substance-Related Disorders

A. Assessment
   1. **Alcohol abuse.** When screening an individual with undetected alcohol problems, use established screening questionnaires, such as CAGE questions (Mayfield, 1974):

DRUG CHART 8-1 Medications Used in Treatment of Alcohol and
                        Heroin Dependence

Pharmacologic Agent	Typical Daily Dosage (Adults)	Rationale for Use
For Alcohol Dependence		
Disulfiram (Antabuse)	125–250 mg/day	Inhibits complete alcohol breakdown in the body; when alcohol is taken with disulfiram, acute hypersensitivity occurs. Symptoms include flushing, severe nausea and vomiting, dizziness, and hypotension. Acts as psychological deterrent to prevent individual from using alcohol. (*Note:* Client must refrain from taking alcohol in any form, including non-beverage alcohol, eg, cough syrups or extracts.)
Naltrexone (ReVia)	50 mg/day	Opioid receptor antagonist blocks brain reward pathway activated by alcohol; reduces pleasurable response to drinking and therefore limits urge to drink.
For Heroin Dependence		
Methadone (Dolophin)	60–120 mg/day	Synthetic narcotic provides noneuphoric state free from physiologic craving for heroin.
Buprenorphine (Buprenex)	12–16 mg/day	Synthetic narcotic; acts in similar manner to methadone.
Levomethadyl acetate (LAAM)	60–90 mg, 3 times/week	Synthetic narcotic with longer half-life than methadone; administered 3 times/week rather than daily.

   a. Have you ever felt you ought to **c**ut down on your drinking?
   b. Have people **a**nnoyed you by criticizing your drinking?
   c. Have you ever felt bad or **g**uilty about your drinking?
   d. Have you ever had a drink in the morning (**e**ye opener) to steady your nerves or get rid of a hangover?
2. Assessment of individuals with a known substance abuse problem (Table 8-4).
   a. Identify symptoms of acute intoxication.
   b. Identify withdrawal symptoms.
   c. Question the individual regarding patterns of use, including types of substances used; frequency of use; amount of use; route of administration. (Note: Clients with a history of substance abuse tend to underestimate use.)

TABLE 8-4
Key Nursing Assessment Questions

QUESTIONS	PROVIDES DATA ABOUT
What substances do you use? How much and how often do you use? What is the method of use (eg, oral, smoked, inhaled, injected)?	Specific substances used and estimate of how severe use has become Note: Underestimation of use is common.
Have you ever experienced withdrawal symptoms? Have you been treated for this in the past?	Presence of physiologic dependence History of previous treatment
Do you believe you have a problem with substance use?	Client acknowledgment of problem or use of denial
Have you had any periods in your life when you did not use substances? How long did this last?	History of drug-free periods; ability to maintain abstinence
Have you experienced any trouble with the law, job losses, or relationship problems associated with substance use?	Losses incurred; extent of effect on social and occupational functioning
Have you ever attempted to harm yourself or another when using substance?	Potential for suicide or acting-out

      d. Perform general physical assessment to determine health status and signs of physical problems related to abuse.

      e. Review past history for presence of previously diagnosed mental illness.

3. Assess client for impact of substance abuse on functioning, including losses incurred (eg, of relationships, jobs, finances, self-respect) and legal problems (eg, DUI, disorderly conduct, selling or using illegal substances).

4. Assess client for treatment history, including hospitalizations, counseling, self-help groups.

5. Assess client for typical emotional responses associated with substance abuse:

      a. Feelings of anxiety, anger, guilt, shame, despair, and depression

      b. Use of common defense mechanisms, including denial (of substance abuse problem), rationalization about use, and projection of blame

6. Assess the effect of the client's substance use on family members, including the extent of family involvement with client, the willingness of the family to participate in the client's treatment, and the family's knowledge base regarding problems of substance abuse (Client and Family Teaching 8-1).

B. Nursing diagnoses

  1. Analysis

      a. Analyze the client's response to screening questionnaires; when substance abuse is suspected, use follow-up assessments.

      b. Analyze extent to which substances have affected the client's social and occupational functioning and general health status.

CLIENT AND FAMILY TEACHING 8-1

Educating Families Who Have a Member with a Substance-Related Disorder

EDUCATING THE FAMILY WITH GENERAL INFORMATION

1. Substance abuse is a disease, not a moral weakness.
2. Substance abuse, when present, affects all family members, not just person with disorder.
3. Symptoms commonly include compulsive need for substance; increasing amount of substance over time with inability to reduce use; and using substance despite multiple problems associated with use.
4. Withdrawal symptoms can occur when intake of substance is reduced or stopped.

EDUCATING THE FAMILY ABOUT TREATMENT

1. Individual can be helped prior to reaching "rock bottom."
2. Options for treatment range from hospital-based programs to handle withdrawal and teach skills necessary for living without substances, to community-based therapy with special drug and alcohol counselor, or self-help groups, such as AA and NA.
3. Family members can encourage individual to get treatment, but cannot make this happen.

EDUCATING THE FAMILY ABOUT HANDLING SYMPTOMS

1. Reality-based statements, such as, "You were unable to work 3 days last week because of your drinking," will help confront denial by the person of problems with substances.
2. Protecting the substance abuser from consequences of their behavior (ie, calling them in sick for work, making excuses to friends) is not helpful and is evidence of codependency.
3. Report any signs of increasing depression or suicidal thoughts by substance abuser or any other family members to mental health system.

EDUCATING THE FAMILY ABOUT SELF-CARE

1. Maintain responsibility for keeping self healthy and functioning in usual roles.
2. Use support groups, such as Alanon and Alateen, or individual counseling.
3. Learn or apply knowledge about managing stress to one's own life.

    c. Analyze the potential for adverse consequences related to withdrawal symptoms.
    d. Analyze the level of depression and potential for suicidal behaviors.
2. Establish individualized nursing diagnoses for the client with a substance-related disorder, including, but not limited to, the following:
    a. Adjustment, impaired
    b. Chronic low self-esteem
    c. Defensive coping
    d. Denial, ineffective
    e. Hopelessness
    f. Individual coping, ineffective

g. Knowledge deficit (specify)
h. Nutrition: less than body requirements, altered
i. Powerlessness
j. Role performance, altered
k. Self-esteem disturbance
l. Social interaction, impaired
m. Spiritual distress
3. Establish nursing diagnoses for the family of the client:
a. Family coping: compromised, ineffective
b. Family process: alcoholism
c. Family process: altered
C. **Planning and outcome identification.** Work with the client, family, or both in setting realistic goals.
1. Establish desired outcome criteria for client with substance-related disorders.
a. The client will acknowledge dependence on abusive substance(s).
b. The client will safely detoxify from substance(s).
c. The client will participate in the treatment program as recommended (in either the hospital or the community).
d. The client will verbalize increased knowledge regarding effect of substances on health and functioning in family and societal roles.
e. The client will maintain sobriety or drug-free state.
f. The client will use adaptive coping measures for handling life stress rather than turning to substances(s).
g. The client will maintain participation in a self-help group (eg, AA, NA), accepting feedback and input from sponsor.
h. The client will establish a life-style that is healthy and free from abusive substances.
i. The client will seek assistance at the first signs of relapse.
2. Establish desired outcome criteria for family members.
a. Family members will verbalize increased knowledge regarding substances and specific effects on individual and family functioning.
b. Family members will seek help from support groups (Alanon and Alateen) or counselor (eg, family therapy).
c. Family members will avoid codependent behaviors.
d. Family members will maintain individual functioning in social and occupational roles despite the success or lack of success of treatment for member with substance-related disorder.
D. **Implementation**
1. During detoxification and withdrawal (see Table 8-2)
a. Monitor vital signs; increased pulse and blood pressure indicate undermedication with benzodiazepine, and decreased blood pressure indicates overmedication with benzodiazepine.
b. Administer scheduled and as-needed (prn) medications for detoxification.
c. Monitor intake and output for client requiring IV fluid replacement.
d. Encourage adequate fluids and nutritious foods.

   e. Maintain standard seizure precautions as indicated by the severity of the client's problem.
2. Maintain attitude of acceptance and a nonjudgmental approach. Be aware of personal biases that will affect nursing care.
3. Teach the client, family, or both about substance abuse (see Client and Family Teaching 8-1).
   a. Inform them about the symptoms of abuse and its consequences on functioning and on general health.
   b. Inform them about the progressive course of dependence.
   c. Inform them about relapse, including warning signs (eg, increased anger and frustration, excuses for poor behavior, increased relationship problems, denying substance problem, and returning to associations with other users).
   d. Inform them about the dangers of IV drug use, including contracting hepatitis B, C, and D, and AIDS.
   e. Emphasize personal responsibility for effecting behavioral change.
   f. Provide information about treatment options (see IV).
4. Encourage the client, family, or both to use self-help groups for support and ongoing assistance (see Table 8-3).
5. Help the client to verbalize and express feelings covered up by the use of substances.
6. Review life-style changes necessary to maintain abstinence or sobriety.
7. Teach and encourage the use of stress management and coping measures (see Chapter 3).
8. Use measures to enhance client self-esteem.
   a. Give appropriate praise and encouragement.
   b. Show respect and maintain client dignity.
   c. Help the client identify and use personal strengths.
   d. Project optimism to counteract helplessness and powerlessness.
E. **Outcome evaluation.** The nurse uses the following criteria to evaluate client outcomes and the effectiveness of nursing implementations.
   1. The client admits substance abuse problem and safely detoxifies from abusive substance.
   2. The client participates in recommended initial treatment program and subsequent follow-up measures.
   3. The client maintains substance-free lifestyle.
   4. The client use adaptive coping measures rather than substance abuse in handling life stress.
   5. The client attends appropriate self-help group and follows 12-step program.
   6. The family members use appropriate support programs and report increased coping of individual members.

STUDY QUESTIONS

1. According to the DSM-IV, the essential difference between substance abuse and substance dependence is that substance dependence
   (1) includes characteristics of tolerance and withdrawal
   (2) includes characteristics of adverse consequences and repeated use
   (3) produces less severe symptoms than that of abuse
   (4) requires long-term treatment in a hospital-based program

2. A family member of a client with a substance abuse problem tells a nurse about calling in sick for the client when the client has had too much to drink and is not capable of working. The family member's behavior can be described as
   (1) caretaking
   (2) codependent
   (3) unhelpful
   (4) supportive

3. When a client abuses a CNS depressant, withdrawal symptoms will be caused by which of the following?
   (1) acetylcholine excess
   (2) dopamine depletion
   (3) serotonin inhibition
   (4) norepinephrine rebound

4. The general classification of drugs belonging to the opioid category is analgesic and
   (1) depressant
   (2) hallucinogenic
   (3) stimulant
   (4) tranquilizing

5. A community nurse practicing primary prevention of alcohol abuse would target which of the following groups for educational efforts?
   (1) adolescents in their late teens and young adults in their early twenties

   (2) elderly men who live in retirement communities
   (3) women working in careers outside the home
   (4) women working in the home

6. A staff nurse has observed a coworker come to work drunk at least three times in the past month. Which of the following would the staff nurse most appropriately do to ensure client safety and obtain necessary assistance for the coworker?
   (1) Ignore the coworker's behavior and frequently assess the clients assigned to the coworker.
   (2) Make general statements in next staff meeting about safety issues.
   (3) Report the coworker's behavior to the appropriate supervisor.
   (4) Warn the coworker that this practice is unsafe.

7. A client being treated in a chemical dependency unit tells a nurse that he only uses drugs when under stress and therefore does not have a substance problem. Which of the following defense mechanisms is the client using?
   (1) compensation
   (2) denial
   (3) suppression
   (4) undoing

8. A nurse is teaching a community group about substance abuse. The nurse would explain that a genetic component has been implicated with which of the following commonly abused substances?
   (1) alcohol
   (2) barbiturates
   (3) heroin
   (4) marijuana

9. A nurse recommends that the family of a client with a substance-related disorder attend a support group, such as Alanon or Alateen. The purpose of these groups is to help family members understand the problem and also
    (1) to change the problem behaviors of the abuser
    (2) to learn how to assist the abuser in getting help
    (3) to maintain focus on changing their own behaviors
    (4) to prevent substance problems in vulnerable family members

10. A nurse is assessing a client who is a chronic alcohol abuser. Which of the following problems is related to thiamin deficiency?
    (1) cardiovascular symptoms, such as decreased hemoglobin and hematocrit
    (2) CNS symptoms, such as ataxia and peripheral neuropathy
    (3) gastrointestinal symptoms, such as nausea and vomiting
    (4) respiratory symptoms, such as cough and sore throat

11. A nurse is assessing a client who abuses barbiturates and anxiolytics. For which of the following common withdrawal symptoms would the nurse assess?
    (1) anxiety, tremors, tachycardia
    (2) respiratory depression, stupor, bradycardia
    (3) muscle aches, cramps, lacrimation
    (4) paranoia, depression, agitation

12. A nurse is teaching an adolescent health class about the dangers of inhalant abuse. Which of the fol lowing is a danger of this type of substance abuse?
    (1) contracting an infectious disease, such as hepatitis or AIDS
    (2) recurrent flashback events
    (3) psychological dependence after initial use
    (4) sudden death from cardiac or respiratory depression

13. Which of the following medications is used in a treatment program for clients abusing heroin to produce a noneuphoric state and to replace heroin use?
    (1) diazepam
    (2) carbamazepine
    (3) clonidine
    (4) methadone

14. A nurse administers bromocriptine (Parlodel) to a client undergoing detoxification for amphetamine abuse. The rationale for this medication is to
    (1) aid in GABA inhibition
    (2) prevent norepinephrine excess
    (3) restore depleted dopamine
    (4) treat psychotic symptoms

15. A nurse is teaching a client about disulfiram (Antabuse), which the client is taking to deter his use of alcohol. Which of the following would the nurse explain would happen if alcohol is taken when using this medication?
    (1) abdominal cramps and diarrhea
    (2) drowsiness and decreased respiration
    (3) flushing, vomiting, and dizziness
    (4) increased pulse and blood pressure

ANSWER KEY

1. The answer is (1). Tolerance (ie, the need to increase the amount of a substance to obtain desired effect) and withdrawal (ie, symptoms occurring when substance is decreased or stopped) are the essential criteria in establishing substance dependence. Both abuse and dependence produce adverse consequences and are characterized by repeated use. Dependence would cause symptoms that are more severe. Answer choice (4) is not necessarily true; after the initial detoxification period, community-based treatment may be appropriate.

2. The answer is (2). Codependency is defined as enabling behaviors that inadvertently promote continued use of a substance by the person abusing substances. The family member's behavior is not an example of caretaking or support. The family member is taking responsibility for the behavior of the other and is allowing the person with the problem to avoid consequences of an abuse problem. The behavior is unhelpful; however, the correct term for this problem is *codependency.*

3. The answer is (4). CNS depressants, when abused, cause depletion of neurotransmitters that are stimulating. When the CNS depressant is stopped, the result is a rebound of excitatory or stimulating neurotransmitters, such as norepinephrine. Acetylcholine, dopamine, and serotonin are not significant in the symptoms of withdrawal from a CNS depressant.

4. The answer is (1). Opiates are both analgesics and CNS depressants because they will decrease the effect of neurotransmitters that are excitatory. Hallucinogenic and stimulant are categories that do not apply to opiates. Although an opiate can provide a tranquilizing effect, the general category would be that of a depressant.

5. The answer is (1). It is known that the high-risk groups for alcohol abuse include individuals between ages 18 and 25 and the unemployed. There is no evidence that elderly men in retirement communities have increased rates of alcohol abuse. Men have a 2 to 3 times increased risk than women of abusing alcohol.

6. The answer is (3). The nurse is obligated by ethical considerations of client safety, as well as by nurse practice acts in many states, to report substance abuse in health care workers. Most health care facilities have an employee assistance program to help workers with substance abuse problems. Ignoring the coworker's behavior would be enabling the behavior (codependency) on the staff nurse's part. Making general statements about safety in a staff meeting avoids dealing with the problem. Warning the coworker is inadequate; it does not ensure client safety or help the person with the problem get necessary help.

7. The answer is (2). Denial is commonly used by individuals who have substance problems. Compensation, suppression, and undoing are incorrect and do not fit the situation described.

8. The answer is (1). Several chromosomes (1, 3, and 7) have been implicated in increased vulnerability to alcohol abuse. Statistics have shown that risk for alcohol abuse in first-degree relatives of alcohol abusers is as high as 50%. Most of the genetic research has been done related to alcohol. Definitive data regarding genetic transmission is not available at this time for barbiturates, heroin, and marijuana.

9. The answer is (3). Family support groups, such as Alanon and Alateen, emphasize the importance of changing one's own behavior rather than trying to change the behavior of the individual with the substance abuse problem. Trying to change the abuser's problem behaviors or learning how to assist the abuser in getting help would be viewed as codependent behaviors, and thus would not be advocated by family support groups. Learning about substance abuse may assist a vulnerable family member to avoid this problem; however, that is not the purpose of these groups.

10. The answer is (2). Wernicke's encephalopathy is a CNS disorder caused by acute thiamin deficiency in people who abuse alcohol. Other symptoms, besides ataxia and peripheral neuropathy, are acute confusion or delirium. Cardiovascular and gastrointestinal symptoms are health problems associated with alcohol abuse, but are not caused by thiamin deficiency. Respiratory problems are not usually directly related to alcohol.

11. The answer is (1). Barbiturates and anxiolytics are CNS depressants, and therefore withdrawal symptoms are related to CNS stimulation from rebounding of neurotransmitters (eg, norepinephrine). Symptoms are increased anxiety and tremors as well as associated vital sign changes, such as tachycardia and hypertension. Respiratory depression, stupor, and bradycardia are most commonly associated with an overdose of barbiturates or anxiolytics. Muscle aches, cramps, and lacrimation are most commonly associated with withdrawal from opiates. Paranoia, depression, and agitation are most commonly associated with withdrawal from CNS stimulants, such as amphetamines or cocaine.

12. The answer is (4). Inhalants are CNS depressants; if taken in an excess amount, they can cause cardiac and respiratory depression. It is impossible to control the inhalant dosage; therefore, death can occur. Contracting an infectious disease, recurrent flashback events, and psychological dependence after initial use are not associated with inhalant abuse.

13. The answer is (4). Methadone maintenance programs are used to provide a heroin-dependent individual with a medically controlled dose of methadone to produce a noneuphoric state that will prevent withdrawal symptoms. This method of treatment is advocated to help heroin abusers avoid criminal activities associated with obtaining heroin; it also prevents diseases associated with IV use of heroin. Diazepam and carbamazepine may be used for withdrawal from alcohol, barbiturates, and anxiolytics. Clonidine can be used in acute withdrawal from heroin to avoid norepinephrine rebound when opiates are stopped.

14. The answer is (3). Amphetamine abuse has the effect on the brain of depleting the neurotransmitter dopamine. When withdrawing from amphetamines, dopamine depletion causes depression, insomnia, and intense craving for the drug. Bromocriptine (Parlodel) is a dopamine agonist that will help restore this neurotransmitter. Aid in GABA inhibition, prevention of norepinephrine excess, and treatment of psychotic symptoms are incorrect rationales for the use of this medication.

15. The answer is (3). Disulfiram (Antabuse) prevents complete alcohol metabolism in the body. Therefore, when alcohol is consumed, the individual has a hypersensitivity reaction. Flushing, vomiting, and dizziness are associated with the incomplete breakdown of alcohol metabolites. Abdominal cramps, diarrhea, drowsiness, decreased respiration, and increased pulse and blood pressure are not associated with the use of disulfiram along with alcohol.

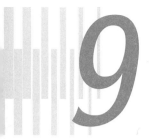

Physical Abuse, Sexual Abuse, and Family Violence

9

Overview

A. Definitions

1. **Violence** is the physical force exerted for the purpose of violating or damaging another person. It is an unjust exercise of power, often resulting in physical injury.
2. **Abuse** is the willful infliction of physical injury, mental anguish, or both.
3. **Family violence** is a pattern of coercive behavior of one family member (or significant other) by another. It includes physical abuse, neglect, psychological abuse, economic abuse, and sexual abuse.
4. An **abuser,** or **perpetrator,** is the person who inflicts violence or abuse on another, and the **victim** is the person who is scapegoat, target, or recipient of the abuse or violence.

B. Types of abuse

1. **Physical abuse** includes beating, hitting, cutting, shooting, burning, and raping.
2. **Neglect** is characterized by withholding or failing to provide personal care, personal needs (eg, food, water, shelter), cleanliness, health care, social contact, and the education and supervision of children.
3. **Psychological abuse** includes:
   a. Verbal assaults and threats of physical harm, usually to intimidate or manipulate
   b. Sarcasm, humiliation, devaluing, and criticism
   c. Inconsistent communication patterns, including withdrawal and silence
   d. Isolation of the victim (eg, preventing the victim from interaction and communication with family and friends)
   e. Violation of personal rights, such as refusing to allow the victim contact with family, friends, and others
4. **Economic abuse** (financial exploitation) includes:
   a. Stealing money or assets of the victim
   b. Denying the victim access to personal finances
   c. Inappropriate use of the victim's money or property
5. **Sexual abuse** is pressured or forced sexual activity, including sexually stimulated talk or actions, inappropriate touching or intercourse, rape, and incest (sexual behavior between blood relatives).

C. Important concepts

1. Family violence is a primary public health issue in the United States. It is estimated that 50% of all Americans have experienced violence in their families.
2. Family violence occurs across many boundaries, affecting all socioeconomic levels, genders, geographic areas, races, religions, and occupations.
3. Family violence also occurs across the lifespan. The victim may be a fetus, an infant, a child, an adolescent, an adult, or an elderly person.

D. Relevant statistics

1. **Child abuse**
   a. In 3 out of 5 families, a child is physically abused by an adult.
   b. Approximately 3 million cases of child abuse are reported each year, and it is estimated that there are 10 to 20 unreported cases for each reported case.
   c. Childhood sexual abuse affects 33% of women and 20% of men before 18 years of age.
   d. Sibling abuse is considered by some experts to be the most common and unrecognized form of family violence.
   e. Child abuse and neglect account for 2000 to 4000 deaths yearly in the United States (Townsend, 1999).

2. **Abuse of women**
   a. One third of all women are abused by a male partner at some time in the relationship.
   b. Family violence accounts for 22% to 35% of women's visits to the emergency room.
   c. Twenty-three percent of all pregnant women seeking prenatal services are victims of abuse.
   d. More injuries to women are incurred through battering than through all rapes, muggings, and automobile accidents combined (Townsend, 1999).
   e. One in seven married women reports rape by her husband.

3. **Abuse of elderly people**
   a. More than 1.5 million older Americans suffer some form of abuse or neglect annually (Dept. of Health & Human Services Report, 1996).
   b. Some experts believe that only 1 in 14 cases is reported, and therefore the full scope of this problem is unknown (Wolfe, 1998).
   c. Both spouses and adult children are often perpetrators of domestic elder abuse. According to one study, 37% of reported cases of abuse were committed by adult children (Wolfe, 1998).

E. Child sexual abuse

1. Child sexual abuse profoundly affects development, causing low self-esteem, self-hatred, difficulty trusting, and poor control of aggressive impulses.
2. There is a high correlation between childhood sexual abuse and adult psychiatric disorders (eg, dissociative disorders, substance abuse disorders) (Walker & Scott, 1998).
3. Victims of child sexual abuse often experience symptoms of post-traumatic stress disorder (PTSD).

F. **Sexual assault** is characterized by use of force in any sexual activity executed against the person's will.

   1. **Characteristics of a sexual perpetrator**

      a. A sexual perpetrator is typically male, between the ages of 25 and 44, and married or cohabiting at the time of the offense.

      b. If the sexual perpetrator has a history of criminal behavior, it is generally crimes against property rather than people.

      c. The majority of perpetrators do not have a history of mental illness (Townsend, 1999).

   2. A **victim of a sexual assault** experiences an overwhelming sense of violation and helplessness following the crime.

      a. The **immediate effect** may be either an *expressed response pattern,* in which the victim expresses feelings of fear, anger, and anxiety, or a *controlled response pattern,* in which the defense mechanism of denial allows the victim to be calm, composed, or subdued.

      b. Long-term effects can include symptoms of PTSD, difficulties with intimate relationships, depressive disorders, and even suicide.

G. **Legal issues in family violence** (Johnson, 1997)

   1. **Child abuse.** All states have mandatory laws for reporting child abuse. Failure to report is a misdemeanor.

   2. **Abuse of women.** Legal protection of battered women varies among states.

      a. Generally, the woman herself must seek legal or civil remedies, such as protective orders, temporary restraining orders, or filing charges against the perpetrator.

      b. When a woman is injured by an abuser using a weapon (eg, gun, knife), the health care provider must report the act of abuse to the police, regardless of the woman's intent to seek legal remedies for the abuse.

   3. **Abuse of elders.** Forty-eight states now have mandatory elder abuse or neglect reporting laws. Nurses and other health care providers must report abuse.

H. **Cycle of violence in families.** Violent acts in families do not occur randomly, but constitute a predictable, three-phase cycle.

   1. **Tension building.** The abuser blames the victim for problems in the abuser's life.

   2. **Serious abusive incident.** The tension in the abuser is relieved by the abusive incident.

   3. **Honeymoon.** The abuser becomes remorseful and promises an abusive incident will not happen again.

I. **Victims of violence** often have physical signs of abuse, and over time behavioral and psychological signs are noted (Tables 9-1 and 9-2). The **characteristics of an abuser or violent perpetrator** are listed in Display 9-1.

J. **Characteristics of family systems in which violence occurs**

   1. One or more members of the family become the focal point for family anxiety and often are blamed for problems.

TABLE 9-1
Physical Signs of Abuse

CHILD VICTIM	BATTERED WOMAN	ELDER VICTIM
Physical Abuse		
Developmental delays	Injuries of head, neck, and shoulder	Malnourishment or dehydration
Bruises, welts		
Sprains, dislocations, fractures	Black eyes	Fecal or urine smell on person
	Injuries during pregnancy	
Cigarette burns	Sprains, dislocations, broken bones	Dirt, fleas, lice on person
Scalding or burns, especially those resembling stocking or glove from immersion of extremity into any hot liquid		Pressure ulcers, sores, skin rashes
	Bruises, welts	
	Patterns left by objects used to inflict injury	Bruises, abrasions, fractures
		Hematomas, grip marks on arms
Internal injuries	Repeated visits to health care facilities, especially emergency rooms	
Injuries in various stages of healing		Multiple injuries in various stages of healing
	Complaints of pain without tissue injury	
Shaken baby syndrome (ie, intracranial and intraocular bleeding without obvious head trauma)	Multiple injuries in various stages of healing	
Dirt, fleas, lice on child		
Sexual Abuse		
Enuresis		
Red and swollen labia and rectum		
Vaginal tears		
Sexually transmitted diseases		
Chronic urinary infections		
Hyperactive gag reflex		

2. The family roles are stereotypic, with rigid traditional sex roles and strong power differential between parents (ie, one parent, usually the male, is the sole authority in the family, and the other parent is treated like one of the children rather than an equal partner).
3. Relationships in the family emphasize control over others.
4. The family may be secretive and isolated from others outside the family.
5. The communication patterns are dysfunctional. Denial, conflict avoidance, double-bind patterns, conditional loving, and rationalization of abuse are common.

K. **Women often choose to remain in an abusive relationship.** Some of these reasons include (Chez, 1994):
1. Belief that there are no alternatives
2. Fear of what will happen if they do leave
3. Inability to support oneself and children

TABLE 9-2
Behavioral and Psychological Characteristics in Victims of Abuse

CHILD VICTIM	BATTERED WOMAN	ELDER VICTIM
Physical Abuse		
Fearful of caregiver	Rationalizes abuse	May have physical or
Seeks affection from others	Fears leaving due to threats	mental impairment
May not cry when approached by examiner or during painful procedure	Relationship with partner is male dominant	Aggressive or very submissive behavior
Behavioral extremes (child is either very aggressive or very submissive)	Isolates from friends and family	Fearful of reporting abuse
	Feelings of inadequacy, accepting self-blame	Dependent on caregiver
Poor academic performance		Feelings of low self-esteem
Regressive behaviors and hyperactivity	Acts so as not to provoke partner	Hopelessness
Self-injurious behaviors	Emotionally and financially dependent on partner	
Runs away, abuses drugs or alcohol	Feelings of powerlessness	
Lack of peer relationships	Use of alcohol or drugs	
	Depression, suicidal thoughts	
	Anxiety, recurrent nightmares	
Sexual Abuse		
Unusual interest in or avoidance of all things of a sexual nature		
Sleep problems, nightmares		
Seductiveness		
Statements that their bodies are dirty or damaged, or fear that there is something wrong with their genital area		
Aspects of sexual molestation in drawings, games, fantasies		

DISPLAY 9-1. **Characteristics of an Abuser or Violent Perpetrator**

- Frequently was abused as child
- Low self-esteem
- Extremely jealous and possessive
- Socially isolated
- Poor impulse control, poor coping measures
- Drug or alcohol abuse
- Rigid and obsessive regarding retaining control
- Narcissistic

4. Fear of being shunned by family and friends

5. Ties (eg, emotional, financial) to abuser, or religious or cultural beliefs

II. Etiology

A. General considerations. No single factor accounts for family violence; multiple factors exist in any situation of family violence or abuse.

B. Genetic theory

    1. Some studies have linked increased aggressiveness with selective inbreeding in mice, suggesting possibility of direct genetic link.

    2. Genetic karyotype XYX has also been implicated in aggressive and deviant behavior (Townsend, 1999).

C. Psychobiologic theory

    1. Research has demonstrated that stimulation of the limbic system has produced evidence of hostile and aggressive responses in humans.

    2. Neurotransmitters, especially norepinephrine, dopamine, and serotonin, all play important roles in facilitating and inhibiting aggression. Dysregulation of these substances is thought to be associated with violence.

    3. Brain disorders, especially tumors in the limbic system and temporal lobe, can predispose a person to violent behavior (Johnson, 1997).

D. Psychosocial and environmental theories

    1. Family theory. Violence occurs in dysfunctional families with problems such as unclear boundaries, enmeshment of individuals and roles, poor coping measures to handle stress, and a multigenerational history of abuse.

    2. Cognitive-behavioral theory. Violence is learned from parents who use abuse as a method of discipline. The abuser acquires the belief that violence and aggression are acceptable and effective responses to real or imagined threats.

    3. Sociocultural theory. Aggressive behavior is a product of one's culture and social structure.

        a. The United States has a long history of violence by one group of people over another.

        b. Current cultural glorification of violence as portrayed in movies, TV shows, video games, and the Internet have all been implicated as contributing factors to aggressive behaviors.

III. Management

A. General considerations. Treatment of abuse victims depends on factors affecting the individual client, such as the type of abuse suffered, presence of physical injuries, age and physical condition of the victim, and the victim's unique family circumstances.

B. Emergency room (ER) treatment. Since 1991, institutions accredited by the Joint Commission on Accreditation of Healthcare Organizations (JCAHO) have been required to adopt the JCAHO's domestic violence standards into their ER protocol.

C. **Crisis intervention services** are helpful to respond to the immediate, short-term problems resulting from abuse. Collaboration with various health team members is important to provide continuity of care.

1. **Public child welfare agencies** are responsible for protecting children from harm and cruelty. The legal system can intervene by awarding temporary or permanent custody of children to individuals (relatives or foster parents) who will provide safe care.

2. Battered women can be referred to a **safe house** or **emergency shelter** to ensure protection for themselves and their children.

3. **Community social service agencies,** including special agencies for elders, can provide a variety of services to ensure safety and support for victims of violence.

D. **Mental health services** can be offered to families who are affected by violence.

1. **Therapeutic support** by means of individual or group counseling for victims of violence is available.

2. **Individual counseling** for the abuser or violent perpetrator is available.

3. **Family therapy** to break the cycle of abuse is available.

E. **Prevention**

1. **Primary prevention** can take place in the community by identifying families at high risk for violence and by promoting educational programs and services that enhance family functioning.

2. **Secondary prevention** involves early detection and treatment for interpersonal violence.

 IV. **NURSING PROCESS OVERVIEW FOR**
Family Violence

A. **Assessment**

1. **Identify assessment data indicative of possible abuse.**

   a. Conduct a thorough examination to determine the nature and extent of the victim's physical injuries (see Table 9-1).

   b. Assess behavioral and psychological characteristics of abuse (see Table 9-2).

2. **Interview the client to validate that abuse has occurred.** Use specific agency protocols for assessment, ensuring the following factors:

   a. Ensure privacy for assessment by questioning the client away from the suspected abuser; this will promote client trust.

   b. Use appropriate language for the client's age and developmental level.

   c. Ask questions that are simple, direct, and as nonthreatening as possible (Table 9-3).

   d. If possible, take meticulous notes (including exact quotes) to record conversations with the client and family.

TABLE 9-3
Key Nursing Assessment Questions

SPECIFIC QUESTIONS	PROVIDES DATA ABOUT
Child Victim	
Do you know why you were brought to the hospital?	Child's perception
How do you feel about being here?	Fears, other feelings of child
Tell me what happened to you.	Child's description of incident
Have you ever been hit with an object?	Past history of abuse
How do your parents (caregivers) discipline you?	Parenting behaviors
Battered Woman	
Are you being threatened or hurt by your partner?	Willingness to acknowledge abuse
Have you ever been injured before?	Past history of abuse
What's the worst episode you remember?	Escalation of violence
Have children been present when you were abused? Have they ever been injured?	Child abuse
Elder Victim	
I notice you have a number of bruises (or other injuries). Could you tell me what happened?	Willingness to acknowledge abuse
You seem frightened by your caregiver; are you?	Validation of observation of relationship
Many patients tell me they have been hurt by someone close to them. Could this be happening to you?	Past history
When you disagree with your caregiver, what happens?	Family dynamics

3. Identify the aspects of family behavior associated with family violence.
   a. Is there a lack of concern about the child or the elder person who is suspected of being abused?
   b. Are there inconsistencies between the nature and extent of injuries and the family's or victim's explanation of what happened?
   c. Was there a delay in seeking help for injuries?
   d. Do the interactions between client and family indicate conflict? Is there screaming and blaming of the victim for the injury?
   e. Is there a history of abusive behavior or substance abuse in a member of the family?
   f. Are there descriptions (by the family) of children as aggressive, antisocial, and prone to injuries?
   g. Is there evidence of increased stress on the family system?
4. **Victims of rape**
   a. Collect assessment data required by law from victims of rape.
   b. Follow protocol of specific agency as well as legal guidelines to ensure unbroken **chain of evidence.**

5. The nurse should assess her own feelings and responses to family violence and abuse.
   a. The nurse's personal memories may be reactivated by issues of violence and abuse.
   b. Negative feelings may emerge, including anger, blame, feeling overwhelmed, frustration, avoidance, fear, and disgust.
   c. Positive feelings may emerge, including hope, support, caring, helpfulness, commitment, and understanding.
   d. The nurse should seek support for self-responses and feelings that interfere with the ability to be therapeutic.

B. Nursing diagnoses
   1. Analyze the client data collected to determine the presence of abuse.
      a. Analyze the family functioning, including evidence of characteristics common in abuser and current stressors affecting family.
      b. Analyze the family members' coping resources and abilities, including use of community resources.
   2. Establish individualized nursing diagnoses for the victim of abuse.
      a. Anxiety (specify level)
      b. Coping: individual, ineffective
      c. Denial, ineffective
      d. Fear
      e. Growth and development, altered
      f. Hopelessness
      g. Injury, risk for
      h. Pain
      i. Post-trauma response
      j. Rape-trauma syndrome
      k. Self-esteem, situational low
      l. Skin integrity, impaired
      m. Spiritual distress
      n. Trauma, risk for
      o. Unilateral neglect
   3. Establish nursing diagnoses for the family.
      a. Family coping: ineffective, compromised
      b. Family processes, altered
      c. Parent/infant, child attachment, altered, risk for
      d. Parenting, altered
      e. Role performance, altered
      f. Violence, risk for: directed at self and others
   4. Establish nursing diagnoses for the abuser.
      a. Coping, individual, ineffective
      b. Knowledge deficit (specify)
      c. Noncompliance
      d. Role performance, altered
      e. Self-esteem disturbance
      f. Social interaction, impaired

g. Spiritual distress

h. Violence, risk for: directed at self/others

C. Planning and outcome identification. Work with the client, family members, health team members, and community resource representatives in setting realistic goals.

1. Establish desired outcome criteria for the victim of abuse.

a. The client will maintain safety.

b. The client will receive treatment for physical and psychological injuries.

c. The client will ventilate feelings by discussing the abusive situation.

d. The client will develop behaviors of a functioning survivor.

2. Establish desired outcome criteria for the family.

a. The family will identify intrafamily violence or abuse.

b. The family will remain free from violence.

c. The family will accept assistance and follow through with community referrals.

d. The family will implement coping measures to prevent further violence.

e. The family will promote healthy growth and development of members.

3. Establish desired outcome criteria for the abuser.

a. The abuser will demonstrate acceptance of responsibility for own behavior.

b. The abuser will establish and maintain impulse controls and coping strategies.

c. The abuser will cope with the legal ramifications of abusive behavior, accepting court-determined punishment.

d. The abuser will cooperate with recommended treatment program.

e. The abuser will refrain from violence against others.

D. Implementation

1. General measures for the victim of abuse

a. Provide first aid or medical treatment as needed.

b. If violence or abuse is imminent, separate the victim from the perpetrator.

c. Provide reports to state protective services for child and elder abuse as required by law. In the case of battered women, reporting is required when injury is from gun, knife, or other weapon.

d. In cases of suspected sexual abuse, follow agency and legal protocols for collection and preservation of evidence in recognized chain of evidence procedure.

e. Ensure sensitive, compassionate care of the victim.

f. Provide support to victim for not tolerating abuse.

g. Listen empathetically to the victim's discussion of current and past abuse.

h. Thoroughly document all injuries and the treatment provided.

i. Collaborate with team approach, including initiating interagency referrals and joint case conferencing.

2. For the child victim

a. Ensure the child's comfort with appropriate introductions and by avoiding touching the child without permission during the interview.

b. Use play activities, including drawings, to encourage disclosure in children who are hesitant or unable to verbalize trauma.

c. Explain all medical tests and procedures in terms a child can understand prior to the procedures.

d. Encourage the child's relationship with the parents; the nurse cannot become a substitute parent to the exclusion of child's natural parents.

3. For the battered woman

a. Communicate acceptance, warmth, and a nonjudgmental attitude; avoid implying in any way that she is at fault for not leaving the abusive situation.

b. Reinforce concern for her safety and her right to be free from abuse.

c. Discuss options available, including shelters, legal protection by reporting abuse, and seeking protection from abuse through a court order.

d. Respect the victim's decisions, including the decision to return to an abusive situation or the decision to not report the abuse. Making decisions for the victim will further erode her self-esteem and reinforce her sense of powerlessness.

e. Help the victim develop a plan to ensure safety, including hiding an extra set of house and car keys; requesting a neighbor to call police if violence begins; having documents such as birth certificate, bank account numbers, social security numbers, and receipts for rent and utilities available; having a list of phone numbers for emergency shelter, legal aid, police, counselor, and support groups.

4. For the elder victim

a. Allow time and be patient in order to promote the elder discussing the situation.

b. Respect the client's dignity and be nonjudgmental.

c. Discuss options for ensuring safety, such as temporary hospital admission, placement in a safe home, and court orders of protection.

d. Provide a list of resources and support services, including adult protective services, public legal services, victim resource agency, local unit on aging, and 24-hour elder abuse hotline.

e. If the elderly person is not competent to make own decisions, guardianship arrangements need to be made (see Chapter 1).

5. For the abuser

a. If the perpetrator is threatening or under the influence of drugs or alcohol, the nurse should call security or police to ensure the safety of oneself and others.

b. Inform the abuser of the duty to report the abuse to the appropriate agency.

c. Enlist the aid of experienced health team personnel (ie, clinical nurse specialist, social worker, protective agency representative, mental health crisis worker) to initiate intervention.

d. In situations of child abuse, the nurse may be aided in being therapeutic with the parents by viewing the abusive parent as a client and the child as a victim of abuse.

    e. If the abuse is acknowledged by the perpetrator, encourage him to accept responsibility for the violent behaviors.

    f. Communicate the belief that violent behaviors can be controlled and that more appropriate functioning is possible.

    g. Encourage and refer the abuser to community resources, such as mental health services, parent education classes, self-help groups (eg, Parents Anonymous), and respite care services for elders.

6. For the family. Promote and encourage healthy family functioning.

    a. Teach the family about the importance of individual responsibility for one's behavior.

    b. Teach the family to acknowledge stressful situations.

    c. Teach the family to develop problem-solving and coping strategies.

    d. Teach the family effective parenting skills.

    e. Teach the family to use community resources and professional assistance in improving functioning.

7. For the community. Be a responsible professional member of the community by promoting social changes that enhance family functioning.

    a. Work to alleviate conditions associated with violence (eg, poverty, inadequate housing, dysfunctional social attitude toward violence, substance abuse). For example, join community volunteer organizations, such as Victim's Resources, or lobby local, state, and federal legislators for changes helpful to families below the poverty level.

    b. Work to develop and maintain resources for families (eg, child care services, respite care for elders, educational programs, support groups). For example, join community volunteer organizations, such as parent-teacher groups or youth athletic leagues.

    c. Support and promote legal and legislative efforts to eliminate family violence.

E. Outcome evaluation. The nurse uses the following criteria to evaluate client outcomes and the effectiveness of nursing implementations.

1. The victim of violence achieves and maintains safety.

2. The victim of violence demonstrates improved self-esteem and self-empowerment.

3. The family affected by violence uses community resources to achieve improved coping.

4. The abuser accepts responsibility for violent behavior and accepts any court-ordered punishment.

5. The abuser refrains from violence against others.

STUDY QUESTIONS

1. An 11-year-old child complains to the school nurse of nausea and dizziness. The child also has a black eye that looks like a new injury. This is the third time in 1 month that the child has visited the nurse. Each time, the child provides vague explanations for various injuries. Which of the following is the school nurse's priority intervention?
   - **(1)** contacting the child's parents and asking about the child's injury
   - **(2)** encouraging the child to be truthful with the nurse
   - **(3)** questioning the teacher about the parent's behavior
   - **(4)** reporting suspicion of abuse to the proper authorities

2. A community nurse is making a home visit to a family of three: a mother, a father, and their child. The community nurse is told by the mother that the father (who is not present) has hit the child on several occasions when he was drinking. The mother further explains that she has talked her husband into going to Alcoholics Anonymous; the mother asks the nurse not to interfere, so her husband won't get angry and refuse treatment. Which of the following is the best response by the nurse?
   - **(1)** The nurse agrees not to interfere if the husband attends an Alcoholics Anonymous meeting that evening.
   - **(2)** The nurse commends the mother's efforts and agrees to let her handle things.
   - **(3)** The nurse commends the mother's efforts and also contacts protective services.
   - **(4)** The nurse confronts the mother's failure to protect the child.

3. A mother reports to a nurse a situation in which her child needed to be disciplined by her husband. The child was slapped in the face for not getting her husband breakfast on Saturday, despite being told on Thursday never to prepare food for him. The nurse analyzes the family system and concludes it is dysfunctional. All of the following factors contribute to this dysfunction *except*
   - **(1)** conflictual relationships of parents
   - **(2)** inconsistent communication patterns
   - **(3)** rigid, authoritarian roles
   - **(4)** use of violence to establish control

4. Which of the following statements about family violence is true?
   - **(1)** Family violence affects every socioeconomic level.
   - **(2)** Family violence is caused by drug and alcohol abuse.
   - **(3)** Family violence predominantly occurs in lower socioeconomic levels.
   - **(4)** Family violence rarely occurs during pregnancy.

5. A nurse is assessing a parent who abused her child. Which of the following risk factors would the nurse expect to establish in this case?
   - **(1)** flexible role functioning between parents
   - **(2)** history of the parent having been abused as a child
   - **(3)** single parent home situation
   - **(4)** presence of parental mental illness

6. A woman is admitted to the emergency room with a fractured arm. The woman explains to the nurse that she was injured when she provoked her husband, who was drunk, and therefore she got hurt when he pushed her. Which of the following best describes a nurse's understanding of the wife's explanation?
   (1) The wife's explanation is appropriate acceptance of her responsibility.
   (2) The wife's explanation is an atypical reaction of an abused woman.
   (3) The wife's explanation is evidence that the woman may be an abuser as well as a victim.
   (4) The wife's explanation is a typical response of a victim accepting blame for the abuser.

7. A community nurse conducts a primary prevention, home visit assessment for a newborn and mother. The mother has three other children, the oldest of whom is 12 years of age. The mother tells the nurse that the 12-year-old child is expected to prepare family meals, to look after the younger children, and to clean the house once a week. Which of the following is the most appropriate nursing diagnosis for this family situation?
   (1) Growth and development, altered, related to performance expectations of child
   (2) Anxiety (moderate), related to difficulty managing home situation

   (3) Parenting, altered, related to role reversal of mother and child
   (4) Social isolation related to lack of extended family assistance

8. The priority nursing implementation for a child or elder victim of abuse is
   (1) assessment of scope of problem
   (2) analysis of family dynamics
   (3) the safety of victim
   (4) teaching coping skills

9. A nurse is conducting an interview with a victim of spousal abuse in the emergency room. Which of the following is the nurse's *first* step?
   (1) Contact the appropriate legal services.
   (2) Ensure privacy for interviewing the victim away from the abuser.
   (3) Establish a rapport with the victim and the abuser.
   (4) Request the presence of a security guard.

10. Which of the following assessments would lead the nurse to suspect that an 8-year-old child is the victim of sexual abuse?
    (1) The child is fearful of the caregiver and other adults.
    (2) The child has a lack of peer relationships.
    (3) The child has self-injurious behavior.
    (4) The child has interest in things of a sexual nature.

11. Which of the following situations would a nurse identify as being at high risk for caregiver abuse?
- **(1)** An adult child quits her job to move in and care for a parent with severe dementia.
- **(2)** An elder with severe heart disease resides in a personal care home and is visited frequently by an adult child.
- **(3)** An elderly parent with limited mobility lives alone and receives help from several adult children.
- **(4)** A wife cares for her husband who is in early stages of Alzheimer's disease and has a network of available support persons.

12. A clinic nurse doing a prenatal assessment suspects that a client has been abused. Which of the following questions would be most appropriate?
- **(1)** "Are you being threatened or hurt by your partner?"
- **(2)** "Are you frightened of your partner?"
- **(3)** "Is something bothering you?"
- **(4)** "What happens when you and your partner argue?"

ANSWER KEY

1. The answer is (4). The nurse is obligated to report suspicion of child abuse to the appropriate protective services. Failure to do so can risk further endangerment of the child, and failure to report is a misdemeanor violation on the part of the nurse. The parents will be contacted and investigation will proceed under the legal authority of the child protective service agency. Although the nurse would expect to establish rapport with the child, encouraging the child to be truthful would send the message that the nurse believes the child is *not* truthful; this intervention is therefore inappropriate. Questioning the teacher may or may not provide validation of the nurse's suspicions; regardless, this intervention does not ensure the child's safety, which is the priority.

2. The answer is (3). The nurse would validate and reinforce the mother's efforts to seek help; however, the nurse must also report the abuse to the appropriate protective services. The priority is to maintain safety of the child. The responses in answer choices **(1)** and **(2)** are inappropriate; the nurse is failing to provide for the child's safety and is not following legal guidelines. In answer choice **(4)**, the nurse is alienating the mother and also is failing to follow legal guidelines and ensure safety.

3. The answer is (1). There is no evidence in this situation that the parents are in conflict; in fact, the mother is describing that the child "needed to be disciplined." Often, in dysfunctional families, one particular child is singled out to be the victim and is the recipient of blame for problems. The inconsistent communication pattern is that the child received conflicting messages regarding preparation of food. The rigid authoritarian roles were shown in that the mother indicates to the nurse that the child needs discipline from the father. This is an example of a rigid role expectation of the father as disciplinarian. Also, the father used violence to retain the position of control.

4. The answer is (1). Family violence occurs in all socioeconomic levels, races, religions, and cultural groups. Although violence is associated with substance abuse, it is not the singular cause. The statement that family violence predominantly occurs in lower socioeconomic levels is false. Abuse often occurs during pregnancy; 23% of all pregnant women seeking prenatal care are victims of abuse.

5. The answer is (2). One of the most important risk factors is a history of childhood abuse in the parent who abuses. Family violence follows a multigenerational pattern. Parents who are flexible in their roles would display a characteristic of healthy functioning. Single-parent households and the presence of mental illness in a parent are not established risk factors for child abuse by a parent.

6. The answer is (4). Accepting self-blame is a common psychological response for a woman who is a victim of abuse. The message from the abuser that violence occurred because the woman provoked the abuser is accepted and owned by the victim. The victim is not responsible for violence. The statements in answer choices **(2)** and **(3)** are not true.

7. The answer is (3). The role of a 12-year-old child in a family should not be that of the parent. In this situation, the child and mother have reversed roles. There is no evidence that the child has altered growth or development, the mother in this situation is not demonstrating signs of anxiety, and there is no evidence in this situation that the family is socially isolated.

8. The answer is (3). The priority implementation when a child or elder is involved in a situation of abuse is establishing the safety of the victim. Legislation exists in most states mandating reporting of such abuse in order to intervene and ensure safety. The question is asking for an implementation, not for the assessment of the problem or an analysis of the family. Teaching coping skills is important; however, the priority implementation is safety.

9. The answer is (2). Privacy, away from the abuser, is important, because the victim may discuss the problem and not fear reprisal from the abuser (especially if the decision is made to return to the situation). The nurse would not be the person to contact legal services; it is up to the woman to make the decision to report abuse. However, if injury is inflicted with a gun, knife, or other weapon, the nurse is legally obligated to report this. The nurse would establish rapport with the victim, but the initial concern of the nurse would not be to establish rapport with the abuser. The situation does not describe the abuser as currently violent or under the influence of substances; therefore, requesting presence of security is not appropriate at this time.

10. The answer is (4). An 8-year-old child is in the latency phase of development; in this stage, the child's interest in peers, activities, and school is priority. Interest in sex and things of a sexual nature would occur appropriately during the age of puberty, not at this time. A child who is the victim of sexual abuse, however, may show unusual interest in sex. The assessments in the other answer choices may indicate abuse, but not necessarily sexual abuse.

11. The answer is (1). In this situation, the adult child has given up her usual role as well as moved her place of residence in order to care for her parent. Caring for someone with severe dementia is very stressful, requiring almost 24-hour vigilance to ensure safety and meet needs. This situation presents high risk for caregiver stress and abuse. The caregivers in answer choice **(2)** are the personnel who work in the personal care home. The adult child does not have primary responsibility and therefore would not be at high risk for severe stress and abuse. In both answer choices **(3)** and **(4)**, the caregivers are receiving support and no one person has primary responsibility. This will decrease risk for severe caregiver stress.

12. The answer is (1). The use of a simple, direct question, asked in an empathic manner, is best to validate presence of an abusive situation. The other questions are indirect and may or may not lead to discussion of an abusive situation. It is appropriate to use direct questioning in the situation of a woman suspected to be the victim of abuse.

10

Childhood and Adolescent Psychiatric Disorders

I. Overview

A. **Statistics.** Mental disorders in children are common and are generally under-diagnosed and undertreated.
   1. Mental health problems occur in 15% to 22% of children and adolescents.
   2. Less than 20% of children and adolescents with a mental health problem receive treatment (Keys, 1998).
   3. Attention deficit-hyperactivity disorder (ADHD) is the most common mental health disorder affecting children; its incidence is estimated at 6% to 9%.

B. **Diagnosis.** The diagnosis of mental disorders in children and adolescents depends on behavior that is inappropriate for age level, deviant when compared to cultural norms, and that creates deficits or impairments in adaptive functioning (Townsend, 1999).

C. **Developmental theory** is basic to understanding infant, childhood, and adolescent disorders. Deviation from developmental norms is an important warning sign of a problem (see Table 2-2).

D. **Common disorders in children**
   1. Specific disorders with **childhood onset** include mental retardation, developmental disorders, elimination disorders, disruptive behavior disorders, and anxiety disorders.
   2. Disorders that occur in children but also have typical adult onset include mood disorders and psychotic disorders.

E. **Symptoms.** Children are not miniature adults, and symptoms of mental disorders may be different in a child or adolescent than in an adult with the same disorder (Table 10-1).

II. Types of Childhood Mental Disorders

A. **Pervasive developmental disorders** are characterized by early problems in three major developmental areas: behavior, social interaction, and communication.
   1. **Mental retardation**
      a. This disorder is characterized by substandard limitations in functioning, manifested by significantly subaverage intellectual functioning (ie, an IQ

TABLE 10-1
Comparison of Symptoms of Mental Disorders in Children and Adolescents
With Those in Adults

DISORDER	CHILD/ADOLESCENT	ADULT
MAJOR DEPRESSIVE DISORDER	Negativism, acting out Physical complaints, weight loss Delays or regression in developmental tasks Sadness, apathy, clinging behavior Nightmares Academic difficulties Intense mood swings Self-loathing, low self-esteem Suicidal thoughts	Depressed mood, sadness, crying Decreased interest in previously enjoyable activities Weight loss or gain Insomnia or hypersomnia Fatigue, loss of energy Decreased ability to concentrate Recurrent thoughts of death, suicide
ANXIETY DISORDERS	Separation Anxiety Disorder Difficulty separating from mother (or other significant caregiver) Worry, increased anxiety about possible harm coming to mother or caregiver Anticipation of separation results in tantrums, crying, screaming, clinging behaviors Refusal to attend school Refusal to sleep at friend's or relative's house	Generalized Anxiety Disorder Excessive worry, apprehension Restlessness, irritability Decreased ability to concentrate Sleep disturbances

less than 70) and related limitations in two or more adaptive skill areas (eg, communication, self-care, activities of daily living, social skills, functioning in a community, self-direction, health and safety, functional academics, leisure and work).

    b. It is manifested before 18 years of age (Johnson, 1997).

2. Autism

    a. This disorder is characterized by marked impairment in social interaction and communication, and a restricted repertoire of activity and interests (Johnson, 1997).

    b. The symptoms of autism include lack of responsiveness to others, withdrawal from social contact, gross impairment in communication, and bizarre responses to the environment (eg, clinging to inanimate objects and repetitive body movements such as hand flapping, rocking, and head banging) (Table 10-2).

TABLE 10-2
Comparison of Autism and Childhood Schizophrenia

	AUTISM	CHILDHOOD SCHIZOPHRENIA
Incidence	4 out of 10,000 births (boys affected 3 to 4 times more often than girls)	Rare
Age of onset	Before 2½ years of age	Between 5 and 10 years of age
Etiologic factors	Genetics, neurotransmitter abnormality, structural brain abnormality	Genetics, pregnancy and birth complications, structured brain abnormalities
Symptoms	Aversion to being held	Delusions
	Repetitive routines	Hallucinations
	Hand flapping and head banging	Regressive behaviors
	Clings to inanimate objects	Thinking disorders
	Language and speech difficulties	
	Mental retardation in 50% of cases	
Treatment	Medication to reduce repetitive movements and behaviors (antidepressants, such as fluvoxamine [Luvox] and clomipramine [Anafranil])	Medication to reduce psychotic symptoms (typical antipsychotics, such as chlorpromazine [Thorazine], and atypical agents, such as olanzapine [Zyprexa])
	Behavioral therapy	Behavioral therapy
	Special education	Individual psychotherapy
	Family education	Family therapy and education

3. **Specific developmental disorders** are characterized by developmental delay that leads to functional impairments in areas such as reading, arithmetic, language, and verbal articulation.

B. **Attention deficit and disruptive behavior disorders**

1. **ADHD** is characterized by developmentally inappropriate degrees of inattention, impulsiveness, and hyperactivity.

   a. According to the DSM-IV, ADHD must be present in at least two settings (eg, at school and at home) and must be present before 7 years of age (DSM-IV, 1994).

   b. Specific characteristics of ADHD are listed in Display 10-1.

2. **Conduct disorder**

   a. This disorder is characterized by repetitive, persistently disruptive, and willfully disobedient behaviors, including violations of age-appropriate norms and social rules. A significant number of children with this disorder develop substance abuse or antisocial personality disorders after 18 years of age.

   b. Examples of behaviors in children with this disorder include stealing, lying, bullying, running away, truancy, substance abuse, setting fires, other forms of vandalism, cruelty to animals, and physical aggression toward others.

DISPLAY 10-1. **Characteristics of ADHD**

Having trouble paying attention to details
Making careless mistakes in schoolwork
Having trouble concentrating on one activity at a time
Talking constantly, even at inappropriate times
Running around in a disruptive way when required to be seated or quiet
Fidgeting and squirming constantly
Having trouble waiting for a turn
Being easily distracted by things going on around them
Impulsively blurting out answers to questions
Often misplacing school assignment, books, or toys
Seeming not to listen, even when directly addressed

ADHD = attention deficit-hyperactivity disorder

3. **Oppositional defiant disorder**
   a. This is a milder form of conduct disorder that includes less extreme behaviors. The behaviors in this disorder do not violate the rights of others to the degree seen in conduct disorder.
   b. The behaviors in this disorder show opposition to authority figures (eg, arguing, defiance, hostility, anger, low frustration tolerance, and the use of alcohol, drugs, or both).
C. **Anxiety disorders** often begin in childhood or adolescence and continue into adulthood.
   1. Obsessive-compulsive disorder, generalized anxiety disorder, and phobias are common in children and adolescents, with symptoms similar to those seen in adults.
   2. **Separation anxiety disorder** is a childhood disorder characterized by the fear of being separated from the person to whom the child is most attached. Symptoms include refusal to attend school, somatic complaints, severe anxiety about separation, and worry about harm coming to a significant caretaker (see Table 10-1).
D. **Schizophrenia.** Childhood schizophrenia is rare, and diagnosis is difficult. Symptoms can mimic pervasive development disorders, such as autism.
   1. Although research on childhood schizophrenia is sparse, some characteristic behaviors have been noted (Antai-Otong, 1995b), including:
      a. Severe cognitive and behavioral disturbances (see Table 10-2)
      b. Social withdrawal
      c. Impaired communication
   2. Schizophrenia in adolescents is more common.
      a. Incidence during late adolescence is high.
      b. Symptoms are similar to those of adults. Initial symptoms may include extreme change in usual behaviors, social isolation, peculiar mannerisms, decreased academic performance, and acting-out behaviors.

E. Mood disorders

1. These disorders are less common in children and adolescents than in adults (Keltner, 1999).

    a. The prevalence in children and adolescents ranges from 1% to 5% for depressive disorders.

    b. The existence of bipolar disorder (manic type) in young children is a matter of some controversy.

    c. Prevalence of bipolar illness in adolescents is estimated at approximately 1%. Symptoms of depression in children are similar to those observed in adults (see Table 10-1).

2. Suicide

    a. Suicide is the third leading cause of death in individuals 15 to 24 years of age. The presence of a mood disorder is a serious risk factor for suicide.

    b. Warning signs for adolescent suicide (Newman, 1999) are listed in Display 10-2.

F. Substance abuse disorders. The symptoms and behaviors are similar to those in adults (see Chapter 8).

1. These disorders are common; it is estimated that 32% of adolescents have a substance abuse disorder (Johnson, 1997).

    a. Rates of alcohol or illicit drug use are higher in boys than in girls.

    b. The greatest risk for developing a substance use disorder is in those 15 to 24 years of age.

    c. Substance use can progress to addiction faster in adolescence; for example, substance use can progress to addiction in 2 years in adolescents compared with 15 to 20 years in adults.

2. Risk factors include a family history of substance abuse, dysfunctional family system, peer pressure, attempt at rebellion, conflicting societal messages about appropriate use and value of substances, poor self-esteem, and lack of or pressure to achieve academic success.

3. Comorbidity with other psychiatric disorders is common, including mood disorders, anxiety disorders, and disruptive behavior disorders.

DISPLAY 10-2. **Warning Signs for Suicide in Adolescents**

        Sudden withdrawal from friends, family, and regular activities
        Violent or highly rebellious behaviors
        Drug or alcohol abuse
        Unusual neglect of personal appearance
        Decline in quality of schoolwork; truancy
        Running away
        Excessive fatigue and somatic complaints
        Poor response to praise or rewards
        Verbal hints, overt threats about suicide
        Giving away prized possessions

4. Warning signs of adolescent substance abuse

a. Decline in social and academic functioning

b. Change from previous functioning, such as developing aggressive behaviors or withdrawing from family interaction

c. Personality changes and low frustration tolerance

d. Associations with other adolescents using substance

e. Hiding or lying about use

III. Etiology

A. **General considerations.** There is no single cause of mental disorders in children and adolescents. Multiple circumstances, including psychobiologic factors, family dynamics, and environmental factors, combine in a complex manner.

B. **Psychobiologic factors**

1. **Genetics and family history** have been implicated in disorders such as mental retardation, autism, childhood schizophrenia, conduct disorders, bipolar disorder, and anxiety disorders.

2. **Structural brain abnormalities.** Research has revealed the presence of structural brain abnormalities and neurotransmitter alterations in patients with autism, childhood schizophrenia, and ADHD.

3. **Prenatal influences,** such as maternal infections, lack of prenatal care, and substance abuse by the mother, all may contribute to neurodevelopmental abnormalities associated with mental disorders. Birth trauma associated with a decreased oxygen supply to the fetus is significant in the development of mental retardation and other neurodevelopmental disorders.

4. **Chronic physical illness or disability** may lead to coping difficulties for the child.

C. **Family dynamics**

1. **Child abuse**

a. Children subjected to ongoing abuse in early childhood have less developed brains (particularly on the left side).

b. Abuse and its subsequent effect on the developing brain are associated with psychological problems, such as depression, memory problems, learning difficulties, impulsivity, and difficulties in relationships (Glod, 1998).

2. **Dysfunctional family system**

a. Relationships characterized by lack of nurturing, poor communication, lack of boundaries between generations, and enmeshment are all implicated in development of mental disorders (see Chapter 14).

b. **Inadequate coping skills** in resolving conflict issues among family members also affects the child's mental health and development.

3. **Poor role modeling.** The lack of adequate parental role models can influence children to adopt dysfunctional behaviors.

D. **Environmental factors**

1. **Poverty.** Inadequate prenatal care, poor nutrition, and lack of necessities associated with insufficient income adversely affect normal growth and development.

2. **Homelessness** among families is increasing at an alarming rate.
   a. Homeless children have multiple health needs that affect their emotional and psychological development.
   b. Studies have indicated an increased rate of minor childhood illnesses, developmental delays, and psychological problems among homeless children when compared with control samples (Townsend, 1999).
3. **Family culture.** Parental behaviors that are dramatically atypical from the surrounding culture can lead to lack of peer group acceptance of the child and psychological difficulties.

IV. Management

A. **Community-based treatment** is more common in today's managed care environment.
   1. **Primary prevention**
      a. A variety of social programs are directed at creating an environment that is health-enhancing for children.
      b. Some examples are early prenatal care; early intervention programs for parents with known risk factors for child rearing problems; and identifying children at risk in programs such as Head Start, to provide education and support for parents of these children.
   2. **Secondary prevention**
      a. Secondary prevention includes early case finding of children with problems in school systems, so that prompt treatment may be initiated. Methods include individual counseling with school guidance programs and community mental health referrals, crisis intervention services for families in traumatic situations, group counseling in the school, and peer counseling programs.
      b. School nurses, community health nurses, and nurses employed in primary practice settings may all contribute to early case finding and initiation of prompt treatment.
   3. **Therapeutic support** for children is provided through individual psychotherapy, play therapy, and special education programs for children who are unable to participate in the normal school system. Behavioral methods of treatment are commonly used to assist the child in developing more adaptive coping methods.
   4. **Family therapy and family education** are important to assist families in acquiring necessary skills and support for making changes that enhance functioning of all family members.

B. **Hospital-based treatment**
   1. **Specialized units** treating children and adolescents are established in psychiatric hospitals. Treatment in these units is usually reserved for clients who have not benefited from less restrictive alternative methods, or for client situations in which the risk for violence to self or others is high.
   2. **Partial hospitalization programs** are also available, providing on-site school programs directed toward the special needs of the child with a mental illness.

   3. Seclusion and restraints for control of disruptive behavior is controversial.
      a. Research indicates that this method can be traumatic for the child and is not effective for learning adaptive responses.
      b. Least restrictive measures include time-out, therapeutic holding, avoiding power struggles, and intervening early to prevent escalating behaviors.
C. Pharmacotherapy
   1. Medications are used as one method of treatment.
   2. Psychotropic medications are used cautiously in children and adolescent clients, because multiple side effects are associated with these drugs (see Chapter 15; Drug Chart 10-1).
      a. The physiologic differences of children and adolescents affect the dose, clinical response, and side effects of psychotropic medications.

DRUG CHART 10-1   **Selected Medications for Treatment of Child and Adolescent Mental Disorders**

Disorder or Specific Behaviors	Medication Classification	Rationale for Use

Childhood schizophrenia
Other psychotic disorders
Acute agitation
Motor hyperactivity and impulsiveness
	Typical antipsychotics
	  Chlorpromazine (Thorazine)
	  Haloperidol (Haldol)
	  Risperidone (Risperdal)
	Atypical antipsychotics
	  Olanzapine (Zyprexa)
		Typical and atypical antipsychotics block dopamine receptor sites and thus decrease psychotic symptoms. Sedative effects of these drugs are useful for hyperactive states. The advantage of atypical antipsychotics is that they have fewer extrapyramidal side effects.

Depression
ADHD
Separation anxiety disorder
Obsessive-compulsive disorder
	Tricyclic antidepressants
	  Imipramine (Tofranil)
	  Clomipramine (Anafranil)
	SSRIs
	  Fluoxetine (Prozac)
	  Sertraline (Zoloft)
	  Fluvoxamine (Luvox)
		Tricyclics are used to alter serotonin and norepinephrine and thus cause mood elevation. They also decrease repetitive behaviors.
		
		SSRIs selectively increase serotonin at synapse and elevate mood.

ADHD	Psychostimulants
	  Methylphenidate (Ritalin)
	  Pemoline (Cylert)
		These alter neurotransmitters and thus increase attention span and the ability to concentrate

ADHD = attention deficit-hyperactivity disorder; SSRI = selective serotonin reuptake inhibitors.

b. The developmental differences in neurotransmitters in children may affect outcome of psychotropic medications, leading to inconsistent results, especially with tricyclic antidepressants.

 V. ### NURSING PROCESS OVERVIEW FOR Childhood and Adolescent Psychiatric Disorders

A. Assessment

1. **Review client history for precipitating stressors and significant data,** including genetic-biologic vulnerability (family history); stressful family and life events; results of mental status exam; history of physical and psychological problems and their treatment; medication history (Table 10-3).

2. Note growth and development patterns of the young child and compare them to standard instruments, such as the Denver Developmental Screening Test and its revised version (Wong, 1997).

3. Note evidence of appropriate developmental task achievement for the child or adolescent (see Table 2-2).

4. Perform physical examination of the child or adolescent, noting normal and abnormal data.

TABLE 10-3
Key Nursing Assessment Questions for Children and Adolescents

SPECIFIC QUESTIONS	PROVIDES DATA ABOUT
Who are the members of your family? Who do you live with?	Family system
What people in your life do you think are supportive and helpful to you?	Quality of relationships with support persons
How does your parent(s) or caregiver discipline you?	·Family discipline patterns
What things do you enjoy doing with your friends?	Positive and negative influences of peer group
Have you experienced any of the following? Parent-child conflict School problems Problems with peers Running away Trouble with legal system Mood swings Feelings of sadness, lack of interest Suspicious or unusual thoughts	Behavior, thoughts, and feelings indicative of specific disorders
What is your experience with alcohol, other drugs, or both?	Drug or alcohol use
What do you think are your strengths, what do you like about yourself?	Self-esteem

5. **Assess behavioral responses** that may indicate childhood or adolescent disorders. Be sure to assess direct interaction, observation of play, and interaction with family and peers.
   a. Is the client displaying aggressive or destructive behaviors?
   b. Does the client have academic problems? Truancy?
   c. Does the client have discipline or conduct problems?
   d. Does the client have problems with peers?
   e. Does the client demonstrate poor impulse control, rebellion, and defiance?
   f. Does the client demonstrate restlessness or hyperactivity?
   g. Does the client demonstrate sexual acting out?
   h. Does the client use or abuse substances, such as alcohol or illicit drugs?
   i. Does the client demonstrate withdrawal or social isolation?

6. **Identify evidence of cognitive disorder.**
   a. Does the client have a lack of reality base or misperception of reality?
   b. Does the client have hallucinations or delusions?
   c. Does the client have language and speech problems?
   d. Does the client have poor attention span or learning difficulties?
   e. Does the client have unusual thought patterns or suspicion of others?

7. **Observe for evidence of a mood disorder.**
   a. Does the client have mood swings?
   b. Does the client have intense emotions (eg, rage, devastation)?
   c. Does the client have a lack of affect?
   d. Does the client have feelings of sadness? Crying? Sense of hopelessness?
   e. Does the client have thoughts of suicide?

8. **Assess the strengths and weaknesses of the client's family system.**
   a. What are the anxiety levels of the family? What coping measures are used?
   b. What is the quality of the relationships in the family? Is there evidence of overt conflict?
   c. Are generational boundaries appropriate or blurred?
   d. Is communication open or poor?
   e. Is the family involved in a larger social system, such as extended family, friends, or community activities? (The implication is that the more isolated the family is from others, the more severe the pathology.)
   f. Does the family have basic knowledge of growth and development?
   g. What are the parenting skills? What are the methods of discipline?

B. **Nursing diagnoses**

1. **Analysis**
   a. Compare the client's growth and developmental level to norms appropriate for age group.
   b. Prioritize the client's physical, behavioral, cognitive, and mood symptoms.
   c. Analyze the relationship of client's symptoms to family system strengths and weaknesses.
   d. Analyze the child or adolescent's self-esteem level.
   e. Determine the client or family's view of the current problem.

2. Establish individualized nursing diagnoses for client and family.
   a. Communication, impaired verbal
   b. Coping, individual, ineffective
   c. Family coping: ineffective: compromised
   d. Family processes, altered
   e. Growth and development, altered
   f. Parent/infant, child attachment, altered, risk for
   g. Parenting, altered
   h. Self-esteem disturbance
   i. Social interaction, impaired
   j. Thought processes, altered
   k. Violence, risk for: directed at self/others

C. Planning and outcome identification
   1. Work with the client and the family in setting realistic goals.
   2. Establish desired outcome criteria for the client, the family, or both.
   a. The client will demonstrate decreased anxiety levels and increased coping skills.
   b. The client will control impulsive or acting-out behaviors.
   c. The client will state improvement in mood.
   d. The client will demonstrate improved attention and the ability to participate in learning activities.
   e. The client will participate in treatment program and follow through with specific referrals.
   f. The client will interact with peer group and establish friendships.

D. Implementation
   1. General implementations
   a. Establish trust.
   b. Listen actively, demonstrating concern and support.
   c. Promote clear, honest, straightforward communication.
   d. Establish position of neutrality; do not take sides of either parent or child.
   e. Support the strengths of the client and the family.
   f. Use the cognitive model to explain relationship between thoughts, feelings, and behavior; that is, thoughts lead to feelings and behavior, but a person does not have to act on feelings or thoughts.
   g. Participate in the treatment plan on the inpatient unit; construct safe, structured environment with the opportunity for the client to increase self-functioning and self-esteem.
   h. Positively reinforce acceptable behavior.
   i. Participate in play therapy, allowing the child to express self through imaginative play.
   j. Collaborate with the client's family, school, and mental health team.
   k. Encourage the use of community support groups for the client and family.
   l. Teach the client and family information about the client's specific disorder and its treatment measures.
   m. Teach the family information about how to nurture the child's emotional health (Client and Family Teaching 10-1).

CLIENT AND FAMILY TEACHING 10-1

Educating Families With a Child or Adolescent Who Has a Mental Disorder

Provide general information about the disorder.

- Mental disorders in children and adolescents occur because of a complex interaction among many factors; there is no single cause.
- Children and adolescents with a mental disorder may respond to treatment, such as therapy for the child, family therapy and education, and medication.
- Prescribed medication, taken as directed, can help stabilize moods and bring about more normal behavior.

Teach the parents about nurturing a child's emotional well being.

- Focus on the "positives" in a child, providing praise when behavior is acceptable.
- When behavior escalates, decrease stimulation in immediate environment and provide a time-out.
- Encourage the child's interests, and accept their limitations.
- Foster a child's self-worth and appropriate independence for age and level of development.
- Set clear, consistent limits and follow them.
- Seek help when overwhelmed by a child's feelings or behaviors or if you are unable to control your own anger and frustration.
- Maintain a parental role; children respond to parents who act like parents, not like friends.
- Strengthen spousal relationships; if separation or divorce occurs, negotiate and collaborate in areas involving the child.
- Maintain one's own interests; overfocusing on a child's problems is not helpful.

Inform the parents about community support groups available for a specific problem experienced by the child or family.

2. **For the child or adolescent with a pervasive developmental disorder**
   a. Create a safe environment, and help the parents to do so at home.
   b. Help the parents decrease their feelings of guilt and blame.
   c. Maintain a consistency of caregivers for the child in the hospital, in school, and at home.
   d. Help the parents and siblings identify and discuss their feelings, issues, and problems associated with living with a child with a severe disorder.
   e. Use diversion if child has increased anxiety or acting-out behaviors. For example, engage the child in physical activity, such as riding a bike, playing with a ball; or engage the child in a pleasurable activity, such as drawing, painting, or playing a favorite game.
   f. Provide the child with familiar objects.
3. **For the child or adolescent with ADHD**
   a. Administer stimulant medication in the morning to maximize effectiveness for daytime activities.
   b. Assist the family to use environmental manipulation to decrease stimuli for behavior control.

c. Assist the family to establish regular scheduled times for eating, sleeping, playing, and doing homework.

d. Collaborate with the client's school, family, and mental health team to ensure proper classroom placement.

4. **For the child or adolescent with conduct disorder or oppositional defiant disorder**

a. Establish firm, consistent limits, describing clearly the consequences of unacceptable behaviors.

b. Assist the parents in defining and maintaining limits.

c. Provide positive feedback for appropriate behaviors.

d. Encourage the client to express anger in an appropriate verbal manner.

e. Use exercise and activity to help the child use excess energy from increased anxiety or anger.

f. Notice cues that behavior is escalating and intervene early.

5. **For the child or adolescent with an anxiety disorder** (see Chapter 3)

a. Maintain a calm manner when the client and parents experience increased anxiety.

b. Teach the client coping measures for handling anxiety.

c. Use cognitive strategies in discussing the client's fears, pointing out reality issues.

d. Assist the client to return to school immediately with family support, if separation anxiety is present.

6. **For the child or adolescent with a mood disorder** (see Chapter 6)

a. Teach client and family about mood disorder, causes, symptoms, and treatment.

b. Capitalize on measures to promote self-esteem.

c. Use cognitive measures in dealing with negative thoughts and feelings.

d. Maintain attitude of hopefulness.

e. Use suicide precautions for client at risk for suicide.

7. **For the child or adolescent with a substance abuse disorder** (see Chapter 8)

a. Teach the client and family information about substances and their effects on physical and psychological well being.

b. Encourage the client and family to attend self-help groups (eg, Alcoholics Anonymous, Narcotics Anonymous, Alateen, Alanon).

c. Foster attitude of hope that the client can achieve and maintain sobriety.

d. Teach coping measures to handle uncomfortable feelings and situations.

E. **Outcome evaluation.** The nurse uses the following outcome criteria to determine effectiveness of nursing interventions.

1. The client and family demonstrate improved coping skills.

2. The client controls impulsive behaviors.

3. The client demonstrates normal mood stabilization.

4. The client participates in educational program at level of ability.

5. The client and family participate in treatment program and accept community referrals.

6. The client interacts socially with peer group.

STUDY QUESTIONS

1. A 9-year-old child is admitted to a psychiatric treatment unit accompanied by both parents. To establish trust and a position of neutrality, which of the following actions would the nurse take?
   (1) The nurse would encourage the parents to leave while interviewing the child alone.
   ✓(2) The nurse would interview the child and parents together, observing interaction.
   (3) The nurse would provide diversion for the child and interview the parents alone.
   (4) The nurse would review the clinical record prior to interviewing the parents.

2. A community nurse is practicing primary prevention for mental disorders in children. Which of the following risk factors would the nurse focus on?
   (1) being raised in single-parent home
   ✓(2) family history of mental illness
   (3) lack of peer friendships
   (4) family culture

3. A school nurse is meeting with the school and treatment team professionals about a child who has been receiving methylphenidate (Ritalin) for 2 months. The meeting is to evaluate the results of the child's medication use. While questioning the teacher, which of the following child behaviors would the nurse ask about to determine medication effectiveness?
   (1) a decrease in repetitive behaviors
   (2) a decrease in signs of anxiety
   (3) an increase in depressed mood
   ✓(4) an increase in concentration on tasks

4. Which of the following behavioral assessments in a child is most consistent with the diagnosis of conduct disorder?
   (1) arguing with adults
   (2) gross impairment in communication
   ✓(3) physical aggression toward others
   (4) refusal to separate from caretaker

5. A child with separation anxiety disorder has not attended school for 3 weeks, and she cries and exhibits clinging behaviors when her mother encourages attendance. The priority nursing implementation by the home-care psychiatric nurse would be
   ✓(1) to assist the child to return to school immediately with family support
   (2) to arrange for a home school teacher to visit for 2 weeks
   (3) to encourage family discussion of various problem areas
   (4) to use play therapy to help the child express her feelings

6. An adolescent hospitalized in a psychiatric unit initiates frequent fights with peers. Which of the following is the most appropriate nursing implementation?
   ✓(1) Anticipate and neutralize potentially explosive situations.
   (2) Ignore minor infractions of rules against fighting.
   (3) Isolate the adolescent from contact with peers.
   (4) Talk to the adolescent each time fighting occurs.

7. The community nurse visits the home of a child recently diagnosed with autism. The parents express feelings of shame and guilt about having somehow caused this problem. Which of the following state-

ments by the nurse would be best to help alleviate parental guilt?

(1) "Autism is a rare disorder. Your other children shouldn't be affected."

✓(2) "The specific cause of autism is unknown. However, it is known to be associated with problems in the structure of and chemicals in the brain."

(3) "Sometimes a lack of prenatal care can be the cause of autism."

(4) "Although autism is inherited from the genes, if you didn't have testing you could not have known this."

8. An adolescent with a depressive disorder is more likely than an adult with the same disorder to exhibit which of the following?

✓(1) negativism, acting out

(2) sadness, crying

(3) suicidal thoughts

(4) weight gain

9. The parents of a child with ADHD tell the nurse they have tried everything to calm their child and nothing has worked. Which of the following *initial* actions is most appropriate by the nurse?

✓(1) Actively listen to the parents' concern before planning interventions.

(2) Encourage the parents to discuss these issues with mental health team member.

(3) Provide literature regarding the disorder and its management.

(4) Tell the parents they are overreacting to the problem.

10. The nurse questions the parents of a child with oppositional defiant disorder about the roles of each parent in setting rules of behavior for the child. The purpose for this type of questioning is to assess which of the following elements of the family system?

(1) anxiety levels

✓(2) generational boundaries

(3) knowledge of growth and development

(4) quality of communication

11. The nurse reinforces the behavioral contract for a child having difficulty controlling aggressive behaviors on the psychiatric unit. Which of the following is the best rationale for this method of treatment?

✓(1) It will assist the child to develop more adaptive coping methods.

(2) It will avoid having the nurse be responsible for setting the rules.

(3) It will maintain the nurse's role in controlling the child's behavior.

(4) It will prevent the child from manipulating the nurse.

12. A nurse is teaching the parents of a child with a pervasive developmental disorder about how to deal with the child when his behavior escalates and he begins throwing things and screaming. Which of the following would the nurse teach the parents?

(1) to accept the child's limitations and ignore this behavior

✓(2) to decrease stimulation in the environment and provide time-out

(3) to seek help when feeling overwhelmed by the child's behavior

(4) to tell the child to calm down and encourage quiet activity

ANSWER KEY

1. The answer is (2). It is important for the nurse to be seen as a neutral intervenor who is interested in the family as an adaptive functioning unit. By conducting the admission interview with the parents and child together, the nurse establishes this neutral role from the beginning. The responses in answer choices **(1)** and **(3)** separate the parents and the child, and thus the nurse does not have the opportunity to establish a position of neutrality. Although the nurse would review the clinical record, this does not demonstrate to the family that the nurse is an advocate for both the parents and the child.

2. The answer is (2). Abnormal genes and family history of mental illness have been implicated in many mental disorders occurring in children and adolescents. There is no evidence that being raised in a single-parent home will increase the risk of a child developing a mental disorder. Children who have problems with peers and withdraw from social interaction may have a mental disorder; however, the nurse noting this problem would be practicing secondary prevention. Family culture is not a risk factor unless parental behavior is dramatically atypical from surrounding culture.

3. The answer is (4). Methylphenidate (Ritalin) is used as a method of treatment for ADHD. Evidence of increased concentration on tasks by a child taking this medication would establish effectiveness of the drug. This medication will not decrease either repetitive behaviors or signs of anxiety. Although this medication is a psychostimulant, it is not used for depression and therefore mood elevation is not a measure of effectiveness in this situation.

4. The answer is (3). Physical aggression toward others is a significant criterion consistent with the diagnoses of conduct disorder. Arguing with adults may indicate a lesser disorder, oppositional defiant disorder. Conduct disorder is a problem that involves violation of social rules. Gross impairment in communication and refusal to separate from caretaker are behaviors that are more consistent with other mental disorders that can affect children.

5. The answer is (1). When a child refuses to attend school as part of separation anxiety disorder, it is important that this behavior not receive any reinforcement. The nurse would intervene by assisting the child to return to school immediately with family support as the priority. Arranging for a home school teacher would reinforce the behavior of not attending school. Although encouraging family discussion of problem areas and the use of play therapy are appropriate interventions to provide treatment for the family, the priority is returning the child to school.

6. The answer is (1). The nurse is responsible for maintaining a safe environment and therefore would observe for signs that an explosive situation is developing and intervene to neutralize the situation and avoid fighting. Ignoring minor infractions of rules against fighting would be incorrect, because fighting on a psychiatric unit would not be a minor infraction and should not be ignored. This could lead to unsafe situations that could escalate out of control. Isolation and seclusion are methods of intervention that can be used as a last resort after less restrictive means are employed. Talking to the adolescent each time a fight occurs does not indicate that the nurse is setting and enforcing clear, consistent rules. The nurse needs to maintain safety and would not allow fighting to occur if it could be avoided.

7. The answer is (2). This statement is factual and does not cast blame on anything the parents did or did not do. The parents are not questioning whether other children will be affected; their concern is directed to the current situation and their feelings about this. The statement in answer choice **(3)** is not true: Lack of prenatal care can be a risk factor in pervasive developmental disorders, but it is not the cause of autism. Although it is thought that there is a genetic component in autism, research has not identified specific genes and there is no diagnostic test for this. The statement in answer choice **(4)** is misleading and would not alleviate guilt.

8. The answer is (1). Adolescents may exhibit behavior that is not typical of an adult with a depressive disorder; negativism and acting out could indicate depression an adolescent. Sadness, crying, and suicidal thoughts are behaviors of both adolescents and adults. The adult may have either weight loss or gain in depression, whereas the adolescent may have weight loss.

9. The answer is (1). The nurse would encourage parents to fully discuss and describe their perception of the problem in order to assess the family system before determining appropriate interventions. In answer choice **(2)**, the nurse has not explored the problem and is deciding before adequate assessment that the mental health team member should be consulted. Providing literature regarding the disorder and its management may be a useful intervention; however, the *initial* action needs to involve a more thorough exploration of the parents' concerns. Telling the parents they are overreacting to the problem is inappropriate, because it dismisses the parents' legitimate concerns and it belittles their feelings.

10. The answer is (2). An important element of assessment for the family system is determining if the parents establish and maintain appropriate generational boundaries, establishing clear rules and expectations as part of the parental role. Although the parents may have anxiety regarding the role of parental rule setting, the nurse's question is not adequate to assess the anxiety levels. The question concerns the roles of the parents and the child in rule setting. It does not provide data regarding knowledge of growth and development or communication quality.

11. The answer is (1). Behavioral therapy is employed for the purpose of developing adaptive behavior that will improve coping. The nurse does not avoid setting rules; it is the responsibility of the nurse to establish and maintain appropriate limits. The nurse works to enhance the child's self-functioning and responsibility for own behavior. The nurse uses behavioral means to assist the child in learning better coping. Although reinforcing behavioral contracts will help prevent manipulative behavior by the child, this is not the best rationale for using behavioral treatment. The goal is improved client behavior.

12. The answer is (2). A child with a pervasive developmental disorder can have bizarre responses to environmental stimuli. By decreasing that stimulating effect and providing a time-out, the child can more readily deescalate the behaviors. Escalating behaviors as described require intervention to promote safety. It is inappropriate to ignore this. The situation requires immediate intervention. The parents should seek help when overwhelmed, but they must intervene when safety is an issue. The response in answer choice **(4)** is inadequate; the child will not be able to calm down without assistance.

Cognitive Impairment Disorders

11

I. Description

A. **Cognitive impairment disorders (CID)** are caused by temporary or permanent damage to neurons, resulting in dysfunction of cognitive processes (ie, higher brain function) including memory, reasoning, orientation, perception, and attention. Personality and behavior are also affected.

1. **Dementia** is a chronic, progressive disorder characterized by severe impairments in cognitive processes and personality and behavioral dysfunctions.
2. **Delirium** is an acute disorder characterized by cognitive impairment, attention deficit, and a reduced level of orientation (ie, the ability to relate to time, place, and person).
3. **Amnestic disorders** are characterized by severe memory impairment and the inability to learn new material; confabulation and apathy may be present.

B. **Common symptoms of CID**

1. Dementia disorders have symptoms such as:
   a. **Aphasia:** the loss of language ability; speech is often impoverished and the client may have difficulty "finding" words.
   b. **Apraxia:** an impaired ability to carry out motor activities despite intact sensory function
   c. **Agnosia:** the failure to recognize or identify common objects despite intact sensory function
   d. **Confabulation:** filling in memory gaps with detailed fantasy believed by the affected individual
   e. **Sundown syndrome:** increased disorientation at night
   f. **Catastrophic reactions:** responses of fear or panic with strong potential to harm self or others
   g. **Perseveration phenomenon:** repetitive behaviors, including pacing and echoing others' words
   h. **Hyperorality:** the need to taste and chew objects small enough to be put in mouth
   i. **Memory losses:** initially, recent memory, and eventually remote memory impairment
   j. **Disorientation** to time, place, and person
   k. **Decreased ability to concentrate** or to learn new material

  l. **Difficulty making decisions**

  m. **Poor judgment:** individual may not be aware of environmental considerations of safety and security

 2. Disorders of delirium are characterized by symptoms such as:

  a. Impaired consciousness and cognition; reduced ability to maintain attention

  b. Disorganized thinking and rambling speech

  c. Disturbance of sleep-wake cycle

  d. Psychomotor changes (eg, either hyperactive and agitated or hypoactive and somnolent)

 3. Amnestic disorders are characterized by symptoms such as:

  a. Impaired ability to learn new information

  b. Inability to recall previously learned information or past events

  c. Profound amnesia may result in disorientation to place and time, but rarely self

  d. Lack of insight into the memory deficits

  e. Apathy, lack of initiative

C. Types of CID. These disorders are classified in the DSM-IV according to their presumed etiology.

 1. Delirium

  a. Delirium due to general medical condition. Multiple different medical conditions can be associated with delirium (see II.A).

  b. Substance-induced delirium is evidenced by history of substance use, physical examination, or laboratory and diagnostic study findings.

  c. Delirium due to multiple etiologies (eg, several different medical conditions or combination of substance use plus medical conditions)

  d. Delirium not otherwise specified, in which insufficient evidence exists to establish definite etiology

 2. Dementia

  a. Dementia, Alzheimer's type (DAT) (Table 11-1)

  b. Vascular (multi-infarct) dementia is characterized by symptoms of dementia within the first year of focal neurologic symptoms. Clients have known risk factors for vascular disease (eg, hypertension, atrial fibrillation, diabetes).

  c. Other types of dementia are associated with general medical conditions, such as Parkinson's disease, Pick's disease, Huntington's chorea, and Creutzfeldt-Jakob disease. Dementia caused by any of these conditions is noted according to the specific disease.

 3. Amnestic disorders

  a. Amnestic disorder due to a general medical condition, which is evidenced by history, physical examination, or laboratory study findings that the memory disturbance is due to direct physiologic consequences of the general medical condition

  b. Substance-induced persisting amnestic disorder, which is evidenced by history of substance use, physical examination, or laboratory study findings

TABLE 11-1
Dementia, Alzheimer's Type: Stages and Related Symptoms

STAGE	BEHAVIOR	AFFECT	COGNITIVE CHANGES
Mild	Difficulty completing tasks Decline in goal-directed activity Lack of attention to personal appearance and ADL Withdrawal from usual social activities Frequently searching for misplaced objects; may accuse others of stealing	Anxious Depressed Frustrated Suspicious Fearful	Recent memory losses (eg, forgets appointments and conversations) Time disorientation Decreased ability to concentrate Difficulty making decisions Poor judgment
Moderate	Socially inappropriate behavior Self-care deficits (eg, with bathing, toileting, dressing, grooming) Wandering and pacing Hoarding objects Hyperorality Sleep-wake cycle disturbance	Labile moods Flat, apathetic Catastrophic agitation Paranoia	Recent and remote memory losses (amnesia) Confabulation Disorientation to time, place, and person Some degree of agnosia, apraxia, and aphasia
Severe	Decreased ability for ambulation and other motor activities Decreased swallowing ability Complete self-care deficits (ie, requires constant care) Absence of caregiver recognition	Flat, apathetic Occasional catastrophic reactions may continue	All cognitive changes continue with increased severity of amnesia, agnosia, apraxia, and aphasia

ADL = activities of daily living

    c. Amnestic disorder not otherwise specified, in which insufficient evidence exists to establish definite etiology

D. Epidemiology

  1. CID is most common among the elderly population.

  2. The severity of symptoms can be affected by physical, psychosocial, environmental, and cultural factors:

    a. Acute and chronic disease processes

    b. Presence of other mental disorder (especially depressive disorders)

    c. Poverty, poor nutrition, or social isolation

    d. Substance abuse or dependence; taking multiple prescription drugs

  3. DAT accounts for 50% to 75% of all diagnosed cases of dementia. It is the fourth leading cause of death in people over 65. Incidence is as follows:

    a. 65 to 75 years of age—5% to 8%

  b. 75 to 85 years of age—15% to 20%
  c. 85 years of age and older—25% to 50%

E. **Diagnosis.** Medical diagnosis of CID is made by careful screening to rule out other possible causes of symptoms. Workup should include:

1. **Mental status examination** and neuropsychological testing
2. **Comprehensive blood work,** including complete blood count (CBC), blood chemistry panel, vitamin B_{12} and folate levels, thyroid panel, and liver and renal function tests
3. **Brain imaging studies,** including computed tomography (CT), positron emission tomography (PET), and magnetic resonance imaging (MRI)
4. **Depressive disorders** in the elderly client may be manifested by symptoms similar to those of CID. Therefore, depressive disorder should be ruled out.

F. **Onset and course**

1. **Delirium** is an acute disorder with rapid onset, which usually can be reversed with prompt treatment.
2. **Dementia** is a chronic disorder with slow onset and generally poor prognosis.
3. **Amnestic disorder** can occur suddenly (eg, severe brain injury and trauma); or it may be chronic (eg, occurring with prolonged substance abuse, chronic neurotoxic exposure, or sustained nutritional deficits). If the disorder is caused by a chronic condition, the course is similar to that of dementia.

II. Etiology

A. **Delirium.** Factors associated with delirium may include:

1. **Acute or chronic illness,** such as congestive heart failure, pneumonia, renal and liver diseases, cancer, and cerebrovascular accidents
2. **Hormonal and nutritional factors,** such as diabetes, adrenal or thyroid imbalances, malnutrition, and dehydration
3. **Sensory impairments** associated with vision and hearing loss as well as sleep deprivation
4. **Medications,** including taking multiple prescribed drugs (especially combinations of drugs with anticholinergic properties)
   a. Drugs interfering with the cholinergic system and the neurotransmitter acetylcholine affect memory, learning, attention, and wakefulness.
   b. Examples of anticholinergic drugs include antipsychotics, antihistamines, some antidepressants, and antiparkinson drugs.
5. **Surgical procedure or trauma,** including blood loss and shock

B. **Dementia.** Factors associated with dementia may include:

1. **Untreated or untreatable acute condition.** If the acute condition that caused delirium is not or cannot be treated, then the possibility exists that the condition will become chronic and hence will be considered a dementia.
2. **Vascular disease** such as hypertension, arteriosclerosis, and atherosclerosis can lead to cerebrovascular accidents. (Treating hypertension can decrease risk of DAT.)

3. **Parkinson's disease:** dementia affects 40% of these patients.
4. **Genetic disorders:** Huntington's chorea or Pick's disease
5. **Prion disease** (protein found in infectious process of Creutzfeldt-Jakob disease)
6. **Infection with the human immunodeficiency virus (HIV)** can affect the central nervous system (CNS), causing HIV encephalopathy or acquired immunodeficiency syndrome (AIDS) dementia complex.
7. **Structural disorders of brain tissue,** such as normal pressure hydrocephalus and injury caused by head trauma

C. **DAT.** Research is ongoing, and no single cause is implicated. It is believed that there are multiple causative factors.
1. **Pathophysiology**
   a. Autopsy has shown presence of **amyloid plaques** (senile or neuritic plaques) in brain tissue or presence of **neurofibrillary tangles** (accumulation of twisted nerve filaments) in neurons.
   b. Presence of both plaques and tangles is associated with nerve cell destruction, loss of connections between neurons, and finally cerebral atrophy.
2. **Genetics.** Presence of abnormal genes alone is insufficient to predict DAT.
   a. **Familial Alzheimer's disease** has an early onset (30 to 40 years of age) and accounts for 20% of all cases of DAT. It has been associated with abnormal genes on chromosomes 1, 14, and 21.
   b. Presence of apolipoprotein E4 (Apo E4) on chromosome 19 occurs two times more often in people with DAT than in the general population.
3. **Toxin model.** Some researchers believe that aluminum accumulation in the brain from exposure to utensils and aluminum products contributes to DAT. Evidence for this theory has been scant.
4. **Neurotransmitter or receptor abnormality.** Loss of acetylcholine (major cholinergic neurotransmitter) is associated with symptoms of CID (dementia). (Increasing acetylcholine levels is current basis for FDA-approved drug therapy for dementia.)

D. **Amnestic disorders.** Factors associated with amnestic disorders include:
1. Head trauma, hypoxia, and acute CNS infections
2. Chronic thiamine deficiency associated with alcoholism (Korsakoff syndrome)

III. Management

A. **Delirium.** Treatment is focused on identifying and treating the underlying cause while supporting the client's physiologic processes and promoting safety. Acute hospital-based care is generally indicated.

B. **Dementia.** Treatment is directed toward a long-term goal of maintaining quality of life for this progressive, degenerative disorder.
1. **Multidisciplinary team approach** includes collaborative efforts from professionals in nursing, medicine, nutrition, psychiatry, psychology, social

work, pharmacy, and rehabilitative specialties (eg, occupational, physical, and activity therapists).

2. **Family focus.** Statistics indicate that 7 out of 10 people with DAT live at home, and 75% of these clients are cared for by family and friends. Thus, a family focus on treatment and management is vital.

3. **Community-focused management**
    a. **Home health visits** are provided by community nurses.
    b. **Adult day care services** provide therapeutic activities, rehabilitative services, recreation, and respite services for family caregivers.
    c. **Residential care facilities** (personal care) provide assisted living for clients.
    d. **Skilled nursing facilities.** Fifty percent of nursing home clients have DAT.
    e. The **Alzheimer's Association** provides support groups, education for community and families, and fundraising and lobbying for research and legislative action.

4. **Pharmacologic intervention**
    a. The **goals of pharmacologic intervention** are to slow the rate of the client's decline with medications that increase acetylcholine levels and help maintain neuronal functioning and to manage behavior and distressing symptoms.
    b. **Experimental therapies** (Drug Charts 11-1 and 11-2)

C. **Amnestic disorders.** Treatment is similar to that of delirium if the amnestic disorder is an acute problem; it is similar to that of dementia if the amnestic disorder is chronic.

DRUG CHART 11-1   **Medications for Symptoms of Dementia***

Classification	Generic/Trade	Usual Daily Dose	Rationale for Use
Anticholinesterase drugs	Tacrine (Cognex)	40 mg/day (10 mg qid)	Anticholinesterase medications interfere with enzyme acetyl-cholinesterase, which acts to break down acetylcholine. Therefore, these drugs allow acetylcholine to remain longer at synapses.
	Donepezil (Aricept)	5 mg/day (once daily)	
	ENA-713 (Exelon)	Currently in clinical trials	
Antioxidants	Vitamine E	400–800 IU/day	Based on combating oxidation process that synthesizes cytotoxic free radicals. There is some evidence that this will delay symptoms.

See Chapter 15 for specific information on side effects and nursing implications.

DRUG CHART 11-2   Medication for Behavior Modification in Dementia*

Indications and Drug Classification	Generic (Trade)	Dosage for Elderly
Anxiety and agitation		
Benzodiazepines (BZA)	Lorazepam (Ativan)	0.25 mg/day; may increase to bid
Non-BZA antianxiety	Buspirone (BuSpar)	15–160 mg/day
Anticonvulsants	Carbamazepine (Tegretol)	200 mg/bid
	Divalprolex (Depakote)	250 mg/bid
Hallucinations and combative behavior		
Antipsychotics		
Typical	Haloperidol (Haldol)	0.25 mg/day or bid
Atypical	Risperidone (Risperdal)	0.5 mg/day or bid
Depression		
Antidepressants (SSRI)	Nefazodone (Serzone)	50 mg/day; can increase to 400 mg/day on bid schedule

Source: Lesseig, D.Z. (1998). Pharmacotherapy for long-term care residents with dementia-associated behavior disturbance. Journal of Psychosocial Nursing and Mental Health Services, 36(2):27–31.

*See Chapter 15 for specific information on side effects and nursing implications.

IV. NURSING PROCESS OVERVIEW FOR CID

A. Assessment

1. **History**. Review client's history and physical examination for characteristic signs and symptoms associated with particular diagnosed disorder(s).
2. **Assess for dementia** using standardized tools, including:
   a. **Mini-Mental Status Exam (MMSE)**
   b. **Short Portable Mental Status Questionnaire**
3. **Rule out depression** by using an appropriate screening tool, such as the Geriatric Depression Scale (Yesavage & Brink, 1983). See Table 11-2 for comparison of symptoms of delirium, dementia, and depression.
4. Ask **key nursing assessment questions** (Table 11-3).
5. **Interview client, caregiver, or family.** Make direct observations about:
   a. **Behavior.** What are the client's self-care and activities of daily living (ADL) abilities? Does the client exhibit socially unacceptable behaviors? Is the client wandering and pacing? Are sundown or perseveration phenomena present?
   b. **Affect.** Does client demonstrate anxiety? Emotional lability? Depression or apathy? Irritability? Suspiciousness? Helplessness? Frustration?
   c. **Cognitive responses.** What is client's orientation level? Does client have recent or remote memory loss? Difficulty in problem solving, organizing, or abstracting? Deficits in judgment? Evidence of aphasia, agnosia, or apraxia?

TABLE 11-2
Comparison of Delirium, Dementia, and Depression in the Elderly Client

	DELIRIUM	DEMENTIA	DEPRESSION
Onset	Acute (hours to days)	Gradual, insidious (months to years)	Can be gradual (weeks to months). Obvious symptoms at least for 2 weeks.
Initial Symptoms	Acute confusion Disorientation (time, place, and person)	Difficulty planning, organizing and completing complex tasks (balancing checkbook, meal planning) Recent memory loss (forgetting appointments, misplacing objects)	Depressed mood Lack of interest in usual activities
Continuing Symptoms	Sensory alterations (illusions, hallucinations) Alteration in sleep/wake cycle Motor changes—agitation or somnolence	Disorientation (time, place) Anxiety, agitation, paranoia (blaming people for stealing misplaced objects) Depressed mood, apathy, loss of spontaneity Lack of attention to grooming, hygiene Lack of regard to safety (leaving stove on, going outside dressed inappropriately) Pacing, wandering Remote memory losses Disorientation to time, place, and person	Complaints of memory loss, poor concentration Feelings of helplessness, hopelessness Sleep problems (hypersomnia, insomnia) Appetite loss, weight loss Physical complaints (headache, muscle aches, GI symptoms) Self-neglect, poor hygiene Thoughts of suicide

6. **Spend time with caregiver or family.**
   a. **Identify primary caregiver** and determine how long care has been provided. (Late stages of DAT can be especially difficult, because family resources may be exhausted.)
   b. **Identify the support systems** available for caregiver and other family members.
   c. **Identify knowledge base** regarding client care and community resources (note areas for teaching).
   d. **Identify spiritual support system** for family.
   e. **Identify specific concerns** about client and caregiver's concerns about self.

TABLE 11-3
Key Nursing Assessment Questions for Clients with Cognitive Impairment Disorder

QUESTIONS	PROVIDES DATA ABOUT
Ask client's name, address, current location, date, time, season, and year.	Orientation status
Ask client to repeat 6 to 7 digits forward.	Attention span
Name three objects (eg, watch, glass, clock) and have client repeat the three objects. Ask client to repeat them again after 5 minutes.	Recent memory
Ask client mother's maiden name, brothers' and sisters' names, and children's and grandchildren's names.	Remote memory
Ask client about any changes in eating or sleeping habits; somatic complaints; irritability; or lack of interest in usually pleasurable things.	Presence of depression
Ask client about usual daily routine of ADL.	Planning and completing ADL

ADL = activities of daily living

B. Analysis

1. After analysis of data assessed, differentiate client priorities.
2. Evaluate client and family coping abilities; evaluate the client's level of anxiety and potential for acting out.
3. Analyze degree of impairment related to specific cognitive disorder.
4. Analyze resources available for client, caregiver, or family

C. Nursing diagnoses

1. **Establish nursing diagnoses of client** including, but not limited to, the following:
   a. Anxiety (specify level)
   b. Coping, individual, ineffective
   c. Thought processes, altered
   d. Home maintenance management, impaired
   e. Nutrition, altered: less than body requirements
   f. Role performance, altered
   g. Confusion, acute
   h. Confusion, chronic
   i. Social isolation
   j. Sensory/perceptual alterations (specify)
   k. Self-care deficit (specify): feeding, bathing/hygiene, dressing/grooming, toileting
   l. Communication, impaired, verbal
   m. Sleep pattern disturbance
   n. Violence, risk for: directed at self/others
2. **Establish nursing diagnoses of caregiver or family.**
   a. Family coping: ineffective: compromised
   b. Family processes, altered
   c. Caregiver role strain

D. Planning and outcome identification

1. Work with client, caregiver, or family in setting realistic goals.
2. Establish desired **outcome criteria** for client, caregiver, or family.
   a. Client will remain safe and free from injury.
   b. Client will demonstrate decreased anxiety levels.
   c. Client will remain oriented at level of ability. If orientation is not possible, client will feel validated and accepted.
   d. Client will maintain existing ability to perform ADL with cues as necessary.
   e. Client will maintain adequate fluids and nutrition.
   f. Client will not harm self or others.
   g. Client will follow scheduled routine of activity and rest.
   h. Client will experience minimal catastrophic reactions.
   i. Caregiver and family will identify and use available support systems.
   j. Caregiver will demonstrate use of measures to prevent burnout.
   k. Caregiver will verbalize confidence in ability to provide care to client.

E. Implementation

1. **Maintain safety.**
   a. Provide emergency measures as necessary (eg, for aspiration, injury, seizures).
   b. Anticipate environmental safety hazards and remove objects of risk; keep surroundings clutter-free.
   c. Minimize risk of cardiovascular problems (eg, anemia, hypertension, angina) with proper diet, medications, exercise, and rest.
   d. Monitor drugs and drug interactions, ensuring safe doses for elderly clients. Pay special attention to medications with anticholinergic properties.

2. **Respond to cognitive deficits.**
   a. Call client by name and introduce yourself. Use short, clear messages. Give directions one at a time.
   b. Support client memory by using calendars, orientation boards, seasonal reminders, signs, and labels as needed.
   c. Avoid stressful demands, and limit client decision-making.
   d. Offer activities within client's ability.
   e. Avoid or limit socially embarrassing situations; support and maintain client's dignity.
   f. Do not reinforce or agree with hallucinations, illusions, or delusions. Respond to and focus on feelings of client.
   g. Use reminiscence techniques to encourage client to capitalize on more intact remote memories. Encourage client to talk about past events; use tape recorder to tape reminiscence and then play back. Use family photo albums to stimulate reminiscence.
   h. Use validation therapy when client no longer responds to reality orientation techniques (Table 11-4).

TABLE 11-4
Reality Orientation and Validation Therapy: Comparison of Techniques

	REALITY ORIENTATION	VALIDATION THERAPY
Purpose	Establish or maintain awareness of current environment	Establish connection between nurse and client by validating emotional memories
Appropriate Use	Client with temporary loss of awareness	Useful when reality orientation is resisted or ineffective
	Useful as first attempt to assist client in becoming aware of current environment	Helpful as calming method when environment is misperceived
Specific Techniques	Establish eye contact, introduce yourself, and state client's name; smile	Establish eye contact, introduce yourself, and state client's name; smile
	Use short, simple sentences providing orienting information	Validate client feelings (eg, "You seem upset")
	Structure environment using clocks, calendars, orientation boards, seasonal decoration, and family pictures	Repeat part of what client said (eg, "You need to fix dinner for your husband ...")
		Reflect what seems to be underlying feelings (eg, "You miss your husband")
		Continue to talk with client about topic (ie, husband)
		As client becomes calmer, redirect her to appropriate current activity

3. **Maintain level of functioning for ADL.**
   a. Promote balance of rest and activity.
   b. Support client in self-sufficiency; use cues and positive reinforcement.
   c. Assist with toileting on structured schedule; use disposable pants as needed to preserve client's dignity.
   d. Maintain balanced diet, and ensure adequate fluids. Offer finger foods if client has difficulty with utensils.
4. **Avoid and minimize catastrophic reactions.**
   a. Maintain consistency of structure and routines.
   b. Decrease environmental stimuli when client is anxious.
   c. Do not approach rapidly or touch client if client is irritable, agitated, or suspicious.
   d. When client is agitated, remain with client and maintain calm, supportive manner.
   e. Use night lights and calm interaction to decrease sundowning.
5. Teach caregiver and family (Client and Family Teaching 11-1 and 11-2).

Home Care of Client with Dementia

- Educate family about dementia: symptoms, progressive nature of disease.
- Provide helpful home care measures:
    Memory aids: use clocks, labels, calendars, lists
    Structure daily routine: regular times for sleeping and awakening, meals, activities, and rest periods
- Educate family about maintaining good nutrition: frequent small meals for clients with poor appetite.
- Educate family about responding to client's memory impairment and losses: attempt to gently reorient client as long as this is not upsetting.
- Educate family about bedtime routines to promote sleep: eliminate caffeine after 2 PM, quiet environment, use night light, toileting prior to bed.
- Educate family about providing directions and instructions with simple words, using gestures if helpful.
- Educate family about safety measures in home: remove or lock up objects or cleaning agents that can cause harm; remove throw rugs, extension cords; paint hot water faucets red; secure doors and windows.
- Educate family that wandering is expected.
    Prepare for this by using identification bracelet.
    Register client with police department (Safe Return program is joint effort of Alzheimer's Association and local police departments).
    Appropriate daily exercise may decrease wandering.
- Educate family about removing client from upsetting situations to prevent catastrophic reactions. Avoid crowds, strangers, confusion, and noise.
- Plan for terminal stage of dementia.
    Loss of ambulation; loss of caregiver recognition; loss of conversation; progression to vegetative state.
    Use of hospice-type approach in late stage: palliative measures; comfort; limited medications and medical interventions.

Prevention of Caregiver Burnout

- Get enough rest.
- Maintain proper nutrition.
- Maintain sense of humor.
- Ask for help from other family members, community agencies, support groups (eg, Alzheimer's Association).
- Take breaks and vacations; use respite services and day-care services.
- Make time for enjoyable activities and hobbies.
- Expect feelings of anger, grief, sadness, and loss as client progresses in disease process.
- Openly talk about feelings, frustrations, and difficulties with supportive persons (eg, family, friends, health care professionals, and support group members).

F. Outcome evaluation
1. Client demonstrates decreased anxiety and increased feelings of security in structured environment. Client maintains maximum degree of orientation within level of ability.
2. Client maintains abilities to perform ADL within structured environment.
3. Client refrains from acting out.
4. Family members use all available support services and community resources.

STUDY QUESTIONS

1. A nurse asks a client with a cognitive impairment disorder what day of the week it is, what the date, month, and year are, and where the client is. The nurse is attempting to assess
   (1) confabulation
   (2) delirium
   √(3) orientation
   (4) perseveration

2. Which one of the following best describes dementia?
   (1) memory loss occurring as part of natural consequence of aging
   (2) difficulty coping with physical and psychological change
   (3) severe cognitive impairment that occurs rapidly
   √(4) loss of cognitive abilities, impairing ability to perform ADL

3. Which one of the following will the nurse use when communicating with a client who has a cognitive impairment?
   (1) complete explanations with multiple details
   (2) pictures or gestures instead of words
   (3) stimulating words and phrases to capture the client's attention
   √(4) short words and simple sentences

4. A 75-year-old client has dementia, Alzheimer's type, and confabulates. The nurse understands that the client
   (1) denies confusion by being jovial
   (2) pretends to be someone else
   (3) rationalizes various behaviors
   √(4) fills in memory gaps with fantasy

5. Which of the following abilities should a nurse expect from a client in the mild stage of dementia, Alzheimer's type?
   (1) remembering the daily schedule
   √(2) recalling events of the past

   (3) coping with anxiety
   (4) solving problems of daily living

6. An 82-year-old man is admitted to the medical-surgical unit for diagnostic confirmation and management of probable delirium. Which of the following statements by the client's daughter best supports the diagnosis?
   (1) "Maybe it's just caused by aging. This usually happens by age 82."
   √(2) "The changes in his behavior came on so quickly! I wasn't sure what was happening."
   (3) "Dad just didn't seem to know what he was doing. He would forget what he had for breakfast."
   (4) "Dad has always been so independent. He's lived alone for years since Mom died."

7. An elderly client with Alzheimer's disease becomes agitated and combative when a nurse approaches to help with morning care. The most appropriate nursing intervention would be
   (1) to tell the client firmly that it is time to get dressed
   (2) to obtain assistance to restrain the client for safety
   √(3) to remain calm and talk quietly to the client
   (4) to call the physician and request order for sedation

8. Which of the following goals is a priority for a client with a DSM-IV diagnosis of delirium and the nursing diagnosis of acute confusion related to recent surgery secondary to traumatic hip fracture?
   (1) The client will complete ADL.
   √(2) The client will maintain safety.
   (3) The client will remain oriented.
   (4) The client will understand communication.

9. Which of the following is not included in the care plan of a client with a moderate cognitive impairment from dementia, Alzheimer's type?
   (1) daily structured schedule
   (2) positive reinforcement for performing ADL
   ✓(3) stimulating environment
   (4) use of validation techniques

10. In clients with a cognitive impairment disorder, the phenomenon of increased confusion in the early evening hours is called
   (1) aphasia
   (2) agnosia
   ✓(3) sundowning
   (4) confabulation

11. An 80-year-old man is accompanied to the clinic by his son. The son tells the nurse that the client's constant confusion, incontinence, and tendency to wander are intolerable. The client has a diagnosed chronic cognitive impairment disorder. The nursing diagnosis most appropriate for the client's son would be
   (1) risk for violence
   (2) sleep pattern disturbance
   ✓(3) caregiver role strain
   (4) social isolation

12. Which of the following outcome criteria is appropriate for the client with dementia?

   (1) Client will return to adequate level of self-functioning.
   (2) Client will learn new coping mechanisms to handle anxiety.
   (3) Client will seek out resources in the community for support.
   ✓(4) Client will follow established schedule for ADL.

13. A family member expresses concern to a nurse about behavioral changes in an elderly relative. Which would cause the nurse to suspect a cognitive impairment disorder?
   (1) decreased interest in activities that were once enjoyed
   (2) fearfulness of being alone at night
   (3) increased complaints of physical ailments
   ✓(4) problems with preparing a meal or balancing a checkbook

14. A nurse notes that a caregiver for a client with dementia persists in correcting the client's misperceptions of reality, even when the client becomes upset and anxious. Which of the following interventions would the nurse teach the caregiver?
   (1) anxiety-reducing measures
   (2) positive reinforcement
   (3) reality orientation techniques
   ✓(4) validation techniques

ANSWER KEY

1. The answer is (3). The initial, most basic assessment for a client with cognitive impairment is level of orientation (ie, awareness of time, place, and person). Confabulation and perseveration may also be symptoms of a cognitive impairment; however, the nurse's questions are not designed to elicit these symptoms. Delirium is a type of cognitive impairment; however, other symptoms are necessary to establish this diagnosis.

2. The answer is (4). Self-care ability is an important measure of the progression of dementia and the loss of cognitive abilities. Difficulty or impaired ability to perform normal activities of daily living (ADL), such as maintaining hygiene and grooming, toileting, making meals, and maintaining a household, are significant indications of dementia. Slowing of processes necessary for retrieval of information is a normal consequence of aging. However, the global statement that memory loss occurs as part of natural aging is not true. Dementia is not normal; it is a disease process. Difficulty coping with changes can be experienced by any client, not just one with dementia. Cognitive impairment occurring rapidly refers to a delirium.

3. The answer is (4). Short words and simple sentences minimize client confusion and enhance communication. Complete explanations with multiple details and stimulating words and phrases would increase confusion in a client with short attention span and difficulty with comprehension. Although pictures and gestures may be helpful, they would not substitute for verbal communication.

4. The answer is (4). Confabulation is a communication device used by patients with dementia to compensate for memory gaps. The remaining answer choices are not correct definitions of confabulation.

5. The answer is (2). Recent memory loss is the characteristic sign of cognitive difficulty in early Alzheimer's disease. Recalling events of the past is usually retained until the later stages of this disorder. Remembering the daily schedule, coping with anxiety, and solving problems of daily living are areas that would pose difficulty in the early phase of Alzheimer's disease.

6. The answer is (2). Delirium is an acute process characterized by abrupt, spontaneous cognitive dysfunction. Cognitive impairment disorders (ie, dementia or delirium) are not normal consequences of aging. Answer choice **(3)** would be characteristic behavior in dementia. Although answer choice **(4)** provides background data about the client, it is unrelated to the current problem of delirium.

7. The answer is (3). It is important to maintain a calm approach when intervening with an agitated client. Telling the client firmly that it is time to get dressed may increase client agitation, especially if the nurse touches the client. Restraints are a last resort to ensure client safety and are inappropriate in this situation. Sedation should be avoided if possible, because it will interfere with CNS functioning and may contribute to client confusion.

8. The answer is (2). Maintaining client safety is the priority goal for an acutely confused client who recently had surgery. All measures to promote physiologic safety and psychosocial well-being would be implemented. This client would not be capable of completing ADL, and safety is a priority over these tasks. When client recovers from the acute confusion, the goals of answer choices **(3)** and **(4)** would be appropriate; at this time, they are not applicable.

9. The answer is (3). A stimulating environment is a source of confusion and anxiety for a client with a moderate level of impairment and therefore is not included in the plan of care. The remaining answer choices are all appropriate interventions that would be part of a plan of care for this type of client.

10. The answer is (3). Sundowning is a common phenomenon that occurs after daylight hours in a client with a cognitive impairment disorder. The remaining answer choices are incorrect responses, although all may be seen in this client.

11. The answer is (3). The son is describing a common problem in a primary caregiver of a client with a cognitive impairment disorder. Although the other nursing diagnoses are possibilities, the scenario does not provide enough information to validate any of these.

12. The answer is (4). Following established activity schedules is a realistic expectation for clients with dementia. All of the remaining outcome statements require a higher level of cognitive ability than can be realistically expected for clients with dementia.

13. The answer is (4). Making a meal and balancing a checkbook are higher level cognitive functions that, when unable to be performed, may signal onset of a cognitive disorder. Although the remaining behaviors may occur, they are not associated only with cognitive impairment and may indicate depression or other problems.

14. The answer is (4). Validation techniques are measures useful in making emotional connections with a client who can no longer maintain reality orientation. These measures are also helpful in decreasing anxiety. Anxiety-reducing measures and positive reinforcements will also be appropriate, but validation techniques will provide both anxiety reduction and positive reinforcement for the client. Reality orientation techniques are not useful when the client can no longer maintain reality contact and becomes upset when misperceptions are corrected.

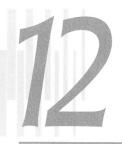

Treatment Modalities:
Crisis Intervention

I. Overview

A. **Definitions**
  1. A **crisis** is an overwhelming reaction to a threatening situation in which an individual's usual problem-solving skills and coping responses are inadequate for maintaining psychological equilibrium.
  2. **Types of crisis** (Table 12-1)
      a. **Developmental crisis** occurs in response to a transition from one stage of maturation to another in the life cycle (eg, going from adolescence to adulthood).
      b. **Situational crisis** occurs in response to a sudden, unexpected event in an individual's life. These events generally revolve around experiences of loss (eg, death of a loved one).
      c. **Adventitious crisis** occurs in response to severe trauma or natural disasters. These crises can affect individuals, communities, and even nations.
  3. **Crisis intervention** is a method of providing assistance to those affected by a crisis, in which the immediate problem is resolved and psychological equilibrium is restored.

B. **General considerations**
  1. Crisis occurs in all individuals at one time or another.
  2. Crisis is not necessarily pathological; it can provide stimulus for growth and learning.
  3. A crisis is time limited and is usually resolved one way or another in a brief period (4 to 6 weeks).
      a. Successful crisis resolution occurs when functioning is restored or enhanced through new learning.
      b. Unsuccessful crisis resolution is when functioning is not restored to pre-crisis level, and the individual experiences decreased levels of functioning.
  4. The individual's perception of the problem determines the crisis. That is, each individual has a unique response to the experience of problems.
  5. **Balancing factors** are important in predicting outcomes for the individual responding to a crisis. Several factors are identified as predictors of good outcomes (Augilera, 1998).
      a. The **perception of precipitating event** is realistic rather than distorted.

TABLE 12-1
Types of Crises

DEVELOPMENTAL (MATURATIONAL)	SITUATIONAL	ADVENTITIOUS
Beginning school	Divorce	Floods
Puberty	Death	Earthquakes
Graduation	Job loss	Wars
Marriage	Academic failure	Crimes of violence
Birth of a child	Diagnosis of serious illness	Rape
Children leaving home		Murder
Retirement		Kidnapping
		Terroristic acts

      b. **Situational supports** (eg, family, friends) are available to the person.
      c. **Coping mechanisms** that alleviate anxiety
  6. Sequence of crisis development
      a. **Precrisis period:** the individual has emotional equilibrium
      b. **Crisis period:** the individual has the subjective experience of upset, failure of usual coping mechanisms, and symptoms are experienced (Table 12-2)
      c. **Postcrisis period:** resolution of crisis

TABLE 12-2
Symptoms Common in Individuals Experiencing Crisis

Physical Symptoms	Somatic complaints (eg, headaches, gastrointestinal symptoms, pain)
	Appetite disturbances (eg, significant loss or gain)
	Sleep disturbances (eg, insomnia, nightmares)
	Restlessness, tearfulness, irritability
Cognitive Symptoms	Confusion, difficulty concentrating
	Racing thoughts
	Inability to make decisions
Behavioral Symptoms	Disorganization
	Impulsive, angry outbursts
	Difficulty carrying out usual role responsibilities
	Withdrawal from social interaction
Emotional Symptoms	Anxiety, anger, guilt
	Sadness, depression
	Paranoia, suspicion
	Helplessness, powerlessness

II. Management of Crisis: Crisis Intervention

A. Assistance

1. **Assistance for an individual affected by a crisis** includes telephone counseling, hotlines, and brief crisis counseling (1 to 6 sessions).
2. **Assistance for groups or communities affected by crisis**
   a. **Mobile crisis teams.** These interdisciplinary teams provide services to groups or communities affected by particular crisis events.
   b. **Disaster response teams.** These teams have an organized plan to provide help to large segments of the population affected by natural disasters.
   c. **Critical incident stress debriefing.** This assistance is directed at groups of professionals, such as hospital personnel, police, and firemen, who have been involved in a crisis situation.

B. Role of the nurse. Nurses provide direct services to people in crisis and serve as members of crisis intervention teams (ANA, 1994).

1. Nurses in acute and chronic hospital settings assist individuals and families responding to the crisis of serious illness, hospitalization, and death.
2. Nurses in community settings (eg, offices, home clinics, schools, businesses) provide assistance to individuals and families in developmental and situational crises.
3. Nurses working with a particular group of clients should anticipate situations in which crises may occur.
   a. **Maternal-child nursing.** The nurse should anticipate crises such as the birth of a premature or stillborn child, miscarriage, and birth anomalies.
   b. **Pediatric nursing.** The nurse should anticipate crises such as the onset of serious illness, chronic or debilitating illnesses, traumatic injuries, or a dying child.
   c. **Medical-surgical nursing.** The nurse should anticipate crises such as the diagnosis of a serious illness, debilitating illness, hospitalization for acute or chronic problems, loss of a body part or function, and death and dying.
   d. **Gerontologic nursing.** The nurse should anticipate crises such as cumulative losses, debilitating illness, dependency, and nursing home placement.
   e. **Emergency nursing.** The nurse should anticipate crises such as physical trauma, acute illness, rape crisis, and death.
   f. **Psychiatric nursing.** The nurse should anticipate crises such as hospitalization for mental illness, life stressors for the seriously mentally ill, and suicide.
4. Nurses collaborate with other health team members to help an individual resolve a crisis situation.

C. Principles of crisis intervention

1. The goal of crisis intervention is to return the individual to the precrisis level of functioning.
2. The emphasis is on strengthening and supporting healthy aspects of an individual's functioning.

3. In crisis intervention, a **problem-solving approach** is used in a systematic manner (similar to nursing process), including:
  a. **Assessing the individual's perception of the problem,** as well as **assessing the strengths and weaknesses** of the individual and family support systems
  b. **Planning specific outcomes** or goals based on priorities
  c. **Providing direct intervention** (eg, providing shelter if the client has been evicted from home, referring client to "safe house" if spousal abuse has occurred)
  d. **Evaluating outcomes** and results of the intervention
4. Maslow's hierarchy. The framework of Maslow's hierarchy of needs can help determine the priorities for an intervention.
  a. **Physical resources** necessary for survival (eg, food, shelter, safety)
  b. **Social resources** necessary for regaining sense of belonging (eg, family support, social network, community support)
  c. **Psychological resources** necessary for regaining self-esteem (eg, positive reinforcement, goal accomplishment)
5. Crisis intervention worker. The role of a crisis intervention worker includes the following functions.
  a. The crisis worker establishes rapport and communicates hope and optimism.
  b. The crisis worker assumes an active, directive role, if necessary.
  c. The crisis worker makes suggestions and offers alternatives (eg, makes referrals to appropriate agencies, such as child welfare agency or medical clinics).
  d. The crisis worker supports the client in choosing alternatives.
  e. The crisis worker collaborates with other professionals to obtain necessary services and resources for client.

 III. **NURSING PROCESS OVERVIEW FOR**
Crisis Intervention

A. Assessment (Table 12-3)
  1. Identify the precipitating event and the circumstances of the crisis.
  2. Determine the client's perception of the crisis, including the underlying needs that the crisis threatens, the degree of life disruption, and the client's symptoms (see Table 12-2).
  3. Determine the presence of balancing factors, including whether the client has a realistic perception of the crisis events, situational supports (eg, family, friends, financial resources, spiritual resources, community supports), and the use of coping mechanisms.
  4. Identify the client's strengths.
B. Nursing diagnoses
  1. Analysis
    a. Analyze the client's unique perception of the crisis and the events precipitating it.

TABLE 12-3
Key Nursing Assessment Questions for Individual Experiencing Crisis

QUESTIONS	PROVIDES DATA ABOUT
"What happened to you?"	Individual's perception of events (realistic or distorted)
"What are your thoughts and feelings about what happened?"	Cognitive, emotional symptoms
"Are you experiencing any physical symptoms or changes in your usual behaviors?"	Physical, behavioral symptoms
"Have you ever experienced anything similar to this in your life? If so, how did you cope at that time?"	Past experience with crisis, coping measures in past
"What do you think are your personal strengths?"	Individual's recognition of strengths
"Who do you feel is supportive or helpful to you in your life?"	Support systems available
"What have you tried to do so far to resolve the crisis?"	Use of coping measures in present situation

    b. Analyze the adequacy of the client's balancing factors and degree of personal, social, and environmental supports.

    c. Analyze the degree to which others are affected by the crisis, such as the client's family, social network, and community.

2. **Nursing diagnoses.** Determine individualized nursing diagnoses for the client, family, community, or any combination thereof, including but not limited to the following:

    a. Body image disturbance

    b. Caregiver role strain

    c. Community coping, ineffective

    d. Coping, individual, ineffective

    e. Denial, ineffective

    f. Family coping: potential for growth

    g. Grieving, dysfunctional

    h. Posttrauma response

    i. Powerlessness

    j. Rape-trauma syndrome

    k. Role performance, altered

    l. Spiritual distress

    m. Violence, risk for: directed at self/others

C. Planning and outcome identification

1. Assist the client, family, community, or combination thereof in setting realistic short-term goals based on returning to precrisis state.

2. Establish desired outcome criteria for the client, family, community, or combination thereof. The affected persons will:

    a. Verbalize the meaning of the crisis situation

  b. Discuss options for resolution
  c. Identify resources available for assistance
  d. Choose a strategy for coping with crisis
  e. Implement necessary measures to bring about crisis resolution
  f. Maintain safety when situation(s) escalates

D. Implementation

  1. Establish rapport by active listening and use of empathic responses.
  2. Encourage the client to fully discuss the crisis situation, and assist the client in verbalizing thoughts and feelings.
  3. Support the client's strengths and use of coping measures.
  4. Use problem-solving approach (see II.C.3).
  5. Intervene to deter any plans for self-harm or suicide.
      a. Recognize warning signs for violence to self (eg, the client stating suicidal threat directly, hinting that others will be better off when she is gone; or the presence of depression). (See Chapter 6.)
      b. Perform a suicide lethality assessment (see Chapter 6).
      c. Remove dangerous objects from the client's immediate environment.
      d. Collaborate with mental health team members to determine whether hospitalization is necessary.

E. Implementation for the client who is angry or violent

  1. Intervene early to prevent the client from acting-out violence toward others.
      a. Recognize verbal signs of escalating anger (eg, shouting, rapid speech, demanding attention, making aggressive statements).
      b. Recognize nonverbal signs of escalating anger (eg, tightened jaw, tense posture, clenched fists, pacing).
  2. Use measures to deescalate the client's anger.
      a. Answer the client's angry questions and demands by providing factual information in a supportive and reassuring manner.
      b. Respond to underlying feelings of anxiety, fear, and frustration. For example, the nurse could say, "It seems to me that you're feeling frustrated about not going home when you expected."
      c. Allow the client to vent anger verbally, recognizing that the nurse may receive displaced anger.
      d. Avoid defending or justifying your own behavior or the behavior of others (eg, treatment team members, hospital policies).
      e. Monitor your own body language, using a relaxed posture with arms hanging loosely at sides.
      f. Provide client control over problem situation by offering alternative solutions for resolution (Zook, 1996).
  3. Respond to the client's violent behavior.
      a. Protect yourself by standing between the client and the exit door, so escape is possible.
      b. Protect others by instructing them to leave the area.
      c. Follow agency protocol, calling violence code.

4. Use principles of managing violence code when needed (eg, if a client is threatening to hurt another client or staff member or if a client is throwing objects or breaking furniture).
   a. Ensure a show of force (minimum of five staff).
   b. Designate one team member as the leader, who will interact with the client and direct the team response.
   c. The team leader stands at the head of the team, with the other members behind in rows of two to three.
   d. If physical restraint is necessary, the team leader decides who will take each limb and who will take the head (to prevent biting).
   e. The team acts as one and accomplishes a smooth, face-down takedown.
   f. Holding regular drills in which these techniques are practiced can ensure safety and avoidance of client and staff injury (Zook, 1996).

F. **Outcome evaluation.** The nurse uses specific outcome criteria in determining the effectiveness of nursing implementations.
   1. The client, family, and community safety is maintained as a result of appropriate intervention in acting-out behavior.
   2. The client identifies a relationship between stressors and symptoms experienced during crisis.
   3. The client evaluates possible solutions to crisis.
   4. The client selects options for solution.
   5. The client returns to a precrisis state or improves the situation or behavior.

STUDY QUESTIONS

1. The school nurse receives a referral from a teacher about a sudden behavior change in a 13-year-old girl. The girl has become increasingly withdrawn and uninterested in her schoolwork. Upon interviewing the girl as well as the teacher, the nurse notes that the girl's behavioral changes correspond with a rapid onset of puberty. Which of the following types of crisis is the girl experiencing?
   (1) adventitious crisis
   (2) developmental crisis
   (3) situational crisis
   (4) natural crisis

2. A nurse is intervening with a client who experienced a crisis following the sudden death of a loved one. Which of the following actions would the nurse take after establishing initial rapport?
   (1) The nurse would ask the client to describe his social support system.
   (2) The nurse would call the client's family to discuss the problem.
   (3) The nurse would encourage the client to describe in detail what happened.
   (4) The nurse would refer the client to a bereavement support group.

3. A nurse working with a client in crisis is assessing the client's balancing factors to predict outcomes for the individual's response to the crisis. Which of the following is the best example of a balancing factor?
   (1) age of the individual
   (2) physical health status
   (3) situational supports available
   (4) type of crisis event

4. The nurse would select which of the following approaches in order to best respond to a client in crisis?
   (1) behavioral approach
   (2) nondirective approach
   (3) problem-solving approach
   (4) supportive approach

5. Which of the following best describes the role of the nurse as a member of a crisis intervention team?
   (1) assistive role
   (2) collaborative role
   (3) educational role
   (4) managerial role

6. For a nurse, which of the following is the goal of crisis intervention?
   (1) for the client to analyze problems in life-style choices
   (2) for the client to improve weaknesses in personal development
   (3) for the client to learn new adaptive measures
   (4) for the client to return to precrisis state

7. A client who has been raped tells the emergency room nurse that the rape was her fault because she walked down the alley on her way to school. Which of the following is the best response from the nurse?
   (1) Accept the client's statement that this was risk-taking behavior.
   (2) Ask the client what other behaviors may have been risky.
   (3) Emphasize that the rapist, not the client, is responsible.
   (4) Suggest that the client discuss this issue later.

8. A client angrily shouts to the clinic nurse, "You better get me in to see the doctor now, or I'll see that you regret it." Which of the following is

the best initial response by the nurse to deescalate this situation?

(1) Call for assistance from security.

(2) Explain to the client the reasons that the doctor is busy.

(3) Firmly tell the client not to shout, but to be patient.

(4) Respond empathetically to the client's underlying frustration.

9. A homeless client with a history of mental illness comes to the clinic and tells the nurse that someone has taken all of the blood pressure pills she received at her last visit to the clinic. The nurse notes that the client is dirty and unkempt and appears to have lost weight since the last visit. Upon questioning, the nurse learns that the client has not been eating regularly because of her fear that the person taking the pills works at the local soup kitchen. Which of the following is the priority nursing intervention in this situation?

(1) Call the local mental health center and make a referral.

(2) Make immediate provisions for the client to eat.

(3) Provide the client with a new supply of medication.

(4) Suggest the client wash up in the clinic bathroom.

10. Which of the following symptoms common in individuals experiencing a crisis would a nurse expect to assess?

(1) feelings of depersonalization, loose associations, flat affect

(2) lack of regard to social norms, apathy, hallucinations

(3) mood swings, feeling of boundless energy, grandiose beliefs

(4) somatic complaints, difficulty performing roles in life, poor concentration

11. When a client is experiencing a crisis, what is the best rationale for the nurse identifying client strengths?

(1) It allows the nurse to better determine the nursing diagnosis.

(2) It helps the nurse understand the client's unique personality.

(3) The nurse can better educate the client if education is based on assessment of strengths.

(4) Reinforcing the client's strengths will aid in coping.

12. The psychiatric nurse hears shouting in the day room and finds a client threatening to kick the television set because the other clients in the room have refused to change the channel. The nurse intervenes by instructing other clients to leave the area. To protect herself while using deescalating measures for the client, the nurse would

(1) position herself between the exit door and the client

(2) stand within an arm's length of the client

(3) stand next to the client with hands at side

(4) sit in a chair next to the client

ANSWER KEY

1. The answer is (2). The definition of a developmental crisis is a crisis that occurs in response to a particular transition from one stage of maturation to another in the life cycle. Puberty marks the transition from childhood to adolescence. An adventitious crisis occurs in response to severe trauma or disaster. A situational crisis occurs in response to sudden, unexpected events in an individual's life. Puberty is neither sudden nor unexpected; it is a normal transition. The response of answer choice **(4)** is not a type of crisis.

2. The answer is (3). It is important for the nurse to assess the individual's perception of the crisis and the events preceding the crisis situation. It is the individual's perception of a problem that determines the crisis. Determining the social support system is important; however, this assessment would occur following the description of the problem. Crisis intervention best occurs in logical, problem-solving sequence and therefore problem description would be the first step. The nurse calling the family to discuss the problem or referring the client to a bereavement support group are interventions that may or may not be appropriate, depending on the client's perception of the problem.

3. The answer is (3). Balancing factors include situational supports available to the client. Other balancing factors include the client having a realistic (rather than distorted) perception of the crisis and having coping mechanisms that are available to alleviate anxiety. The age and physical health status of the individual are factors that may or may not be influential in predicting outcomes for an individual client; they are not considered balancing factors. The type of crisis event would not be a balancing factor. The individual's realistic perception of a specific crisis would be the important determination.

4. The answer is (3). The problem-solving method is used in a systematic manner as part of crisis intervention. The behavioral approach or the nondirective approach would not be selected as part of crisis intervention. Although a supportive approach (eg, supporting client strengths) is part of crisis intervention, the overall method guiding the nurse is the problem-solving approach.

5. The answer is (2). The nurse works as a member of a health team and therefore needs to collaborate with other professionals in helping the individual resolve the crisis. The nurse may assist the client and may also teach the client; however, the question is asking for the nurse's role as a team member. The nurse may or may not be in a managerial role on the team.

6. The answer is (4). Crisis intervention is designed to enable the individual, group, or community to return to the precrisis state of equilibrium as soon as possible by resolving immediate problem(s). Analyzing problems in life-style choices and improving weaknesses in personal development are goals that would be more appropriate for a longer-term therapeutic intervention, in which the focus is not on immediate problem solutions but on insight development. Although new adaptive measures may be learned as a result of a crisis intervention approach, this is not the goal.

7. The answer is (3). The client's feeling of self-blame is a response to the rape-trauma crisis. This is not a realistic perception of the event and, therefore, the nurse points out reality (ie, telling the victim that the rapist is responsible). The responses in answer choices **(1)** and **(2)** would serve to reinforce the client's perception that her own behavior was a cause of the rape. Because this is not true, the nurse needs to reinforce the reality of this situation. The response in answer choice **(4)** avoids the client's distress and is nonsupportive to the situation.

8. The answer is (4). The nurse is using the intervention of responding to underlying feelings (ie, frustration) as part of the therapeutic approach to a client who is angry. This approach will help to deescalate anger. The client is not yet at the point of acting-out anger in a physical manner, and therefore calling the security force would be premature. The goal would be for the nurse to help the client deescalate rather than having security intervene. Defending the physician is inappropriate in this situation. This response would further escalate the client's anger. It is important to respond to the client's underlying feelings. If the nurse firmly tells the client not to shout and to be patient, the client is likely to see this as nonsupportive and authoritarian. The client would likely continue to escalate the anger level.

9. The answer is (2). The nurse uses principles of Maslow's hierarchy of needs in determining priority for intervention. Therefore, it is most essential that the nurse make immediate provisions for the client to eat, because this basic need is currently unmet. All of the remaining interventions would be appropriate during crisis intervention; however, providing for the client's nutrition is the priority.

10. The answer is (4). The client who is in crisis has difficulty performing usual roles in life because of the acute distress experienced. Somatic symptoms and poor concentration are also common because of the influence of the physiologic stress response. All of the remaining symptoms would commonly occur with the onset of a mental illness. They are not typical of the response of an individual to a crisis.

11. The answer is (4). An important principle of crisis intervention is the strengthening and supporting of healthy aspects of an individual's functioning. This is important because the client needs to resolve the crisis and individual strengths aid coping. The remaining responses would be correct as general statements of rationale for a nurse assessing client strengths. However, in the situation of a crisis, the best rationale for the nurse identifying strengths is to aid in coping and therefore resolving crisis.

12. The answer is (1). The nurse stands between the client and the exit door to allow for quick exit from the area if the client attempts physical aggression. The client can easily reach out and physically harm the nurse. Standing within an arm's length of the client would not be self-protective. Standing or sitting next to the client could be misinterpreted as a threat and the client may lash out.

13

Treatment Modalities: Group Therapy

Definitions

A. Group. A group is a collection of individuals whose association is based on shared common interests, values, goals, or purpose.

B. Group dynamics are the underlying forces working to produce behavior patterns in groups. These forces include group roles, stages of group development, and group norms.

C. Group process is the meaning of verbal and nonverbal interactions within group and includes:

1. Content of communication (ie, what is said verbally)
2. Relationships among members
3. Seating arrangements
4. Speaking patterns or tones
5. Body language and gestures
6. Group themes, which may be overtly or covertly expressed

D. Therapeutic groups. These groups focus on group relations, interactions among members, and here-and-now issues in living and behaving (eg, relationship conflicts, problems coping with one's job, health problems).

E. Group psychotherapy. In this group, the focus is on encouraging members to analyze and improve interpersonal functioning. A specific theoretical framework may be used in conducting these groups. (See Chapter 2 for discussion of these theoretical frameworks). Some common frameworks may include:

1. Psychoanalytic group therapy
2. Interpersonal group therapy
3. Cognitive-behavioral group therapy

II. **Group Dynamics**

A. Groups can be curative. Yalom (1985) identified 11 curative factors that individuals can achieve through interpersonal interactions within the group (Display 13-1).

DISPLAY 13-1. **Curative Factors in Groups as Identified by Yalom (1985)**

1. Installation of hope: belief that problems can be solved
2. Universality of experience: support by others with similar problem
3. Information imparted; knowledge shared
4. Altruism: concern and support for others
5. Corrective experience of primary family group: re-experience and resolve early conflicts
6. Development of socialization: learn and develop new skills
7. Initiative behaviors: role modeling
8. Interpersonal learning: perceptions of self by members
9. Group cohesiveness: sense of belonging
10. Catharsis: sharing positive and negative feelings
11. Existential factors: self-direction of one's life

B. **Development.** Groups proceed in typical stages of development.
   1. **Orientation stage.** In this stage, member anxiety may be high, superficial sharing occurs, expectations of group are established, and group norms are specified.
   2. **Working stage.** In this stage, members increase their self-disclosure, develop cohesiveness, and work productively on goals or purpose of group.
   3. **Termination stage.** In this stage, members share feelings of sadness or loss, may reexperience initial anxiety, and summarize group experience.
C. **Group roles.** Groups typically have roles that members play within the group. These roles can overlap and change among members, depending on the situation. They may also be helpful or impede group.
   1. The **initiator** suggests innovative ideas and starts interactions.
   2. The **coordinator** organizes and integrates the progress of the group.
   3. The **evaluator** appraises group performance.
   4. The **information seeker** elicits facts.
   5. The **gatekeeper** screens input and maintains open communication.
   6. The **encourager** praises and accepts.
   7. The **harmonizer** maintains peace through compromise and alternatives.
   8. The **commentator** processes the group interactions.
   9. The **blocker** inhibits group advancement.
   10. The **recognition seeker** seeks self-praise.
   11. The **monopolizer** controls by endless talking.
   12. The **self-confessor** discloses personal information inappropriately.
D. **Group norms.** The group norms refer to implicit or explicit rules of conduct defining member behavior.
   1. **Productive norms** (eg, agreeing that all members' opinions are valued, only one member speaking at a time) will enhance group function.

2. **Nonproductive norms** (eg, not allowing disagreements or accepting absenteeism and tardiness) will inhibit group function.

E. **Leadership.** The leadership of groups can be shared (eg, by co-leaders or co-therapists), or the leader can be one individual. The following are commonly identified leadership styles (Table 13-1).

1. Authoritarian
2. Democratic
3. Laissez-faire

F. **Setting.** Group therapy can occur in both inpatient and outpatient community settings. Brief inpatient stays and managed care directives provide a financial incentive for using group methods of treatment.

G. **Role of the nurse.** In group therapy, the role of the nurse is a function of the educational level and experience of the nurse. The American Nurses Association (ANA) has set standards for specific roles of nurses working with groups.

1. The psychiatric-mental health generalist registered nurse works with therapy groups on a problem representing an immediate difficulty related to health or well-being (eg, medication teaching groups, stress management groups) (ANA, 1994).

2. The psychiatric-mental health clinical specialist or nurse practitioner works in the role of group therapist, using her knowledge of behavior at the interpersonal, intrapersonal, and group levels (ANA, 1994).

TABLE 13-1
Leadership Behavior and Its Effect on Group Function

LEADERSHIP STYLE	CHARACTERISTICS OF LEADER	EFFECT ON GROUP MEMBERS
Authoritarian	Exerts total control Makes all decisions Discourages members sharing Task oriented	Can become frustrated and angry May scapegoat members May exhibit passive-aggressive behavior (eg, absenteeism)
Democratic	Encourages member involvement Fosters collaboration, cohesiveness Promotes open communication	Feel individual is valuable Develop loyalty Work productively
Laissez-faire	Functions as resource/consultant Provides minimal direction Promotes minimal interpersonal interactions	Feel lost or without direction Become disorganized May be apathetic

III. Types of Groups

A. Psychotherapy groups

B. Therapeutic groups

1. **Support groups** provide acceptance and empathy for members, reinforce existing strengths, and reduce anxiety. Some examples of these groups include post-traumatic stress groups, cancer support groups, and Recovery, Inc.

2. **Activity groups** (eg, art, music, and dance groups) facilitate communication and interaction.
   b. These groups encourage expression of feelings in ways other than verbally.
   c. These groups enhance self-esteem.

3. **Education groups** (eg, medication management, stress management)
   a. These groups provide information on topics of interest.
   b. They empower self-management of behaviors.

4. **Socialization groups** (eg, clubs, hobby groups) help members improve interaction skills and plan activities for mutual enjoyment.

5. **Reality-orientation groups** (eg, current events group)
   a. These groups assist clients who have cognitive impairments.
   b. They use a variety of environmental reminders (eg, clocks, television, radio, newspapers, magazines).

6. **Community meeting groups** (eg, inpatient groups on a particular psychiatric unit)
   a. These groups explore common concerns and focus on problems in group living situations.
   b. They discuss and clarify rules, requests, and privileges.
   c. They encourage self-direction by client(s).

C. Self-help groups. Members (rather than mental health professional leadership) run the group.

1. Members share the same problem (eg, an addiction), which is the chief focus in the group work.

2. These groups offer strategies for coping.

IV. NURSING PROCESS OVERVIEW FOR Group Therapy

A. Assessment

1. Assess the individual client behaviors in the group.

2. Assess group processes, noting factors such as:
   a. Seating preferences
   b. Communication patterns (eg, who talks, to whom communication is directed, how often an individual speaks)
   c. Nonverbal patterns of communication (eg, tone of voice, body language)
   d. Response to group norms
   e. Roles assumed by members

B. Nursing diagnoses

1. Recognize the effects of behavior of group and self on group members. For example, a member may realize what behavior of others will trigger an emotional response in self.
2. Analyze group dynamics and group processes.
3. Determine individualized nursing diagnoses for client(s) within group, including but not limited to:
   a. Anxiety
   b. Communication, impaired verbal
   c. Coping, individual, ineffective
   d. Decisional conflict (specify)
   e. Health maintenance, altered
   f. Knowledge deficit (specify)
   g. Post-trauma response
   h. Self-esteem disturbance
   i. Social interaction, impaired
   j. Therapeutic regimen: individual, ineffective management

C. Planning and outcome identification

1. Work with group members in setting realistic goals.
2. Establish desired outcome criteria for group and individual members.
   a. Members will participate in group activities.
   b. Members will demonstrate concern for individual members of the group.
   c. Members will focus on the identified purpose related to the specific type and task of group.
   d. Members will improve communication and socialization skills.
   e. Members will learn effective management of therapeutic regimens.
   f. Members will demonstrate improved individual coping behaviors.

D. Implementation

1. During **orientation phase**
   a. The nurse should be directive and active in establishing the contract for meeting schedules, purpose, and goals for the group.
   b. The nurse should encourage open communication and feedback from all members.
   c. The nurse should discuss and establish group norms of behavior.
2. During **working phase**
   a. The nurse should assume the appropriate role as leader, depending on the type of group.
   b. The nurse should listen, observe, and provide therapeutic feedback.
   c. The nurse should comment on behavior that enhances or hinders group progress.
   d. The nurse should recognize conflicts and discuss them in an open manner.
   e. The nurse should foster self-esteem building.
   f. The nurse should focus on here-and-now issues and problems of members.
   g. The nurse should provide appropriate information in educational group.
   h. The nurse should ensure participation of all members.

3. During **termination phase**

   a. The nurse should assume a supportive role in assisting members to identify and discuss termination feelings.

   b. The nurse should encourage evaluation of group and individual members' progress.

   c. The nurse should refer those whose needs were unmet by the group for further evaluation and treatment.

E. Outcome evaluation

   1. Group as a whole

   a. The group exhibits shared allegiance and responsibility.

   b. The group demonstrates active participation by all members.

   c. The group accomplishes the goals or purpose of the group.

   d. The group communicates among members and not just between leaders and members.

   2. Individual members

   a. Individual members demonstrate use of communication skills.

   b. Individual members apply problem-solving skills to one's own life.

   c. Individual members report improved coping and behavior.

   d. Individual members state effective ways to manage therapeutic regimen.

STUDY QUESTIONS

1. During a support group meeting, one of the members continually interrupts when others are talking and offers solutions to problems addressed. Which of the following is the *best* way for the nurse leader to intervene?
   (1) by asking the group to address this behavior
   (2) by ignoring the interruption
   (3) by telling the client who is speaking to proceed
   (4) by reviewing the established group norms

2. The nurse group leader assesses communication and relationships among members, seating arrangements, and group themes. In doing this, which of the following is the nurse leader analyzing?
   (1) group behavior
   (2) group norms
   (3) group process
   (4) group roles

3. The nurse assesses that a number of parents in a child-care clinic have misconceptions about child development in relationship to discipline. In which of the following types of groups would the nurse address this issue?
   (1) an activity group
   (2) an education group
   (3) a self-help group
   (4) a support group

4. Clients involved in a psychotherapy group identify negative cognitions and work toward changing thoughts in order to influence behaviors. Which of the following is the theoretical framework of this group psychotherapy?
   (1) cognitive-behavioral framework
   (2) interpersonal framework
   (3) psychoanalytic framework
   (4) self-help framework

5. The community nurse is working with a support group and notes a high rate of absenteeism and minimal participation by members. Which of the following leadership styles is the nurse most likely using in this situation?
   (1) authoritarian
   (2) democratic
   (3) laissez-faire
   (4) progressive

6. When working with a caregiver support group in the community, the nurse establishes expectations of the group and discusses norms of group behavior. Which of the following stages is this group in?
   (1) orientation
   (2) reorganization
   (3) working
   (4) termination

7. The effectiveness of a therapy group during termination needs to be evaluated. Which of the following would be the *best* way to determine this?
   (1) by asking members to discuss this
   (2) by eliciting the opinion of the leader
   (3) by measuring members' participation in problem-solving
   (4) by referring to adherence of group norms

8. Community meetings are held as part of the therapeutic milieu approach on an inpatient psychiatric unit. The purpose of these meetings would be
   (1) to encourage expression of feelings in ways other than verbal
   (2) to provide information on topics of interest
   (3) to focus on issues arising from group living
   (4) to provide direction from the treatment team

9. The nurse group leader of a support group in a partial hospitalization community program notes that the group atmosphere has become negative and nonaccepting of members. Which of the following nursing interventions would be best?
    (1) asking members to be more accepting
    (2) ignoring this observation until the group decides to discuss it
    (3) selecting the most prominent offenders for private discussion
    (4) sharing this observation with group

10. The nurse initiates a medication management teaching group for clients recently prescribed antidepressant medications. Which of the following would be the most appropriate nursing diagnosis for the individuals in this group?
    (1) Anxiety
    (2) Decisional conflict (taking antidepressants)
    (3) Coping: individual, ineffective
    (4) Therapeutic regimen: individual, ineffective management

ANSWER KEY

1. The answer is (1). Assisting the group to look at this behavior helps members to explore and resolve disruptive interpersonal actions and facilitates group process. Ignoring this behavior would miss an opportunity for the group to examine and resolve problems in the group. Telling the client who is speaking to proceed or reviewing the established group norms would hinder group development because the nurse is taking control.

2. The answer is (3). Group process encompasses the verbal and nonverbal interactions within the group, which are represented by communication, seating, and content of group themes. Group behavior is a part of group process. Group norms refer to implicit or explicit rules of conduct defining members' behavior. Group roles are various aspects of behavior that individuals may assume within a group.

3. The answer is (2). An education group is best designed to impart information on topics of common interest to a group. Activity groups encourage nonverbal expression of feelings and would be inappropriate for this situation. Self help groups are member run rather than planned by mental health team members. The parents in this situation have misconceptions that can best be addressed by education. Support groups are designed to provide acceptance and empathy for members, not to impart identified knowledge.

4. The answer is (1). Cognitive behavior groups use this theoretical framework as described. Interpersonal group framework would involve emphasis on interpersonal sharing and fostering communication between members to improve functions in interpersonal situations. Psychoanalytic group framework would involve development of insight into problem areas through examination of early developmental issues. Self-help group framework is member run and involves sharing specific problems common to all members and offering suggested solutions.

5. The answer is (1). When the leader style is authoritarian, the group may demonstrate passive-aggressive behavior, such as absenteeism and minimal participation. Democratic leadership leads to loyalty and productive group work. Laissez-faire leadership may contribute to disorganized group functioning and apathy. Answer choice (4) does not describe a leadership style.

6. The answer is (1). The orientation phase of a group sets expectations of purpose or goals and specifies group norms. Reorganization does not describe a stage of group development. Working and termination are other phases of group development consisting of productive work (working stage) and summarizing group experiences (termination stage).

7. The answer is (3). Evaluation of effectiveness of a group would include the determination of members' participation in the problem-solving process. Groups that are effective will have accomplished this goal. Asking the members to discuss effectiveness would be appropriate during the working phase of the group, but it would not provide evaluation data. Although eliciting the opinion of the leader is valuable, measuring participation would provide objective data. Adhering to group norms is a part of the group process that is best determined during the working phase of the group.

8. The answer is (3). Community encompasses both clients and staff, and meetings are held on a regular basis to provide a means of focus on important issues related to living together in a group situation. Encouraging expression of feelings in ways other than verbal describes the purpose of an activity group. Providing information on topics of interest describes the purpose of an educational group. Providing direction from the treatment team is not consistent with a community approach, in which self-direction is encouraged.

9. The answer is (4). The nurse would facilitate group process by commenting on behavior that hinders group functioning. Asking members to be more accepting or selecting the most prominent offenders for private discussion are not correct, because in these cases the nurse is assuming responsibility for directing a solution to the problem. Ignoring the negative, nonaccepting atmosphere until the group decides to discuss it avoids dealing with an important issue to group functioning.

10. The answer is (4). *Therapeutic regimen: individual, ineffective management* is the appropriate nursing diagnosis for individuals who participate in group learning about treatment. *Anxiety* and *Decisional conflict* are nursing diagnoses that do not apply to this situation. There is no evidence that the clients in this situation are anxious or conflicted about taking antidepressants. *Coping: individual, ineffective* is a nursing diagnosis but it would not be the focus of the group.

14 Treatment Modalities: Family Therapy

I. Overview

A. **Family.** A family is a social system composed of two or more persons who coexist and have strong emotional attachments, regular interaction, and shared concerns and responsibilities.

1. A **nuclear family** is composed of a mother and father (married or unmarried) and their child or children (by birth or adoption).
2. An **extended family** is a broad group of people related by blood and marriage, including grandparents, uncles, aunts, and cousins.
3. A **single-parent family** is composed of a parent and child or children (by birth or adoption).
4. A **blended family** is a married or unmarried couple, one or both of whom were married previously, and includes his, her, or their child or children.
5. An **alternative family** is composed of persons with or without blood or marital ties who live together to achieve common goals.

B. **System.** A system is a set of elements that have reciprocal interactions or relationships. The family is considered a system.

1. A **suprasystem** is a broad system composed of multiple smaller systems (eg, neighborhood, community, cultural group, nation).
2. A **subsystem** is composed of smaller subsets of the family (eg, siblings, parents, parent-child, intergenerational relatives).
3. **Boundaries** are parameters defining who is inside and outside the system. Boundaries may be **open** (allowing free interchange), **closed** (restricting interaction), or **diffuse** (unclear). Diffuse boundaries may change the definition of who is inside or outside the system.
4. **Homeostasis** is maintenance of system continuity, constancy, and equilibrium. All systems, including family systems, strive to maintain homeostasis.

II. Concepts: Family Systems

A. **Members of interdependent family systems**

1. Change in any one part of a family system affects all other parts and the system as a whole.
2. Roles, behaviors, and relationships among family members are maintained in relative constancy.

3. **Coalitions** (eg, a dyad between two people) formed among members of the system may become problematic. For example, an intergenerational dyad may hinder intergenerational communication.

4. **Triangles** are considered an emotional configuration involving three family members or two family members and an issue (eg, a conflictual relationship between spouses can be calmed by pulling in a child to deflect attention away from the spousal conflict).

B. **Differentiation** (the process of becoming an individual and developing autonomy) occurs within the family system.

1. A **low level of differentiation** is characterized by a person being governed by emotions, acting impulsively, and having difficulty sharing and giving in a relationship.

2. A **moderate level of differentiation** is characterized by less emotional functioning; however, the individual may tend to view the world in "black or white" or "either/or" terms. Relationships may be lasting, but in times of anxiety, fusion or loss of self-functioning may occur.

3. A **high level of differentiation** is characterized by a person having a balance between emotions and intellect. The individual views the world in its contextual nature, with an understanding regarding multiple perspectives. Relationships are characterized by mutual respect for the uniqueness and differences of others.

C. **Relationships within a family may be characterized by the following:**

1. **Mutual respect** and encouragement for differences and uniqueness of each individual

2. **Enmeshment, or fusion,** which is overinvolvement among members with the expectation that the individuals in a family think and act alike

3. **Disengagement,** which is underinvolvement among members and estrangement of individuals in the family

4. **Schismatic parental relationship,** which occurs when overt conflict exists and the child or children must "take sides"

5. **Skewed parental relationship,** which occurs when one spouse is dysfunctional, leading to an imbalance of roles and functioning in family

D. **Developmental stages.** Families proceed through predictable developmental stages corresponding to the life cycle. Each phase may be characterized by a particular set of adjustments that can be stressful for the family. The stages include:

1. Coupling or marriage (relationship negotiation)
2. Childbearing (adjusting to parenting)
3. Preschool-age children (coping with toddlers)
4. School-age children (interacting with wider social system)
5. Teenage children (coping with independence)
6. Empty nest (spousal relationship renegotiation)
7. Retirement (redefining self)
8. Aging (handling losses)

E. Functioning in society. Families function within the larger societal system and perform the following tasks:

1. **Physical maintenance of members,** including provision of food, shelter, and clothing
2. **Physical and emotional resource allocation,** including allocation of expenses, goods, space, and emotional support
3. **Division of labor,** including financial responsibilities, household management, and child rearing
4. **Socialization of members,** including physical, emotional, social, and spiritual guidance
5. **Entry and release of members,** including birth, adoption, moving out, visitation, living-in
6. **Order,** including conforming to family or societal rules, standards, and norms
7. **Interaction with larger systems,** including interacting with church, school, neighborhood, community, and society
8. **Cultural transmission,** including that of values, beliefs, roles and functioning, and traditions

F. Characteristics. Families can be characterized as functional or dysfunctional in terms of common characteristics (Table 14-1).

III. Family Therapy

A. Goal. The goal of family therapy is to bring about beneficial change in individual members by focusing on the family as a whole.

B. Objectives

1. Use the family's strengths to assist the family in identifying problems, setting goals for change, and solving problems.
2. Foster open communication among family members.
3. Assist one or more family members to differentiate.
4. Use a historical view of family membership and functioning across generations to understand current problems.
   a. Take a family history.
   b. Construct a family genogram, which is a pictorial representation of the family over time and includes births, deaths, marriages, and other significant events (Fig. 14-1).

C. Types

1. **Family systems therapy**
   a. Murray Bowen (1978) is the theorist responsible for family systems therapy.
   b. **Approach.** Assist the individual(s) within the family to avoid being dominated by emotional reactivity and to achieve a higher level of differentiation of self.

TABLE 14-1
Comparison of Functional and Dysfunctional Family Systems*

CHARACTERISTICS	FUNCTIONAL FAMILY	DYSFUNCTIONAL FAMILY
Role definitions	Clearly defined as to who does what, when, where, and how	Unclear definitions result in important tasks not being accomplished
	Flexible in response to need; members can fill in or take over as necessary	Rigid in response to need; unable to fill in or take over when necessary
Boundaries	Clearly defined among family subsystems as well as suprasystems	Unclear or diffuse; difficult to determine subsystems
	Open boundaries encourage multiple exchanges from family to larger systems	Closed boundaries discourage interactions from family with larger social systems
Belief systems	Beliefs are supported by facts and reality	Beliefs are based on stereotypes, myths, and biases
	Family members are able to identify and discuss differences	Family members may not be cognizant of belief patterns and are not open to discussion
Communication	Clear, direct, congruent verbal and nonverbal communication	Confusing, indirect communications; may be incongruent verbal and nonverbal communication
		May have double-bind patterns; recipient is a victim and cannot win (eg, "Do what I tell you— be more independent.")
Differentiation	Encourages individuation of members	Discourages individuation of members
	Respects differences	Is threatened by differences
Resolving problems	Defines and names problems, explores alternative solutions, evaluates solutions	Unable to define problems and cannot generate alternative solutions
	Uses necessary resources for assistance	Ineffective use of resources for assistance

These differences are illustrated for clarification purposes; any given family may have aspects of both functional and dysfunctional characteristics.

2. **Structural therapy**
   a. Salvador Minuchin (1974) is the theorist responsible for structural therapy.
   b. **Approach.** Encourage change in the family organization to modify each family member's position in the group.
3. **Interactional therapy**
   a. Virginia Satir (1964) is the theorist responsible for development of interactional therapy.

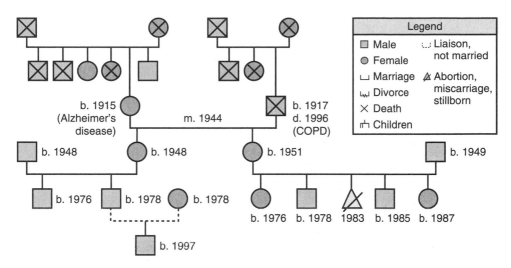

FIGURE 14-1
Family genogram.

    b. **Approach.** Identify invisible, unspoken laws governing family relationships and use communication theory to promote improvement in relationships.

D. Role of the nurse in family therapy

    1. Psychiatric-Mental Health Nurse Specialist (APRN or CNS). The nurse prepared at this level can function as a family therapist, using family theory to provide services such as family diagnosis or psychotherapeutic intervention (ANA, 1994).

    2. Psychiatric-Mental Health Nurse Generalist (RN,C). The nurse at this level typically applies the nursing process to families, including:

      a. Assessment of family roles, functions, and needs as well as establishing standard North American Nursing Diagnosis Association (NANDA) nursing diagnoses

      b. Education of families regarding illnesses, resources, and treatment regimens as well as working with members to provide effective illness management

      c. Use of techniques of therapeutic communication to assist families to improve communication

      d. Collaboration with other health team members to enhance family functioning and improve the health of it members; this collaboration includes referrals, acting as case manager, and team membership (Frisch, 1998)

 IV. **NURSING PROCESS OVERVIEW FOR**
Family Therapy

A. Assessment (Table 14-2)

    1. Determine membership in family.

    2. Identify family developmental stage as well as internal and external stressors.

TABLE 14-2
Key Nursing Assessment Questions for Families

QUESTIONS	PROVIDES DATA ABOUT
"Who are the members of your family?"*	Family boundaries Family genogram
"Where do the family members live?"	Shared and nonshared living arrangements
"To what particular culture or ethnic group does your family belong?"	Cultural and ethnic identification and practices
"Are there any particular health practices or customs that are important to your family?"	
"Who provides significant support to members of your family?"	Internal and external resources
"What would you say are the special strengths of your family?"	Family perception of strengths
"Describe the usual communication patterns of your family."	Communication patterns
"Describe the current issues or problems affecting your family."	Family perception of problems

If applicable, collect data for family genogram (see Figure 14-1).

3. Determine ethnic and cultural beliefs and practices relative to health.
4. Review significant aspects of the family history.
5. Collect data for construction of family genogram.
6. Identify family strengths, support systems, and communication patterns.
7. Determine the family perception of the problem.

B. **Nursing diagnoses**
   1. Analyze characteristics of the family as functional or dysfunctional.
   2. Analyze internal and external stressors on family functioning in relation to current problem(s).
   3. Determine nursing diagnoses applicable to the family, including:
      a. Family coping: ineffective: compromised
      b. Family coping: ineffective: disabling
      c. Family coping: potential for growth
      d. Family processes, altered

C. **Planning and outcome identification**
   1. Work with family members to establish realistic goals.
   2. Establish desired outcome criteria.
      a. Family members will use resources both within and outside the family to cope with problems.
      b. Family members will communicate clearly, using congruent verbal and nonverbal messages.

    c. Family members will assume clearly defined roles and responsibilities according to the situation.

    d. Family members will encourage individual growth and autonomy of members.

D. Implementation

1. Develop an alliance with family based on trust.
2. Remain neutral and objective; avoid taking sides.
3. Focus on here-and-now problems and relationships.
4. Model clear, congruent verbal and nonverbal communication.
5. Assist the family to define "who owns the problem" and who is responsible for resolution.
6. Assist the family to develop effective communication skills, such as active listening and the use of "I" messages.

    a. For example, instead of saying "You should be more responsible about being on time," the statement, "When I waited for an hour and you weren't home, I was really worried," is an "I" message and is preferable.

    b. An "I" message lets the other person know exactly how their behavior affected the well-being of the speaker. This type of message is less likely to cause anger and defensiveness because it encourages each person to be responsible for their own feelings. "You" messages are generally accusatory and may create conflict.

7. Support and enhance existing coping skills of family.
8. Provide education regarding:

    a. The biologic nature and signs and symptoms of mental illness

    b. Rationale for treatment recommendations

    c. Monitoring psychotropic medications

    d. Problem-solving techniques

9. Refer the family to a qualified family therapist when problems are beyond the scope of nursing intervention at the generalist level.
10. Collaborate with mental health team and family regarding recommendations for treatment and follow-up.
11. Encourage family members to take time for leisure pursuits and maintenance of community involvements to prevent caregiver burnout.

E. Outcome evaluation

1. Family members successfully use available resources for coping with problems.
2. Family members demonstrate clear, congruent communication.
3. Family members fulfill roles and responsibilities.
4. Family members demonstrate autonomous, differentiated behaviors.

STUDY QUESTIONS

1. The school guidance counselor refers a family with an 8-year-old child to the mental health clinic because of the child's frequent fighting in school and truancy. Which of the following data would be a priority to the nurse doing the initial family assessment?
   (1) the child's performance in school
   (2) family education and work history
   (3) family perception of current problem
   (4) the teacher's attempts to solve problem

2. When interacting with a mother and father who are divorcing, the nurse notes that the major theme of parental disagreement is the behavior of their 13-year-old daughter. The father states that the daughter is irresponsible and lacks respect for his authority, whereas the mother cites the belief that a strict, authoritarian father rules the daughter. Which of the following family systems concepts is this situation an example of?
   (1) differentiation of child
   (2) enmeshed relationship of parents
   (3) skewed relationship of parents
   (4) triangulation of child

3. A 19-year-old client is admitted to a psychiatric inpatient facility for treatment of major depression. The nurse learns that the client's father has been on total disability for 3 months since an accident and that the mother has recently experienced relapse of a chronic alcohol problem. The nursing diagnosis established is *Family coping: ineffective-compromised related to situation stressors*. Which of the following is the most appropriate goal (outcome criterion) for intervention?

   (1) Establish independence of the client from the family system.
   (2) Ensure the mother's compliance with alcohol treatment.
   (3) Identify ownership of problem as belonging to parents.
   (4) Use family and external resources to cope with problems.

4. The parents of a client with schizophrenia express feelings of responsibility and blame for the client's problems. Which of the following would the nurse providing family education do?
   (1) Acknowledge parents' responsibility.
   (2) Explain the biologic nature of schizophrenia.
   (3) Provide referral to a support group.
   (4) Teach the parents various ways they must change.

5. The nurse collecting family assessment data asks, "Who is in your family and where do they live?" Which of the following is the nurse attempting to identify?
   (1) boundaries
   (2) ethnicity
   (3) relationships
   (4) triangles

6. The school nurse is conducting a class on parent-child relationships to encourage functional family development. Which of the following things would the nurse teach the class about family resolution of conflict situations?
   (1) Children need to be encouraged to accept parental advice.
   (2) Conflict generally does not arise in functional families.
   (3) Discussion of conflict in a clear, direct way is important.
   (4) Solutions to conflicts should be provided by a neutral party.

7. According to family systems theory, which of the following best describes the process of differentiation?
   (1) cooperative action among members of a family
   (2) development of autonomy within the family
   (3) incongruent messages wherein the recipient is a victim
   (4) maintenance of system continuity or equilibrium

8. A nurse is interacting with a family that is composed of a mother, a father, and a hospitalized adolescent who has a diagnosis of alcohol abuse. The nurse agrees with the adolescent's view about family rules. Which of the following implementations is most appropriate?
   (1) The nurse should align with the adolescent who is the family scapegoat.
   (2) The nurse should encourage parents to adopt more realistic rules.
   (3) The nurse should encourage the adolescent to comply with parental rules.
   (4) The nurse should remain objective and encourage mutual negotiation of issues.

9. A 16-year-old has returned home following hospitalization for treatment of anorexia nervosa. The family nurse doing a home visit is told by the parents that their child has always done everything to please them and they cannot understand the current stubbornness about eating. The nurse analyzes this family situation as characteristic of
   (1) differentiation
   (2) disengagement
   (3) enmeshment
   (4) scapegoating

10. A family is in treatment with a family therapist for multiple problems. The nurse collaborating with the therapist learns that members of the family expect that everyone should think alike about important issues and discourage disagreement. The role of the nurse when interacting with this family would include:
   (1) assisting each member to use "I" communication messages
   (2) encouraging members to comply with therapist recommendations
   (3) determining how family perceives the problems
   (4) providing literature on effective family functioning

ANSWER KEY

1. The answer is (3). The family's perception of the problem is essential because change in any one part of a family system affects all other parts and the system as a whole. Each member of the family has been affected by the current problems related to the school system and the nurse would be interested in this here-and-now data. The child's performance in school and the teacher's attempts to solve the problem are relevant and may be collected; however, priority would be given to the family's perception of the problem. The family education and work history may be relevant, but would not have priority.

2. The answer is (4). The concept of triangles in a family system refers to the emotional configuration involving three family members or two members and an issue. In this situation, the conflict between the spouses is handled by deflecting attention away from spouses and onto the child. Differentiation is the process of developing autonomy within the family system. Enmeshed relationship between spouses refers to overinvolvement with the expectation that everyone in the family think and act alike. A skewed relationship between spouses refers to one spouse who is dysfunctional and therefore roles are imbalanced.

3. The answer is (4). There are several problems currently facing this family, including the father's disability, the mother's relapse, and the child's hospitalization. Mobilizing and using resources from both inside the family (strengths) and outside the family (support systems) will constitute the most appropriate outcome for the nursing diagnosis. Autonomy or differentiation of self takes place within the family system and does not mean that independence from the family system occurs. Ensuring the mother's compliance with alcohol treatment and identifying ownership of the problem as belonging to the parents are incorrect responses, because each member of the family is involved in the current problems.

4. The answer is (2). The parents are feeling responsible and this inappropriate self-blame can be limited by supplying them with the facts about the biologic basis of schizophrenia. Acknowledging the parents' responsibility is neither accurate nor helpful to the parents to reinforce blame. Support groups are useful; however, the nurse needs to handle the parents' self-blame directly instead of making a referral for this problem. Teaching the parents various ways they must change would reinforce the parental assumption of blame; although parents can learn about schizophrenia and what is helpful and not helpful, the approach suggested in this option implies the parents' behavior is at fault.

5. The answer is (1). Family boundaries are parameters defining who is inside and outside the system. The best method of obtaining this information is asking the family who they consider to be members. The question the nurse asks would not elicit information regarding ethnic or cultural data, and different questions would need to be asked to elicit information related to the nature of the family relationship.

6. The answer is (3). In families, the ability to discuss difficult issues openly among members reflects healthy behavior. Communication needs to be reciprocal between parents and children. Healthy, functional families are defined not by the absence of conflict but by the manner in which it is handled. The family needs to work out solutions, not have solutions provided by another.

7. The answer is (2). Differentiation is the process of becoming a self, developing autonomy while staying in contact with the family system. Cooperative action among family members does not refer to process of differentiation, although individuals who have a high level of differentiation would be able to accomplish cooperative action. Incongruent messages in which the recipient is a victim describes double-bind communication. Maintenance of system continuity or equilibrium is homeostasis.

8. The answer is (4). The nurse who wishes to be helpful to the entire family must remain neutral and not take sides. Taking sides in a conflict situation in a family will not encourage negotiation, which is important for problem resolution. If the nurse aligned with the adolescent, then the nurse would be blaming the parents for the child's current problem; this would not help the family problem. If the nurse encouraged the parents to adopt more realistic rules or encouraged the adolescent to comply with parental rules, then the nurse is deciding who is correct and the family does not have the opportunity to come to resolution on their own. Learning to negotiate conflict is a function of a healthy family.

9. The answer is (3). Enmeshment is a fusion or overinvolvement among family members whereby the expectation exists that all members think and act alike. The child who always acts to please parents is an example of how enmeshment affects development. Often, the child who develops anorexia nervosa exerts control only in the area of eating behavior. The remaining answer choice responses are not appropriate to the situation described.

10. The answer is (1). Use of "I" communication messages will allow each member to begin to identify and discuss differences. This process is healthy and will encourage differentiation. The family therapist does not "tell" the family what to do; however, the therapist helps members find solutions to their own problems. Determining how the family perceives the problems is appropriate during assessment and would have been part of the data collection done initially. Literature is helpful in educating the family; however, this situation calls for a nursing action that will stimulate differentiation of members.

15

Treatment Modalities: Somatic Therapies

I. Psychopharmacology: An Overview

A. **Psychotropic (psychoactive) medications** exert their effect in the brain, altering emotions and affecting behaviors. There are two primary mechanisms of action:
   1. Altering amounts of neurotransmitters at the synapse
   2. Binding to specific receptor sites at presynaptic and postsynaptic neurons
B. **Neurotransmitters** are chemical messengers that carry inhibiting or stimulating messages from one neuron to another across the space (synapse) between them.
   1. **Receptor sites** are channels or specially tailored protein molecules located on presynaptic and postsynaptic cell membranes (see Chapter 2).
   2. **Selected neurotransmitters** that can be altered by psychotropic medications include:
      a. **Dopamine,** which is primarily affected by antipsychotics
      b. **Serotonin,** which is primarily affected by antidepressants and antipsychotics
      c. **Norepinephrine,** which is affected by mood-stabilizing agents, antidepressants, antipsychotics, and psychostimulants
      d. **Gamma-aminobutyric acid (GABA),** which is primarily affected by antianxiety agents
      e. **Acetylcholine,** which is affected by anticholinesterase agents, antipsychotics, and antidepressants
C. **Psychotropic medications in the treatment of mental illness**
   1. Many mental illnesses (eg, schizophrenia, depression, anxiety disorder) once thought to be purely psychological have been found to be associated with chemical imbalances of neurotransmitters in the brain.
   2. Psychotropic medications are used to relieve behavioral and emotional symptoms of mental illness.
D. **Electroconvulsive therapy (ECT) in the treatment of mental illness**
   1. ECT is used primarily for clients with depression.
   2. **Procedure**
      a. Short-acting anesthesia is used to induce unconsciousness. The client's vital signs, oxygenation, and cardiac functioning are carefully monitored before, during, and following ECT.

b. An electric current (70 to 150 volts) is applied through the brain for 0.5 to 2 seconds, producing a seizure that lasts 30 to 60 seconds.
c. Following ECT, the client is monitored according to routine postoperative protocols.
3. ECT treatments are administered 2 to 3 times per week for a total of 6 to 12 treatments.

E. **Medicinal herbs in the treatment of mental illness**
1. Two popular over-the-counter herbal preparations are available for clients who choose an alternative method for treating symptoms of mental illness.
a. **St. John's wort** is reported to alleviate mild depression.
b. **Ginkgo biloba** is reported to improve memory.
2. Herbs are currently not regulated in the United States. However, their use has increased dramatically as Americans seek alternatives to traditional medicine.
3. The National Institutes of Health (NIH) is currently (1999–2001) conducting a study to determine the effectiveness of St. John's wort in the treatment of depression (Greenwald, 1998).

II. Antipsychotics (Neuroleptics) (Table 15-1)

A. **Standard antipsychotic agents**
1. **Indications**
a. **Psychotic symptoms** (eg, hallucinations, delusions, paranoid thinking, poor reality contact), which may occur in clients with schizophrenia, bipolar disorders, and cognitive impairment disorders
b. **Acute agitation, rage, and hyperactive states,** which can occur in clients with a variety of mental disorders
c. Treatment of **intractable vomiting, hiccoughs, and vertigo**
2. **Mechanism of action.** Antipsychotics block selected dopamine receptors in the striatal and limbic areas of the brain, an action believed to reduce psychotic symptoms.
a. Antipsychotics also affect other receptors, including those for histamine, serotonin, norepinephrine, and acetylcholine.
b. The effect on these receptors accounts for the multiple side effects.
3. **Pharmacokinetics**
a. The serum is 18 to 40 hours. The drug accumulates in fatty tissue, which accounts for the persistence of the drug's effect when the drug is stopped.
b. A wide variation exists among doses recommended for an individual client. Dosage titration is important for targeting specific changes in an individual client's symptoms.
c. Tolerance does not develop with these drugs.
d. Oral absorption is significantly affected by foods and stomach acidity level. Antipsychotic agents should be taken at least 2 hours after eating and should not be used concurrently with antacids or histamine$_2$ (H$_2$) blocking agents (eg, Cimetidine).

TABLE 15-1
Antipsychotic (Neuroleptic) Drugs

GENERIC	TRADE	USUAL DAILY DOSAGE (ADULT)
High-Potency Typical Neuroleptics*		
Thiothixine	Navane	6–30 mg
Trifluoperazine	Stelazine	2–30 mg
Haloperidol†	Haldol	1–15 mg
Perphenazine	Trilafon	3–24 mg
Fluphenazine†	Prolixin	2.5–20 mg
Moderate-Potency Typical Neuroleptics‡		
Loxapine	Loxitane	25–250 mg
Molindone	Moban	40–225 mg
Mesoridazine	Serentil	30–150 mg
Low-Potency Typical Neuroleptics§		
Chlorpromazine	Thorazine	50–800 mg
Thioridazine	Mellaril	50–800 mg
Chlorprothixene	Taractan	50–400 mg
Atypical Neuroleptics		
Clozapine	Clozaril	300–900 mg
Risperidone	Risperdal	6–16 mg
Pimozide	Orap	2–10 mg
Olanzapine	Zyprexa	10–15 mg
Sertindole	Serlect	15–20 mg
Quetiapine	Seroquel	50–400 mg

*Low-dose range; increased extrapyramidal symptom (EPS) response and seizure risk; low incidence of anticholinergic effects.

†These medications can be given in an oil suspension (decanoate) that is administered intramuscularly and has delayed onset and prolonged action. Administration may be 1 to 2 times weekly or up to 1 time per month.

‡Mild-dose range; moderate EPS response; moderate hypotensive and anticholinergic effects.

§High-dose range, low EPS response; increased sedation, hypotensive, and anticholinergic effects.

4. Use across the lifespan
   a. Antipsychotic agents are prescribed for adults and children. Caution is needed when administering these agents to elderly clients with decreased kidney and liver function, because side effects are intensified. Low doses are recommended for elderly clients.
   b. Not recommended for use during pregnancy and lactation.
5. Contraindications
   a. Known allergic response to any antipsychotics
   b. Central nervous system (CNS) depression
   c. Parkinson disease

d. Blood dyscrasias
e. Hepatic disease
f. Acute narrow angle glaucoma
g. Benign prostatic hypertrophy

6. **Interactions**
   a. There are additive anticholinergic effects when antipsychotics are taken with antihistamines, antidepressants, antiparkinsonian agents, and other drugs with anticholinergic effects.
   b. There are additive hypotensive effects when antipsychotics are taken with other agents that lower blood pressure (eg, beta blockers, calcium channel blockers, antianginal nitrate preparations).
   c. Caffeine and nicotine will interfere with therapeutic effects, and intake of these substances should be minimized (ie, no more than 10 cigarettes or 200 mg of caffeine daily [roughly equal to two cups of coffee]).

7. **Common side effects** (Table 15-2)
   a. Anticholinergic effects, including dry mouth, blurred vision, urinary retention, and constipation
   b. Cardiovascular effects, including postural hypotension and tachycardia
   c. Sedation, drowsiness, and lack of alertness
   d. Photosensitivity, including sunburn and rash
   e. Weight gain
   f. Endocrine changes, including amenorrhea and gynecomastia
   g. Extrapyramidal effects (Table 15-3)

8. **Side effects.** The following are serious but uncommon adverse effects of antipsychotic agents (Table 15-4; see also Table 15-3).
   a. Agranulocytosis (white blood cell level less than 2000)
   b. Acute dystonic reaction, characterized by severe, sudden muscle spasms
   c. Tardive dyskinesia, characterized by involuntary mouth, tongue, and facial movements
   d. Seizures
   e. Hepatotoxicity, which may be characterized by jaundice, nausea, and abdominal pain
   f. Neuroleptic malignant syndrome (NMS), which is a severe reaction that can be fatal (see Table 15-4)

B. **Atypical antipsychotic agents**

1. **Mechanism of action.** Atypical antipsychotics block dopamine receptors in the limbic system and affect serotonin receptors in the cortical areas of the brain.

2. **Advantages over typical antipsychotics**
   a. Atypical antipsychotic agents reduce positive symptoms (eg, hallucinations, delusions) of schizophrenia, but also lessen the negative symptoms (eg, blunted affect, apathy, and social withdrawal).
   b. These agents cause decreased (or no) extrapyramidal system (EPS) effects, because they do not affect dopamine in striatal areas.
   c. These agents do not cause tardive dyskinesia.

TABLE 15-2
Managing Common Side Effects of Psychotropic Medications

SIDE EFFECTS	NURSING IMPLEMENTATIONS
Anticholinergic Effects	
Dry mouth	Suggest use of sugarless gum/candy, rinse mouth frequently with water (avoid commercial mouthwash, which will increase dryness).
Blurred vision*	Caution client to avoid driving or operating heavy machinery until vision problem subsides.*
Urinary retention†	Teach client to report sensation of bladder fullness or incomplete emptying. Assess client for bladder distention.†
Constipation	Encourage client to drink 6–8 glasses of water daily, add fiber to diet, and exercise regularly.
Cardiovascular Effects	
Postural hypotension	Teach client to change positions slowly, especially when going from lying to standing position. Assess client's blood pressure; may take lying, sitting, and standing pressures to validate postural changes.
Arrhythmias	Teach client to report sensations of racing pulse or heartbeat, feeling of lightheadedness and dizziness. Assess pulse (radial and apical).
Central Nervous System Effects	
Headache	This effect may be temporary until client becomes accustomed to medication. Teach client to check with healthcare provider before taking any OTC medications—acetaminophen and some NSAIDs may be contraindicated.
Drowsiness, fatigue, decreased mental alertness	Teach client to take prescribed dose at bedtime (for those medications taken once daily). Teach client to use caution when driving or operating machinery while this effect persists.
Gastrointestinal Effects	
Nausea, decreased appetite, diarrhea	Teach client to take medications with meals. Advise eating 6 small meals rather than 3 larger ones. Maintain normal fluid intake. Report continued diarrhea to healthcare provider.
Weight gain, appetite increase	Teach client to eat adequate calories for maintaining normal weight. Encourage regular program of exercise; discourage frequent snacking with high caloric foods.
Endocrine Effects	
Amenorrhea in women	Teach client to continue to use appropriate measures for birth control since pregnancy can still occur.
Gynecomastia in men	Teach client that this effect can occur; encourage client to discuss effect of this on body image.
Sexual dysfunction (anorgasmia in women, erectile dysfunction in men	Teach client to report to healthcare provider any changes in sexual desire or functioning. Medication may be decreased or changed.

*Eye pain can indicate attack of acute narrow angle glaucoma. Teach client to notify physician of acute eye pain.
†Client with benign prostatic hypertrophy can be susceptible to acute urinary retention requiring catheterization. Instruct client to notify physician about this problem.

TABLE 15-3
Extrapyramidal Symptoms (EPS) of Psychotropic Drugs

EFFECT	TREATMENT	NURSING IMPLEMENTATIONS*
Pseudoparkinsonism: Drooling, lack of facial responsiveness, shuffling gait, and fine intention tremors.	Symptoms treated by antiparkinson (anticholinergic) drugs, such as: • Trihexyphenidyl (Artune) • Benztropine (Cogentin) • Biperiden (Akinston)	1. Assess for this effect. 2. Administer antiparkinson drugs if prescribed. 3. Notify physician and obtain order for antiparkinson agents, if not prescribed.
Acute dystonic reaction: Muscle spasms of jaw, tongue, neck, or eyes. Laryngeal spasms possible.	Stop drug. Antidotes are: • Diphenhydramine (Benadryl, 25–50 mg, IM or IV). • Benztropine (Cogentin, 1–2 mg IM or IV).	1. Recognize this as emergency. 2. Withhold any further doses. 3. Alert physician if no standing order for antidote. 4. Administer antidote if order available. 5. Reassure client.
Akathesia: Motor restlessness	Add antiparkinson agents as described above. May reduce dose of antipsychotic if symptom persists.	1. Assess for this effect. 2. Administer anticholinergic drugs. 3. Reassure client.
Tardive dyskinesia: Involuntary movements of mouth, tongue, and face. Movements may extend to fingers, arms, and trunk.	Stop drug or continue at lower dose. Change to another medication. No antidote available.	1. Assess for this effect. 2. Recognize that elderly client is more susceptible. 3. Notify physician if this occurs.

*The nurse would utilize standard assessment tool in order to detect signs of EPS reactions. An example of such a tool is the Abnormal Involuntary Movement Scale (AIMS).

IM = intramuscularly; IV = intravenously.

3. **Pharmacokinetics.** The use of these agents across the lifespan, indications, contraindications, and interactions are similar to those of typical antipsychotic agents (see II.A.3–6).

4. Common side effects are similar to those of typical antipsychotics and include the following:
   a. Seizures
   b. Agranulocytosis is associated primarily with clozapine, with an incidence of 1% to 2%. The United States Food and Drug Administration currently mandates weekly testing of white blood cell count for the first 6 months while taking this drug. Biweekly testing can then be instituted if counts are acceptable.

TABLE 15-4
Managing Serious Side Effects of Psychotropic Medications

SIDE EFFECT	SYMPTOMS	TREATMENT	NURSING IMPLEMENTATIONS
Agranulocytosis	1. White blood cell (WBC) level <2000 2. Sore throat, low-grade fever, malaise, sores in mouth	1. Stop drug. 2. Reverse isolation for client safety.	1. Monitor results of complete blood counts (CBC), being alert to decreasing WBC. 2. Suspect this problem if client has symptoms described and notify physician. 3. Withhold any further doses. 4. Protect client with decreased WBC from infection.
Seizures	Tonic-clonic seizure activity	1. Reduce dose or stop drug. 2. Add anticonvulsant medication to prevent further seizures.	1. Provide for client safety during any seizure activity. 2. Notify physician. 3. Administer anticonvulsant as prescribed.
Hepatotoxicity	1. Abnormal liver function series (elevated enzymes) 2. Fever, nausea, jaundice, and abdominal pain	1. Stop drug. 2. Treat symptoms with bedrest, good nutrition, and adequate fluids.	1. Monitor client for symptoms. 2. Monitor results of liver function studies. 3. Notify physician if hepatotoxity is suspected. 4. Ensure adequate rest, nutrition, and fluids for client affected.

(continued)

III. Antidepressants (Table 15-5)

A. Tricyclic antidepressants (TCAs)
1. Indications
a. TCAs are used to treat depression, including symptoms of depressed mood, loss of interest in activities or pleasure, altered sleep patterns, and somatic complaints.
b. TCAs are used to treat the anxiety symptoms that may occur as part of depressive disorder.

TABLE 15-4
Managing Serious Side Effects of Psychotropic Medications *(Continued)*

SIDE EFFECT	SYMPTOMS	TREATMENT	NURSING IMPLEMENTATIONS
Neuroleptic malignant syndrome (NMS)	1. Occurs as result of massive dopamine blockade in brain and CNS. 2. Altered consciousness, severe hypthermia (102°F and above), diaphoresis, tachycardia, and EPS reactions.	1. Stop drug. 2. Administer drug that will stimulate dopamine receptors, such as bromocriptine (Parlodel). 3. Administer IV fluids, hypothermia measures, and antiarrhythmic medications.	1. Monitor client for any symptoms of NMS. 2. Withhold any further doses. 3. Notify physician. 4. Prepare to transfer client to intensive care unit in medical-surgical unit of hospital.
Serotonin syndrome (SS)	1. Occurs as result of use of antidepressants that will increase serotonin bioavailability. 2. Severe hypothermia, altered muscle tone (hyperreflexia), altered consciousness, tachycardia, diaphoresis	1. Stop drug. 2. Administer drug that is serotonin receptor antagonist, methysergide (Sansert) or cyproheptadine (Periactin). 3. Administer IV fluids, hypothermia measures, and antiarrhythmic medications.	1. Ensure that SSRIs and MAOIs are not used concurrently and monitor appropriate washout period when switching between these groups. 2. Monitor client for these symptoms. 3. Withhold any further doses. 4. Notify physician. 5. Prepare to transfer client to intensive care unit.

    c. TCAs are also used to treat anxiety disorders (especially panic attacks), phobic disorders, and obsessive-compulsive disorder.

2. Mechanism of action. TCAs block reuptake of several neurotransmitters (ie, nonselective action) at presynaptic neurons. Neurotransmitters affected include serotonin, norepinephrine, acetylcholine, and dopamine.

3. Pharmacokinetics

    a. The serum half-life is 20 to 126 hours, and therefore TCAs can be taken once daily.

    b. **Therapeutic blood levels** are established for TCAs, so that effectiveness can be associated with a blood level to establish optimal dose for an individual client.

    c. Tolerance does not develop with these drugs; however, taking three times the maximum dose can be lethal, and therefore caution is important in prescribing for suicidal patients.

TABLE 15-5
Antidepressants

GENERIC NAME	TRADE NAME	USUAL DAILY DOSE (ADULT)
Tricyclics (TCAs)*		
Amitriptyline	Elavil	75–300 mg
Amoxapine	Ascendin	150–450 mg
Clomipramine	Anafranil	75–250 mg
Desipramine	Norpramin	75–300 mg
Doxepin	Sinequan	100–300 mg
Imipramine	Tofranil	75–300 mg
Maprotiline	Ludiomil	100–200 mg
Nortriptyline	Aventyl, Pamelor	50–150 mg
Protriptyline	Vivactil	20–60 mg
Trimipramine	Surmontil	75–300 mg
Monoamine Oxidase Inhibitors (MAOIs)[†]		
Phenelzine	Nardil	45–90 mg
Isocarboxazid	Marplan	30–50 mg
Tranylcypromine	Parnate	20–60 mg
Moclobemide	Manerix	300–600 mg
Selective Serotonin Reuptake Inhibitors (SSRIs)[‡]		
Fluvoxamine	Luvox	100–300 mg
Fluoxetine	Prozac	40–80 mg
Paroxetine	Paxil	20–50 mg
Sertraline	Zoloft	50–150 mg
Atypical Antidepressants[§]		
Bupropion	Wellbutrin	150–300 mg
Mirtazapine	Remeron	15–45 mg
Nefazodone	Serzone	200–400 mg
Venlafaxine	Effexor	75–300 mg
Trazodone	Desrel	150–300 mg

Drugs causing potentially fatal interactions with TCAs include antiarrhythmics, MAOIs, and SSRIs.

[†]*Drugs causing potentially fatal interactions with MAOIs include vasoconstrictors, decongestants, meperidine and other narcotics, TCAs, and SSRIs.*

[‡]*Drugs causing potentially fatal interactions with SSRIs include MAOIs and TCAs.*

[§]*Drugs causing potentially fatal interactions with atypical antidepressants include MAOIs.*

    d. **Therapeutic effectiveness** takes 2 to 4 weeks; the client may become discouraged and discontinue taking the drug if not taught about this.

4. Use across the lifespan

    a. TCAs are prescribed for adults and the elderly. They are used with caution in elderly clients because of the potential cardiac effects.

    b. Although widely used for children and adolescents, none of the antidepressants have been approved by the FDA to treat depression in those younger than 18 years of age (Mohr, 1998).

    c. TCAs are not recommended during pregnancy and lactation.

5. Contraindications

    a. **Cardiovascular disease.** This can be a serious problem; thus a baseline electrocardiogram (ECG) is recommended prior to TCA treatment, especially in the elderly client.

    b. Glaucoma

    c. Benign prostatic hypertrophy

    d. Liver and renal diseases

6. Interactions

    a. There may be additive anticholinergic effects when TCAs are taken with antihistamines, antipsychotics, antiparkinsonian agents, and other drugs with anticholinergic effects.

    b. There may be additive serotonergic effects (see Table 15-4) when TCAs are combined with other categories of antidepressant drugs.

    c. There may be additive sympathomimetic effects when TCAs are combined with drugs causing adrenergic stimulation; the combination may cause tachycardia and hypertension.

    d. There may be additive hypotensive effects when TCAs are combined with drugs that lower blood pressure (eg, beta blockers, calcium channel blockers, and antianginal nitrate preparations).

    e. Bleeding may be increased when TCAs are combined with warfarin (Coumadin).

7. Common side effects (see Table 15-2)

    a. Anticholinergic effects, including dry mouth, blurred vision, urinary retention, and constipation

    b. Cardiovascular effects, including hypotension, hypertension, arrhythmias, prolonged QRS complex, and heart failure

    c. Photosensitivity

    d. Gastrointestinal effects, including anorexia and nausea

    e. Central nervous system effects, including sedation and fatigue

8. Serious adverse effects (see Table 15-4)

    a. **TCA overdose** (Table 15-6)

    b. **Serotonin syndrome,** which is characterized by hypothermia, hyperreflexia, tachycardia, diaphoresis, and decreased level of consciousness

    c. Agranulocytosis (white blood count less than 2000)

    d. Seizures

TABLE 15-6
Tricyclic Antidepressant Overdose (Anticholinergic Toxicity)*

SYMPTOMS	TREATMENT
Sedation	1. Monitor vital signs and electrocardiogram
Ataxia	2. Maintain patent airway
Agitation	3. Cathartics or gastric lavage with activated charcoal
Stupor	4. Medications that are cholinergic stimulants such as
Coma	physostigmine (Antilirium)
Convulsions and respiratory depression	

*Blocking cholinergic action (ie, blocking acetylcholine from exerting its effect on the body) can result from overdose of tricyclic antidepressants.
(Keltner, N., Schwecke, L., & Bostrom, C. [1999]. Psychiatric nursing [3rd ed.]. St. Louis: Mosby.)

B. Monoamine oxidase inhibitors (MAOIs) (see Table 15-5)

1. **Mechanisms of action.** MAOIs inhibit the enzyme monoamine oxidase, which is responsible for breaking down excess serotonin and norepinephrine at the synapse. When this enzyme is inhibited, the neurotransmitters remain active at the synapse.

2. **Pharmacokinetics**
   a. The serum half life is unknown for these drugs.
   b. The enzyme monoamine oxidase is also active in the liver, inhibiting the liver's activity. This effect leads to elevated levels of other drugs that are normally metabolized in the liver.
   c. Therapeutic effectiveness is reached in 2 to 4 weeks.

3. Use across the lifespan and indications for use are similar to that for TCAs (see II.A.3–4).

4. **Contraindications**
   a. Cardiovascular disease or history of stroke
   b. Hyperthyroidism
   c. Pheochromocytoma
   d. **Elective surgery.** MAOIs should be discontinued at least 2 weeks before surgery because of risk for severe hypotension when anesthesia is given to a person taking MAOIs.

5. **Interactions**
   a. There may be additive serotonergic effects when an MAOI is combined with any other antidepressant (see Table 15-4).
   b. There may be additive anticholinergic effects when combined with drugs that have anticholinergic side effects.
   c. There may be additive sympathomimetic effects when an MAOI is combined with drugs that stimulate the sympathetic nervous system (eg, epi-

nephrine, norepinephrine, amphetamines, over-the-counter cold preparations) (Table 15-7).

    d. There may be additive sympathomimetic effects when an MAOI is combined with foods containing tyramine (see Table 15-7).

  6. Common side effects (see Table 15-2)

    a. Anticholinergic side effects

    b. Cardiovascular side effects

    c. Central nervous system stimulation, resulting in anxiety, agitation, restlessness, and insomnia. Teach the client to report this effect to health care provider, who may discontinue MAOI.

  7. Serious side effects (see Table 15-4)

    a. Agranulocytosis

    b. Hepatic toxicity

    c. **Hypertensive crisis** (see Table 15-7). Symptoms include severe occipital headache, nausea, vomiting, elevated blood pressure, photophobia, dilated pupils, and arrhythmia. Treatment is directed at measures to decrease blood pressure, such as oral administration of nifedipine (Procardia) or intravenous administration of phentolamine (Regitene).

C. Selective serotonin reuptake inhibitors (SSRIs) (see Table 15-5)

  1. Mechanism of action. SSRIs specifically affect the neurotransmitter serotonin by preventing its reuptake at the synapse. Because other neurotransmitters are not affected, these drugs do not have the same side effects as antipsychotic agents, TCAs, and MAOIs.

TABLE 15-7
Substances that Interact with MAOIs

FOODS*	BEVERAGES*	DRUGS†
Products containing brewer's yeast	Beer	Over-the-counter cold and cough preparations
Broad beans	Coffee	Over-the-counter drugs for allergies
Pickles, sauerkraut	Tea	
Bananas, figs, raisins	Chianti wine	Prescribed drugs such as psychostimulants
Cheddar or aged cheese, yogurt		Drugs used as substances of abuse such as cocaine, amphetamines
Chicken liver, pickled herring, smoked salmon, snails		
Chocolate, licorice, soy sauce		

MAOIs = Monoamine oxidase inhibitors

*Foods and beverages containing tyramine in combination with an MAOI can cause hypertensive crisis. These substances need to be avoided.

†Medications containing ephedrine, epinephrine, phenylephrine, and phenylpropanolamine will have an addictive effect with norepinephrine levels already elevated by the MAOI.

2. Pharmacokinetics
a. The serum half-life is 20 to 168 hours and therefore can be given once daily.
b. Tolerance does not develop, and these drugs have a low potential for overdose.
c. Therapeutic effectiveness occurs in 2 to 4 weeks.
3. Use across the lifespan and indications for use are similar to those for TCAs.
4. Contraindications
a. Hypersensitivity reactions
b. Severe hepatic or renal disease
c. Seizures
d. Diabetes mellitus
5. Interactions
a. There may be additive CNS depression when combining SSRIs with alcohol, antihistamines, and opioids.
b. There may be additive serotonergic effects when SSRIs are combined with other antidepressants (eg, TCAs, MAOIs). Discontinue use for a 5-week period when switching from an SSRI to a MAOI (termed *wash-out period*).
c. SSRIs may increase risk of toxicity from other drugs (eg, digitoxin, phenytoin, lithium, warfarin).
6. Common side effects (Table 15-8)

TABLE 15-8
Common Side Effects of SSRIs

SIDE EFFECT	NURSING IMPLEMENTATION
Insomnia	• Take dose early in the day • Eliminate caffeine • Use relaxation measures before bed
Headache	• Client may use analgesics as prescribed (check with health care provider for OTC drugs) • If severe headaches, may require drug discontinuation
Weight loss	• Encourage client to eat adequate calories to maintain weight • **Caution** with use of these drugs with client with an eating disorder
Sexual dysfunction (anorgasmia in women, ejaculatory dysfunction in men)	• Teach client to report any problem with sexual function to health care provider • If this persists, may switch to another antidepressant

SSRIs = Selective serotonin reuptake inhibitors.

D. Atypical antidepressants

1. **Mechanism of action.** These drugs do not have a well-explained mechanism of action, although they are thought to act similarly to the TCAs. An advantage over the TCAs is fewer side effects, particularly fewer anticholinergic and cardiovascular effects.

2. **Pharmacokinetics** for each drug in this category is unique to the drug. Consult a pharmacology text for greater details.

3. **Use across the lifespan and indications for use** are similar to that of TCAs.

4. **Contraindications and interactions**
   a. **Bupropion (Wellbutrin)** may cause seizure disorder.
   b. **Nefazodone (Serzone)** may cause additive cardiotoxicity with drugs used for allergies, such as terfenadine (Seldane) and astemizole (Hismanal).
   c. **Trazodone (Desyrel)** may increase risk of digitalis toxicity when taken with digoxin preparations.
   d. **Venlafaxine (Effexor)** has the potential for increased blood pressure, so clients with known hypertension should not take.

5. **Common side effects**
   a. **Bupropion (Wellbutrin)** may increase seizure risk. It contains the same active ingredient found in Zyban, which is used in smoking cessation; therefore, it should not be used with this drug.
   b. **Nefazodone (Serzone)** is associated with a risk of hypotension.
   c. **Trazodone (Desyrel)** is associated with a risk of priapism (prolonged painful penile erection).
   d. **Venlafaxine (Effexor)** is associated with a risk of hypertension.

E. Nontricyclic selective norepinephrine reuptake inhibitors (SNRIs)

1. **Mechanisms of action.** The SNRIs act selectively to prevent reuptake of norepinephrine at the synapse. These drugs are currently under development, and mirtazapine (Remeron) is currently the only FDA-approved SNRI.

2. **Common side effects** include insomnia, dry mouth, constipation, and tachycardia (see Tables 15-2 and 15-8).

IV.   Mood Stabilizers (Table 15-9)

A. Lithium carbonate (Eskalith, Lithane)

1. **Indications**
   a. Treatment of the manic cycle of bipolar disorder
   b. Prevention of recurrent episodes of mania and depression characteristic in bipolar disorder
   c. Treatment of schizoaffective disorder and episodes of acute hyperactivity associated with other mental disorders

2. **Mechanism of action** is poorly understood. Lithium is thought to normalize reuptake of neurotransmitters, including serotonin, norepinephrine, dopamine, and acetylcholine. Unlike most of the psychotropic medications, lithium exerts its action intracellularly rather than at the synapse.

TABLE 15-9
Mood Stabilizers

CLASSIFICATION	GENERIC NAME	TRADE NAME	USUAL DAILY DOSAGE (ADULT)
Antimanic	Lithium carbonate	Eskalith, Lithane	Acute manic 1800–2400 mg Maintenance 300–1200 mg
Anticonvulsants	Carbamazepine	Tegretol	2–20 mg
	Valproic acid	Depakene, Depakote	500–1500 mg

3. **Pharmacokinetics**
   a. The serum half-life is approximately 24 hours.
   b. Lithium is metabolized by the kidneys and is similar in chemical structure to sodium, competing at various body receptor sites with sodium. If sodium intake is reduced or serum sodium levels are depleted, lithium will be reabsorbed rather than excreted by the kidney and may reach toxic levels in the body.
   c. The blood level of lithium has a narrow therapeutic range (0.6 to 1.2 mEq/L). Blood levels greater than 1.5 mEq/L are considered toxic.
   d. Upon initiation of lithium, blood is drawn either daily or every 2 to 3 days until a therapeutic level is identified for the individual client.
   e. When symptoms are resolved for an individual client, the lithium dose is decreased for maintenance treatment to one-half to two-thirds the acute dose. Blood levels are then monitored every 2 to 3 months or when a problem is suspected.
4. **Use across the lifespan**
   a. Lithium is prescribed for children and adults. Elderly clients are particularly sensitive to toxicity because of decreased renal function.
   b. It is not recommended for use during pregnancy and lactation.
5. **Contraindications**
   a. Hypersensitivity response to lithium
   b. Renal disease
   c. Thyroid disease
6. **Interactions**
   a. There is an increased risk of lithium toxicity with multiple medications, including anesthetics, angiotensin-converting enzyme (ACE) inhibitors, nonsteroidal anti-inflammatory drugs (NSAIDs), tetracycline, and thiazide diuretics.
   b. There is an increased risk of lithium toxicity when sodium intake is less than 2 g/day; when fluids and sodium are lost due to excessive exercise, dehydration, or gastrointestinal illness; and when fluid intake is less than 6 to 8 glasses of water daily.
   c. Decreased levels of lithium may occur when taken with multiple medications, including acetazolamide, theophylline preparations, mannitol and other osmotic diuretics, sodium bicarbonate, and xanthines.

7. **Common side effects** (see Table 15-2)
   a. Gastrointestinal effects, including nausea, anorexia, and diarrhea
   b. Fatigue and lethargy
   c. Weight gain
   d. Polyuria (usually benign)
8. **Lithium toxicity is associated with elevated blood levels of the drug.**
   a. Mild toxicity (lithium level 1.5 to 2.0 mEq/L) is characterized by apathy, diminished concentration, mild ataxia, muscle weakness, hand tremors, and muscle twitching.
   b. Moderate toxicity (lithium level 2.0 to 2.5 mEq/L) is characterized by severe diarrhea, nausea and vomiting, moderate ataxia, mild confusion, slurred speech, tinnitus, frank muscle twitching, and tremors.
   c. Severe toxicity (lithium level above 2.5 mEq/L) is characterized by nystagmus, muscle fasciculation, deep tendon hyperreflexia, decreased level of consciousness, tonic-clonic seizures, coma, and death (Table 15-10).
9. **Treatment of lithium toxicity includes:**
   a. Withholding any further doses (even if toxicity is only suspected)
   b. Obtaining immediate serum lithium level to confirm toxicity level
   c. Monitoring vital signs, electrolyte levels, blood urea nitrogen, and creatinine
   d. Intravenous therapy with normal saline
   e. Hemodialysis, if indicated for severe toxicity
10. **Other potential serious side effects include:**
    a. **Thyroid impairment.** Thyroid function studies are monitored every 3 to 6 months for clients on long-term lithium therapy.
    b. **Renal impairment.** Renal function studies are monitored every 3 to 6 months for clients on long-term lithium therapy.

B. **Anticonvulsants** (see Table 15-5)
   1. **Mechanism of action** is not well understood in treatment of bipolar disorder. It is thought to inhibit "kindling" activity in the brain; that is, it interrupts the automatic stimulating sequences of neurotransmission. It will also stimulate GABA, which helps produce a calming effect.

TABLE 15-10
Preventing Lithium Toxicity

* Restrict caffeine intake.
* Maintain adequate water intake (6–8 glasses/day).
* Maintain adequate sodium intake (2 g/day).
* Drink fluids with necessary electrolytes when exercising (ie, sports drinks).
* Contact health care provider for severe gastrointestinal symptoms.
* Inform all health care providers about lithium therapy, especially when surgical intervention planned.
* Contact health care provider if symptoms indicating toxicity occur.
* Maintain appointments to monitor blood levels as prescribed.

2. **Pharmacokinetics**
   a. The serum half-life for carbamazepine (Tegretol) is 15 to 30 hours, whereas valproic acid (Depakote) is about 8 hours.
   b. Blood levels can be monitored for both drugs and can be associated with symptom improvement in the individual client.
3. **Use across the life span and indications for use** are similar to lithium.
4. **Contraindications** include cardiovascular disease, hepatic impairment, hypersensitivity reactions, and blood dyscrasias.
5. **Interactions**
   a. **Carbamazepine**
      (1) There may be increased carbamazepine levels with erythromycin, cimetidine, propoxyphene, isoniazid, calcium channel blockers, and the SSRIs.
      (2) Decreased carbamazepine levels may occur with divalproex, phenytoin, and phenobarbital.
      (3) Carbamazepine can decrease levels of medications, including oral contraceptives, warfarin, theophylline preparations, antipsychotics, divalproex, anticoagulants, and doxycycline.
   b. **Valproic acid**
      (1) There may be increased valproic acid levels with aspirin.
      (2) It potentiates the effect of alcohol, warfarin, and aspirin.
      (3) There is an increased seizure risk when used with phenytoin or clonazepam.
      (4) Effects of phenobarbital, primidone, and MAOIs are increased.
      (5) There is an increased CNS depressant effect when combined with antihistamines, antidepressants, opioids, and sedative hypnotics.
6. **Common side effects** (see Table 15-2)
   a. CNS effects include drowsiness, fatigue, and sedation
   b. Gastrointestinal effects, including nausea, vomiting, and indigestion (especially with valproic acid)
   c. Photosensitivity, including sunburn and rash
   d. Visual disturbances, including blurred vision
7. **Serious side effects** (see Table 15-4) include hepatic toxicity and agranulocytosis.

 V. **Antianxiety Agents (Anxiolytics) and Sedative-Hypnotics** (Table 15-11)

A. **Benzodiazepines (BZAs)**
   1. **Indications**
      a. BZAs are the drug of choice for treatment of anxiety and sleep disorders.
      b. They are also used in acute alcohol withdrawal, preoperative sedation, seizure disorders, short-term treatment of acute mania, and as muscle relaxants.
      c. They are also used for treatment of agitation and hyperactivity in cognitive impairment disorders.

TABLE 15-11
Antianxiety (Anxiolytic) Drugs

GENERIC	TRADE	USUAL DAILY DOSAGE (ADULT)
Anxiolytic Benzodiazapines		
Chlordiazepoxide	Librium	15–100 mg
Diazepam	Valium	4–40 mg
Oxazepam	Serax	30–120 mg
Chorazepate	Tranxene	15–60 mg
Lorazepam	Ativan	2–6 mg
Aprazolam	Xanax	0.75–4 mg
Clonazepam	Klonopin	0.5–20 mg
Prozepam	Centrax	20–60 mg
Sedative-Hypnotic Benzodiazapines*		
Temazepam	Restoril	15–20 mg
Triazolam	Halcion	125–250 mg
Zolpidem	Ambien	10–20 mg
Flurazepam	Dalmane	15–30 mg
Antihistamines		
Hydroxyzine	Atarax, Vistaril	50–100 mg
Diphenhydramine	Benadryl	25–50 mg
Other		
Buspirone	BuSpar	15–60 mg

*Dosages given for benzodiazapines used as sedative-hypnotics are the usual hypnotic doses (not daily doses).

2. **Mechanism of action.** BZAs depress subcortical levels of the CNS, particularly the limbic system and reticular formation. They will potentiate the action of GABA, thereby producing a calming effect (Townsend, 1999).

3. **Pharmacokinetics**
    a. The serum half-life for drugs in this group vary widely (eg, 5 to 30 hours for oxazepam and 30 to 100 hours for chlorazepate).
    b. The onset of action for drugs in this group also varies, thus leading to the use of some of these drugs as anxiolytics whereas others are primarily used as sedative-hypnotics (see Table 15-11).
    c. BZAs produce tolerance to their effects within days, and continued use (weeks to months) may lead to dependence. Abrupt cessation can precipitate withdrawal reactions (see Chapter 8).

4. **Use across the lifespan**
    a. These agents are prescribed for adults.
    b. They are prescribed for children and the elderly with caution because of increased risk for CNS depression.
    c. They are not recommended for use during pregnancy or lactation.

5. **Contraindications**
    a. Alcohol or substance abuse problems (cross-tolerant with alcohol)

    b. Hepatic or renal impairment

    c. Hypersensitivity reactions

    d. Central nervous system depression

6. Interactions

    a. Increased sedation and CNS depression may occur when these agents are combined with alcohol, barbiturates, narcotics, antipsychotics, antidepressants, antihistamines, neuromuscular blocking agents, cimetidine, and disulfiram.

    b. Decreased effectiveness may occur when these agents are combined with nicotine and caffeine.

7. Common side effects (see Table 15-2)

    a. CNS effects, including sedation, fatigue, headache, and motor incoordination (Table 15-12).

    b. Gastrointestinal effects, including nausea and dry mouth

8. Serious side effects

    a. Withdrawal syndrome, if abruptly discontinued (see Chapter 8)

    b. Respiratory depression with high doses or deliberate overdose (Table 15-13)

    c. Paradoxical behaviors of restlessness, talkativeness, and insomnia can occur.

B. Antihistamines (see Table 15-11)

  1. Indications. These medications are used primarily for the relief of allergic symptoms. However, they are also used for:

    a. Anxiety symptoms associated with a variety of mental disorders

    b. Sleep induction

  2. Mechanism of action. Antihistamines produce CNS depression and sedation as a side effect of their therapeutic activity of blocking histamine. Because of their relative safety, especially in the elderly, they can be used as anxiolytics.

  3. Pharmacokinetics

    a. The serum half-life is 2.4 to 7 hours, so that it can be used to induce sleep (ie, sedative-hypnotic use).

    b. Unlike BZAs, these drugs are not associated with tolerance and dependence.

  4. Use across the lifespan

    a. These agents are prescribed for adults, children, adolescents, and the elderly.

    b. They are not recommended for use during pregnancy and lactation.

TABLE 15-12
Safe Use of Benzodiazepines

- Do not drive or operate machinery.
- Do not abruptly stop taking drug as this can cause acute withdrawal to occur.
- Do not take with alcohol or any other sedative drugs.

TABLE 15-13
Benzodiazepine (BZA) Overdose*

SYMPTOMS	TREATMENT

Somnolence
Confusion
Diminished reflexes
Hypotension
Coma
	1. Induce vomiting or use of gastric lavage.
	2. Monitor vital signs and electrocardiogram.
	3. Maintain patent airway.
	4. Medications include:
	  • Levarterenol (Levophed) for hypotension
	  • Physostigmine (Antilirium) for acute diazepam poisoning.
	  • Flumazenil (Mazicon), a BZA blocker, acts to reverse CNS depression of BZAs.

BZAs taken alone in therapeutic doses are relatively safe; however, if combined with alcohol or other central nervous system depressants, results can be fatal.

5. **Contraindications**
   a. Hypersensitivity response
   b. Hepatic disease
   c. Narrow angle glaucoma
   d. Seizure disorders
   e. Prostatic hypertrophy
6. **Interactions**
   a. Additive CNS depression may occur with alcohol, opioids, and other sedative-hypnotics.
   b. Additive anticholinergic effects may occur with TCAs, guanidine, MAOIs, and other drugs causing anticholinergic responses.
7. **Common adverse effects**
   a. CNS effects, including drowsiness, fatigue, and dizziness
   b. Anticholinergic effects, including dry mouth, blurred vision, urinary retention, and constipation
8. **Serious adverse effects** include postural hypotension (see Table 15-2)

C. **Buspirone (BuSpar)** (see Table 15-11)
   1. **Indications**
      a. It is primarily prescribed for treatment of generalized anxiety disorder.
      b. It may be used for children and the elderly who have disruptive or aggressive behaviors.
   2. **Mechanism of action.** This non-BZA anxiolytic does not act on GABA, but exerts its effects on serotonin receptors. Its specific action is not well understood, but it will reduce anxiety.
   3. **Pharmacokinetics**
      a. The half-life is 2 to 7 hours.
      b. A lag time exists before buspirone exerts its antianxiety effect. It may take 10 days to 2 weeks before effectiveness occurs. Teach the client to continue taking medication for this time.
      c. Tolerance and dependence are not associated with this drug.

4. **Use across the lifespan**
   a. It is prescribed for children, adults, and the elderly.
   b. It is not recommended for use during pregnancy and lactation.
5. **Contraindications** include hypersensitivity reactions and hepatic disease.
6. **Interactions**
   a. Hypertension can occur when used with MAOIs.
   b. Increased sedation may occur with alcohol.
   c. There is an increased risk of hepatic toxicity when used with trazodone.
7. **Common side effects** (see Table 15-2)
   a. CNS effects include dizziness, drowsiness, headache, fatigue, and weakness.
   b. Gastrointestinal effects include dry mouth, nausea, and diarrhea or constipation.
   c. Cardiovascular effects include palpitations and hypotension or hypertension.
   d. Endocrine effects include amenorrhea.

VI. Other Medications

A. **Psychostimulants** (Table 15-14)
   1. **Indications**
      a. Children and adults with attention deficit-hyperactivity disorder (ADHD)
      b. Adults with narcolepsy
   2. **Mechanism of action.** Psychostimulants act directly on neuronal synapses to increase release of norepinephrine, serotonin, and dopamine. The increased amount of norepinephrine available at the synapse accounts for the CNS excitation produced. How psychostimulants work paradoxically to decrease hyperactive and impulsive behaviors in children with ADHD is not well understood.
   3. **Pharmacokinetics**
      a. The serum half-life for both methylphenidate (Ritalin) and dextroamphetamine (Dexedrine) is relatively short (ie, 2 to 6 hours). Therefore, several doses are required during the day.
      b. The serum half-life for pemoline (Cylert) is longer (ie, 9 to 14 hours) and therefore once-daily dosing is sufficient.

Table 15-14
Psychostimulants

GENERIC	TRADE	USUAL DAILY DOSE (CHILDREN AND ADULTS)
Methylphenidate	Ritalin	10–60 mg
Dextroamphetamine	Dexedrine	5–40 mg
Pemoline	Cylert	56.25–75 mg

    c. Psychostimulants have a high potential for tolerance and abuse. Withdrawal can occur if medications are abruptly discontinued (see Chapter 8).

  4. Use across the lifespan

    a. These are prescribed for children and adults with ADHD.

    b. It is used infrequently in the elderly client.

    c. It is contraindicated during pregnancy and lactation.

  5. Contraindications

    a. Substance abuse

    b. Seizure disorders

    c. Hepatic disease

    d. Cardiovascular disease

    e. Tourette syndrome and other abnormal movement disorders

  6. Interactions

    a. Use with MAOI or vasopressors may cause hypertensive crisis.

    b. There is an additive sympathomimetic effect with other drugs stimulating sympathetic nervous system.

    c. Excessive use of caffeine can cause additive CNS stimulation.

    d. Antipsychotics can decrease CNS stimulation.

  7. Common side effects (see Table 15-2)

    a. CNS effects, including headache, insomnia, agitation, and irritability

    b. Cardiovascular effects, including hypertension and palpitations

    c. Gastrointestinal effects, including nausea, vomiting, anorexia, and diarrhea

  8. Serious side effects include seizures and hepatotoxicity (see Table 15-4).

B. Anticholinesterase drugs (Table 15-15)

  1. Indications. These agents are used for the treatment of mild to moderate cognitive impairments associated with Alzheimer disease and other cognitive impairment disorders.

  2. Mechanism of action. These drugs inhibit the enzyme acetylcholinesterase, which normally acts to break down acetylcholine at the synapse. Therefore, increased amounts of acetylcholine are present at the synapse and this effect is thought to lessen the memory impairments in Alzheimer disease.

  3. Pharmacokinetics

    a. The serum half-life of tacrine (Cognex) is short (ie, 2 to 4 hours), requiring doses 3 times daily.

    b. The serum half-life of donepezil (Aricept) is 70 hours, therefore requiring only one dose daily.

TABLE 15-15
Anticholinesterase Drugs

GENERIC	TRADE	USUAL DAILY DOSE (ADULT)
Tacrine	Cognex	40–160 mg
Donepezil	Aricept	5–10 mg

    c. Tolerance does not occur with these drugs.

4. Use across the lifespan

    a. It is prescribed for the adult or elderly client with cognitive impairment.

    b. It is generally not prescribed in children.

    c. It is not recommended during pregnancy and lactation.

5. Contraindications include cardiovascular disease (especially sick sinus syndrome) and hepatic disease.

6. Interactions

    a. There is an increased risk of bleeding when used with NSAIDs.

    b. There is an increased risk of theophylline toxicity when used with theophylline preparations.

    c. There is a potentiation of action of drugs that are cholinergic stimulants (ie, bethanechol).

    d. Nicotine decreases blood levels of these drugs.

7. Common side effects (see Table 15-2)

    a. CNS effects, including dizziness and headache

    b. Gastrointestinal effects, including nausea, vomiting, diarrhea, and anorexia

    c. Cardiovascular effects, including bradycardia

8. Serious side effects include hepatatoxicity and gastrointestinal bleeding (see Table 15-4).

 VII. NURSING PROCESS OVERVIEW FOR
Somatic Therapies

A. Assessment

  1. Review data collected on client receiving somatic therapy, including:

    a. History and physical examination

    b. Laboratory and diagnostic studies, including complete blood count, blood chemistry study, thyroid profile, and liver and renal function studies

    c. Baseline electrocardiogram

    d. Baseline vital signs

    e. Medication and allergy history

    f. Target symptoms for which medication has been prescribed

  2. Assess the client, family, or both for knowledge regarding psychotropic medications prescribed, including:

    a. The expected beneficial effect and when it is most likely to occur

    b. The dose frequency and instructions regarding food and fluids

    c. The minor side effects and the measures taken to counteract them

    d. The major side effects and appropriate action (eg, stop further doses, contact health care provider)

    e. The foods, beverages, and other medications that the patient should avoid

  3. Assess client, family, or both for knowledge regarding ECT therapy, including:

    a. Expected beneficial effect and when it is most likely to occur

    b. Necessity for signing informed consent

    c. Pretreatment routine.

       (1) NPO for at least 4 hours before treatment

       (2) Baseline vital signs

       (3) Removal of jewelry, glasses, contact lenses, and dentures

       (4) Pretreatment medications used to decrease secretions (atropine sulfate), to induce light coma (methohexital), and to prevent musculoskeletal complications from seizure activity (succinylcholine).

    d. Posttreatment routine

       (1) Frequent monitoring of vital signs

       (2) Safety precautions (eg, siderails, no food or fluid until gag reflex returns)

       (3) Reassurance and appropriate reorientation for post-ECT initial confusion

B. Nursing diagnoses

1. Analyze available client data, indicating any risk factors for client while taking medication or receiving ECT therapy.

2. Determine appropriate nursing diagnosis, including but not limited to:

    a. Anxiety

    b. Health-seeking behaviors (specify)

    c. Injury, risk for

    d. Knowledge deficit (specify)

    e. Therapeutic regimen: families, ineffective management

    f. Therapeutic regimen: individual, ineffective management

C. Planning and outcome identification

1. Work with the client and family in establishing realistic goals.

2. Establish desired outcome criteria for client receiving psychotropic medications or ECT therapy.

    a. The client and family will verbalize expected benefits from treatment.

    b. The client and family will safely self-administer medications.

    c. The client and family will utilize measures to counteract minor side effects.

    d. The client and family will contact health care provider if major side effects are encountered.

    e. The client and family will follow prescribed laboratory and other testing to monitor medications and any side effects.

D. Implementation

1. Reinforce the client's and family's accurate knowledge regarding medications or ECT therapy.

2. Teach the client and family any additional information necessary to safely take prescribed medications or ECT therapy.

3. Monitor the client for any side effects of medications.

4. Institute appropriate nursing action for any side effects experienced by client (see Tables 15-2 and 15-4).

5. Monitor the client for symptom improvement.

6. Monitor the client's vital signs, level of consciousness, and presence of gag reflex following ECT therapy.

7. Reorient the client after ECT therapy.

E. Outcome evaluation

1. The client experiences beneficial effect from medication or ECT therapy.

2. The client safely self-administers prescribed medications.

3. The client uses appropriate measures to counteract any minor side effects.

4. The client and family contact health care provider when any major side effects are experienced.

5. The client complies with prescribed laboratory or other testing to ensure safety while taking medications.

STUDY QUESTIONS

1. A client who is on lithium therapy is visited by the home health nurse to have blood drawn for a routine lithium level. A nurse assesses that the client is apathetic, has difficulty responding to questions, walks with an unsteady gait, and has fine hand tremors. Which of the following would the nurse suspect the client is experiencing?
   (1) an expected reaction to lithium therapy
   (2) pseudoparkinson syndrome caused by lithium therapy
   (3) a medical problem unrelated to lithium therapy
   (4) toxic effects of elevated lithium levels

2. A client refuses to remain on psychotropic medications following discharge from an in-patient psychiatric unit. Which of the following would the community mental health nurse providing follow-up care first assess about this client?
   (1) income level and living arrangements
   (2) involvement of family and support systems
   (3) reason for in-patient admission
   (4) reason for refusal to take medications

3. A nurse is assessing postural blood pressures for a client taking risperidone (Risperdal) for chronic schizophrenia. Which of the following results would cause the nurse to withhold the next dose of this drug?
   (1) sitting blood pressure (BP) of 124/84 mm Hg; standing BP of 104/60 mm Hg
   (2) sitting BP of 112/60 mm Hg; standing BP of 104/60 mm Hg

   (3) sitting BP of 130/80 mm Hg; standing BP of 128/78 mm Hg
   (4) sitting BP of 150/90 mm Hg; standing BP of 146/88 mm Hg

4. A nurse understands that the therapeutic effects of the typical antipsychotic medications are associated with which of the following neurotransmitter changes?
   (1) decreased dopamine
   (2) increased acetylcholine
   (3) stabilization of serotonin
   (4) stimulation of GABA

5. Sertraline (Zoloft), an SSRI, is prescribed for a client with major depression. After 1 week, the client complains of no improvement and refuses to take the medication from the nurse. Which of the following would be the nurse's first response?
   (1) charting the client's refusal to take this dose
   (2) informing the client's physician about noncompliance
   (3) informing the client that 2 to 4 weeks is needed for a positive response
   (4) reviewing the client's symptoms on admission and current complaints

6. Which of the following would be most important for the nurse to teach the client taking the monoamine oxidase inhibitor phenelzine (Nardil)?
   (1) the avoidance of foods and beverages containing tyramine
   (2) the importance of maintaining regular follow-up visits
   (3) the possible adverse effects, such as hypertension
   (4) the rationale for the therapeutic effect of mood elevation

7. A client who is taking the antipsychotic medication chlorpromazine (Thorazine) complains of dry mouth and constipation. Which of the following would be the appropriate nursing action?
    (1) Advise the client to chew sugarless gum and eliminate gas-forming foods.
    (2) Encourage the client to rinse mouth with water and add fiber to diet.
    (3) Consult with the client's physician about changing antipsychotic medication.
    (4) Question the client about the amount and type of daily exercise.

8. A client taking fluphenazine (Prolixin) experiences an acute dystonic reaction. Which of the following prn medications would the nurse administer to this client?
    (1) acetaminophen (Tylenol), 325 mg orally
    (2) diphenhydramine (Benadryl), 25 mg intramuscularly
    (3) milk of magnesia, 30 ml orally
    (4) thiothixene (Navane), 6 mg intramuscularly

9. Assessment of a client who is taking haloperidol (Haldol) reveals a temperature of 102°F, blood pressure of 180/92 mm Hg, and profuse diaphoresis. Which of the following adverse effects would the nurse suspect?
    (1) agranulocytosis
    (2) extrapyramidal reaction
    (3) hepatotoxicity
    (4) neuroleptic malignant syndrome

10. A nurse teaches a client who is taking the benzodiazepine oxazepam (Serax) to avoid excessive intake of

(1) cheese
(2) coffee
(3) sugar
(4) shellfish

11. Which of the following principles should the nurse understand to plan care for the client receiving anxiolytic medication?
    (1) Enhanced psychomotor coordination is expected.
    (2) Increased mental alertness is a common effect.
    (3) Medications that are CNS depressants will potentiate sedative response.
    (4) Consumption of foods containing tyramine can cause hypertension.

12. To prevent lithium toxicity from occurring, the nurse would teach the client to maintain adequate intake of
    (1) fruits and vegetables
    (2) low-fat diet
    (3) protein and vitamin C
    (4) water and sodium

13. Which of the following best explains why tricyclic antidepressants are used with caution in the elderly?
    (1) central nervous system effects
    (2) cardiovascular system effects
    (3) gastrointestinal system effects
    (4) serotonin syndrome effects

14. Which of the following is the most serious side effect of the atypical antipsychotic clozapine (Clozaril)?
    (1) agranulocytosis
    (2) anticholinergic effects
    (3) postural hypotension
    (4) pseudoparkinsonism

15. A client is admitted to the emergency room following a suicide

attempt by overdosing on the tricyclic antidepressant imipramine (Tofranil). In addition to monitoring vital signs and the electrocardiogram, the nurse would be prepared to provide for which of the following as priority?
(1) frequent stimulation
(2) electrolyte replacement
(3) patent airway
(4) quiet environment

16. A nurse would know that MAOI antidepressants are contraindicated with medications containing which of the following?
(1) aspirin
(2) acetaminophen
(3) codeine
(4) norepinephrine

17. When a nurse suspects a client is experiencing either neuroleptic malignant syndrome or serotonin syndrome as a result of psychotropic medications, which of the following actions takes priority?
(1) ensuring adequate fluids
(2) maintaining bed rest
(3) monitoring client for expected symptoms
(4) withholding further drug doses

18. A nurse is working with a client who has overdosed on a benzodiazepine. Which of the following would the nurse prepare to administer?
(1) carbamazepine (Tegretol)
(2) diphenhydramine (Benadryl)
(3) flumazenil (Mazicon)
(4) physostigmine (Antilirium)

19. A nurse is working with the family of a client who is taking tacrine (Cognex). Which of the following symptoms would the nurse teach the family to be alert for in order to detect early signs of liver problems?
(1) constipation and bloating
(2) dizziness and fatigue
(3) frequent belching and heartburn
(4) nausea and abdominal pain

20. A nurse is teaching the family of a child who taking the psychostimulant methylphenidate (Ritalin). To manage the common side effects of nausea and anorexia, which of the following would the nurse recommend?
(1) Discourage frequent snacking with high-calorie foods.
(2) Eat adequate calories to maintain normal weight.
(3) Offer six small meals rather than three large meals.
(4) Take prescribed medication at bedtime.

21. Which of the following nursing interventions would be the priority for a client immediately after receiving an ECT treatment?
(1) assessing vital signs and reorienting
(2) applying restraints to prevent injury
(3) administering previously held medications
(4) encouraging intake of fluids and nutritious food

ANSWER KEY

1. The answer is (4). The symptoms described—apathy, difficulty concentrating, ataxia, and tremors—are those that occur because of elevated lithium levels and their effect on the CNS. These symptoms indicate the client is experiencing mild toxicity. This client's reaction is not an expected response; the goal of monitoring blood levels of lithium is to prevent toxicity. Also, these are not the symptoms of pseudoparkinsonism (nor does lithium cause pseudoparkinsonism).

2. The answer is (4). The first area for assessment would be the client's reason for refusing medication. The client may not understand the purpose for the medicine, may be experiencing distressing side effects, or may be concerned about the cost of the medicine. In any case, the nurse cannot provide appropriate intervention before assessing the client's problem with the medication. The patient's income level, living arrangements, and involvement of family and support systems are relevant issues following determination of the client's reason for refusing medication. The nurse providing follow-up care would have access to the client's medical record and should already know the reason for in-patient admission.

3. The answer is (1). The significant blood pressure decrease with position change is an indication of the side effect of postural hypotension. The prudent nurse would withhold the next dose and notify the physician. The other blood pressure readings do not indicate postural hypotension.

4. The answer is (1). Excess dopamine is thought to be the chemical cause for psychotic thinking. The typical antipsychotics act to block dopamine receptors and therefore decrease amount of this neurotransmitter at the synapses. The typical antipsychotics do not increase acetylcholine, stabilize serotonin, or stimulate GABA.

5. The answer is (3). The client may not understand that therapeutic effects of the antidepressants take at least 2 to 4 weeks. If the client continues to refuse medication even after the appropriate teaching, the nurse would then chart refusal and inform the physician. The response in answer choice (4) is not relevant to the situation described.

6. The answer is (1). The most important teaching for a client taking a monoamine oxidase inhibitor (MAOI) is that foods and beverages containing tyramine need to be avoided to prevent a severe hypertensive reaction. Medications containing psychostimulating drugs also must be avoided; however, the choices do not include this response. Follow-up care is important; however, the priority teaching issue is dietary restrictions. If client is unaware of these restrictions, a hypertensive response can be experienced before any follow-up appointment. The response in answer choice (3) is vague. The fact that hypertension can occur is true; however, the client is not being informed how to avoid this. The client may or may not want details regarding how mood elevation is achieved with an MAOI. For many clients, knowledge that their mood will elevate is sufficient. The details about how this occurs is not a priority.

7. The answer is (2). Rinsing the mouth with water (rather than mouthwash, which is drying) will help eliminate the problem of dry mouth. Adding fiber to the diet will facilitate the passage of a normal stool and help avoid constipation. Chewing sugarless gum will help with dry mouth; however, eliminating gas-forming foods is not the treatment for constipation. Changing medications because of experiencing these common side effects is not indicated. The client should be instructed in measures to counteract the side effects. Exercise is important and it can help stimulate peristalsis; however, the problem of dry mouth is not addressed in this response.

8. The answer is (2). Diphenhydramine (Benadryl) is the antidote for acute dystonia. The dose needs to be given intramuscularly because a client in acute dystonia often has difficulty swallowing. The remaining medications would not treat an acute dystonic reaction and are prescribed as-needed for other reasons; for example, acetaminophen would be prescribed for headache, milk of magnesia for constipation, and thiothixene for agitation.

9. The answer is (4). Neuroleptic malignant syndrome is characterized by high temperatures, elevated blood pressure, diaphoresis, tachycardia, and extrapyramidal symptoms. The other reactions are all serious adverse effects of the typical antipsychotics (eg, haloperidol). However, the symptoms of the client are those of neuroleptic malignant syndrome.

10.   Coffee, which contains caffeine, is psychostimulating and will counteract the intended effect of relaxation, which will be produced by the effect of oxazepam on the neurotransmitter GABA. There is no reason for the client to avoid cheese, sugar, or shellfish while taking oxazepam.

11. The answer is (3). The nurse needs to teach the client about the serious effects of potentiation of CNS depression that can occur when taking other medicines that have the same body reaction as the anxiolytics. Other medications would include any of the sedative-hypnotic medicines, alcohol, and any barbiturates. Enhanced psychomotor coordination and increased mental alertness are the opposite reactions expected of anxiolytic medications; therefore, these statements do not apply. Hypertension when consuming tyramine-containing foods is a side effect of the MAOI antidepressants, not the anxiolytics.

12. The answer is (4). When sodium or water is depleted in a client taking lithium, the potential for lithium toxicity increases; lithium will be reabsorbed by the kidney to replace depleted sodium and counteract water loss. The remaining responses are unrelated to prevention of lithium toxicity.

13. The answer is (2). The TCAs affect norepinephrine as well as other neurotransmitters, and thus have significant cardiovascular side effects. Therefore, they are used with caution in the elderly client who by virtue of age and other medical conditions may have increased risk factors for cardiac problems. The remaining side effects would apply to any client taking a TCA and are not particular to an elderly person.

14. The answer is (1). The incidence of agranulocytosis associated with clozapine therapy is 1% to 2%. Therefore, clients taking this drug must be screened weekly for the first 6 months of therapy for evidence of decreased white blood count (less than 2000). Anticholinergic effects and postural hypotension can occur; however, they are not considered a serious side effect. Pseudoparkinsonism is not usually associated with clozapine, and this lack of extrapyramidal side effects is one of the advantages of the atypical antipsychotics.

15. The answer is (3). Symptoms of TCA overdose include sedation, ataxia, stupor, and sometimes convulsions and respiratory depression. Therefore, maintaining a patent airway is an essential component of nursing care for this client. Although the nurse would assess the client's level of consciousness and provide stimulation in order to do so, this is less essential than maintaining an airway. Intravenous therapy and electrolyte replacement may be indicated, especially if the client has been treated with gastric lavage. However, this would not be as important as an airway. A quiet environment may be indicated if the client has any agitation; however, airway patency precedes this measure.

16. The answer is (4). MAOIs act to inhibit the enzyme responsible for breaking down neurotransmitters, including norepinephrine. Therefore, if medicine containing norepinephrine is taken along with the MAOI, the potential for a hypertensive crisis is increased. Norepinephrine acts peripherally to cause vasoconstriction, and therefore increases blood pressure. The remaining medications are not contraindicated.

17. The answer is (4). The nurse must withhold any further doses of psychotropic medications if either neuroleptic malignant syndrome or serotonin syndrome is suspected. Withholding the medications will help to avoid increasing the severity of these reactions. These remaining actions are important, but the priority is preventing symptom worsening by stopping the psychotropic drug.

18. The answer is (3). Flumazenil (Mazicon) is the antidote for a benzodiazepine overdose; it acts to reverse the CNS depression caused by overdose. The remaining drugs will not reverse CNS depression.

19. The answer is (4). Nausea and abdominal pain may occur if the client is developing early liver problems. Jaundice would also be an important symptom; however, it may occur later as liver dysfunction increases. Constipation, bloating, and frequent belching and heartburn may indicate gastrointestinal problems, but not liver dysfunction. Dizziness and fatigue may indicate a problem with the CNS.

20. The answer is (3). A client (especially a child) may have increased response of nausea and lack of appetite when presented with large meals. Offering smaller portions more frequently can help stimulate appetite. The remaining responses would not help address this problem.

21. The answer is (1). The client will be monitored in the same manner as any postoperative client coming out of anesthesia. Applying restraints is not necessary and may cause agitation. Medications, fluids, and food will be given *after* the swallowing and gag reflexes return.

Comprehensive Test Questions

1. Which of the following nursing implementations is the best for facilitating communication with a psychiatric client who speaks a foreign language?
   (1) to rely on nonverbal communication
   (2) to select symbolic pictures as aids
   (3) to speak in universal phrases
   √ (4) to use the services of an interpreter

2. A nurse is working with a client who is from a culture that uses the services of a special healer. The client requests this healer's services when hospitalized on a psychiatric inpatient unit. Which of the following nursing implementations is congruent with culturally sensitive nursing care?
   (1) explaining to the client that this is inappropriate for a hospital setting
   √ (2) facilitating the client's request
   (3) reflecting to the client that this means an unhealthy reliance on magical healing
   (4) referring the client to the physician

3. A nurse and client are talking comfortably about the client's progress as well as feelings about the therapeutic relationship. Which phase of the therapeutic relationship is this typical of?
   (1) assessment
   (2) orientation
   (3) working
   √ (4) termination

4. A client tells the nurse, "People think I am no good, if you know what I mean." Which of the following responses by the nurse is most therapeutic?
   (1) "People don't always mean what they say about you. Perhaps you are too sensitive."
   (2) "I think you're a good person. So you see, at least there is one person who doesn't feel that way."
   √ (3) "I'm not sure what you mean. Tell me more about that."
   (4) "What is the reason people don't think you're good?"

5. A team treatment plan for a psychiatric client utilizes a contract approach as well as a system in which privileges are based on client participation in therapeutic activities. The theoretical framework that is being implemented in this situation is a
   √ (1) behavioral framework
   (2) educational framework
   (3) interpersonal framework
   (4) psychodynamic framework

6. A nurse explains to a mental health care technician that a client's obsessive-compulsive behaviors are related to unconscious conflict between id impulses and the superego (or conscience). On which of the following theories does the nurse base this statement?
   (1) behavioral theory
   (2) cognitive theory
   (3) interpersonal theory
   √ (4) psychoanalytic theory

7. A community mental health nurse is working with a family who has a member with chronic persistent men-

tal illness. The family expresses concern about the client's ability to properly manage a small inheritance received from a relative. The nurse would respond to the family concerns using which of the following legal principles as a basis?

(1) ANA Code of Ethics
(2) autonomy
(3) confidentiality
(4) commitment

8. A client admitted to a psychiatric facility under an involuntary procedure has refused to take medication prescribed for psychotic symptoms. The treatment team meets to discuss this situation. Which statement made during this discussion reflects the ethical principle of beneficence?

(1) "Because the client really needs the medication for self-protection, an order to give the drug as an injection should be obtained."
(2) "The client has the right to refuse medications, so other treatment options should be explored."
(3) "The client has been involuntarily committed and therefore does not have the right to refuse."
(4) "The family should be consulted and asked to provide consent for the medication."

9. A nurse is observed as routinely responding to clients in an autocratic, controlling manner and with little consideration for their dignity and rights. After attempts to directly acknowledge the situation with the nurse in question, the nurse's colleagues plan to meet with the supervisor to express their concern about this unprofessional behavior. The plan to go to the supervisor is

(1) appropriate, because peer review is a professional activity needed to maintain quality care
(2) appropriate, because the nurse is probably looking for limits to be set on this behavior
(3) inappropriate, because it is up to the supervisor to evaluate the nurse
(4) inappropriate, because each nurse is responsible only for his or her own practice

10. A client with depressive symptoms is given prescribed medications and talks with his therapist about his belief that he is worthless and unable to cope with life. On which of the following frameworks of psychiatric care is this treatment plan based?

(1) behavioral framework
(2) cognitive framework
(3) interpersonal framework
(4) psychodynamic framework

11. A nurse who explains that a client's psychotic behavior is unconsciously motivated understands that the client's disordered behavior arises from which of the following?

(1) abnormal thinking
(2) altered neurotransmitters
(3) internal needs
(4) response to stimuli

12. A nurse observes that a mother is highly anxious when caring for her infant. Which of the following theorists would state that the mother's anxiety is communicated and internalized by the infant?

(1) Freud
(2) Sullivan
(3) Maslow
(4) Erikson

13. A client with depression has been hospitalized for treatment after taking a leave of absence from work. The client's employer expects the

client to return to work following inpatient treatment. The client tells the nurse that, "I'm no good, I'm a failure." According to cognitive theory, these statements reflect

(1) learned behavior

(2) punitive superego and decreased self-esteem

(3) faulty thought processes that govern behavior

(4) evidence of difficult relationships in the work environment

14. Which one of the following actions represents a nurse using Selye's general adaptation theory?

(1) teaching clients stress-reduction techniques

(2) helping clients develop awareness of stressors

(3) examining life events that require adaptation

(4) explaining to clients how the body responds to stress

15. A nurse observes a client pacing in the hall. Which of the following may the nurse say to help the client recognize anxiety?

(1) "I guess you're worried about something, aren't you?"

(2) "Can I get you some medication to help calm you?"

(3) "Have you been pacing for a long time?"

(4) "I notice that you're pacing. How are you feeling?"

16. A client who is a Vietnam War veteran suffers from nightmares and flashbacks about his war experience. He has been diagnosed with post-traumatic stress disorder. Which of the following nursing diagnoses would be most appropriate?

(1) fear, related to intrusive images from past experiences

(2) ineffective individual coping: compromised, related to failure to establish role responsibilities

(3) anxiety, related to fear of the unknown

(4) self-esteem disturbance, related to past experiences of inadequacy in combat

17. A client is diagnosed with hypochondriasis. During a discussion with a nurse, the client makes all of the following statements. Which one of these statements is most typical of a client with this diagnosis?

(1) "I feel tired all the time."

(2) "I think I have stomach cancer."

(3) "Nobody understands my problems."

(4) "I haven't been able to concentrate."

18. The nurse describes a client as anxious. Which of the following statements about anxiety is true?

(1) Anxiety is usually pathological.

(2) Anxiety is directly observable.

(3) Anxiety is usually harmful.

(4) Anxiety is a response to a threat.

19. A client with a phobic disorder is treated by systematic desensitization. The nurse understands that this approach will do which of the following?

(1) help the client execute actions that are feared

(2) help the client develop insight into irrational fears

(3) help the client substitute one fear for another

(4) help the client decrease anxiety

20. A client with obsessive-compulsive disorder is hospitalized on an inpatient unit. Which of the following nursing responses is most therapeutic?

(1) accepting the client's obsessive-compulsive behaviors

(2) challenging the client's obsessive-compulsive behaviors

(3) preventing the client's obsessive-compulsive behaviors

(4) rejecting the client's obsessive-compulsive behaviors

21. Which of the following symptoms would a nurse assess in a client with generalized anxiety disorder?

(1) blank affect, echolalia, feelings of unreality

(2) sadness, lack of hope, poor self-esteem

(3) suspicion, withdrawal from others, anger

(4) restlessness, sleep disturbance, difficulty concentrating

22. A 45-year-old woman with a history of depression tells a nurse in her physician's office that she has difficulty with sexual arousal and is fearful that her husband will have an affair. Although the nurse should assess all of the following factors, which would be least significant in contributing to the client's sexual difficulty?

(1) education and work history

(2) medications used

(3) physical health status

(4) quality of spousal relationship

23. A nurse is planning care for a client with borderline personality disorder who exhibits mood instability and frequent emotional outbursts. Which of the following factors would the nurse identify as *most* essential for care?

(1) dealing with what is verbalized rather than underlying feelings

(2) isolating the client when intense emotions are experienced

(3) maintaining calm, matter-of-fact response to client emotions

(4) promoting group interactions in which the client can ventilate

24. Which of the following client outcomes would the nurse evaluate as indicating successful treatment for a client with an antisocial personality disorder?

(1) charming behavior when around authority figures

(2) decreased episodes of impulsive behaviors

(3) statements of self-satisfaction

(4) statements indicating no remorse for behavior

25. A nurse is working in a medical clinic in which alternative medicine is utilized as adjunct to traditional treatment. The nurse is working with a client with an autoimmune disorder. Which of the following would this nurse teach the client to help increase the client's sense of control over symptoms?

(1) pathophysiology of disease process

(2) principles of good nutrition

(3) side effects of medications

(4) stress management techniques

26. A nurse is assessing a client with anorexia nervosa. In addition to weight loss, which of the following would the nurse expect to find?

(1) bradycardia, lanugo, amenorrhea

(2) fluid retention, tachycardia, hypertension

(3) irregular menses, diarrhea, dental caries

(4) tachycardia, intolerance to heat, skin rashes

27. Which of the following nursing diagnoses is most appropriate for a client with anorexia nervosa who expresses feelings of guilt about not meeting family expectations?

(1) anxiety

(2) body image disturbance

(3) defensive coping

(4) powerlessness

28. Which of the following nursing implementations would be most appropriate for a client with anorexia nervosa during initial hospitalization on a behavioral therapy unit?

(1) Emphasize the importance of good nutrition to establish normal weight.

(2) Ignore the client's mealtime behavior and focus instead on issues of dependence and independence.

(3) Help establish a plan using privileges and restrictions based on compliance with refeeding.

(4) Teach the client information about the long-term physical consequences of anorexia.

29. In planning care for the client with a somatoform disorder, the nurse would avoid which of the following?

(1) evaluating physical symptoms

(2) reinforcing secondary gains

(3) limiting manipulative behavior

(4) teaching relaxation techniques

30. A nurse is evaluating therapy with the family of a client with anorexia nervosa. Which of the following would indicate that the therapy was successful?

(1) The parents reinforce increased decision making by client.

(2) The parents clearly verbalize their expectations for the client.

(3) The client verbalizes that family meals are now enjoyable.

(4) The client tells the parents about feelings of low self-esteem.

31. A nurse is working with a client with somatoform disorder. Which of the following outcome goals would the nurse typically establish for this client?

(1) The client will recognize signs and symptoms of physical illness.

(2) The client will cope with physical illness.

(3) The client will take prescribed medications.

(4) The client will express anxiety verbally rather than by physical symptoms.

32. Which of the following is the most distinguishing feature of a client with an antisocial personality disorder?

(1) attention to detail and order

(2) bizarre mannerisms and thoughts

(3) submissive and dependent behaviors

(4) disregard for social and legal norms

33. For which of the following reasons is evaluation especially difficult in clients with personality disorders?

(1) These clients are often withdrawn even after therapy and may not share results openly.

(2) Typically, few changes in these clients' behavior may be identified over time.

(3) Nurses may reject these clients because of irritating behaviors.

(4) These clients improve rapidly and wish to move on with their lives.

34. A client is admitted to the psychiatric unit with a diagnosis of major depressive disorder. The nurse would assess for which of the following physiologic signs of depression?

(1) complaints of restlessness and anxiety

(2) complaints of rapid heart rate and dizziness

(3) significant appetite and sleep pattern changes

(4) significant increase in thirst and urinary frequency

35. Which of the following methods would a nurse use to determine a client's potential risk for suicide?
   (1) Wait for the client to bring up the subject of suicide.
   (2) Observe the client's behavior for cues of suicide ideation.
   (3) Question the client directly about suicidal thoughts.
   (4) Question the client about plans for the future.

36. A client with dysthymic disorder reports to a nurse that his life is hopeless and will never improve in the future. Using a cognitive approach for intervening in this distorted belief, which of the following would the nurse do?
   (1) Agree with the client's painful feelings.
   (2) Challenge the accuracy of the client's belief.
   (3) Deny that the situation is hopeless.
   (4) Present a cheerful attitude.

37. A client with a bipolar disorder exhibits manic behavior. The nursing diagnosis is *Altered thought processes* related to difficulty concentrating, secondary to flight of ideas. Which of the following outcome criteria would indicate improvement in the client?
   (1) The client verbalizes feelings directly during treatment.
   (2) The client verbalizes positive self-statements.
   (3) The client speaks in coherent sentences.
   (4) The client reports increased feelings of calm.

38. A client with major depression has not verbalized about problem areas to staff or peers since admission to a psychiatric unit. Which of the following activities would the nurse recommend to help this client express himself?
   (1) art therapy in a small group
   (2) basketball game with peers on unit
   (3) reading self-help book on depression
   (4) watching a movie with the peer group

39. A home health psychiatric nurse visits a client with chronic schizophrenia who was recently discharged from a prolonged stay in a state hospital. The client lives in a boarding home, reports no family involvement, and has little social interaction. The nurse plans a referral to a day treatment program in order to assist the client with which of the following?
   (1) management of hallucinations
   (2) medication teaching
   (3) social skills training
   (4) vocational training

40. A client with paranoid schizophrenia often directs brief, hostile verbal outbursts toward the nursing staff. Which of the following nursing actions is the most therapeutic way to address this problem?
   (1) Administer antipsychotic medications as needed when verbal outbursts occur.
   (2) Minimize the outbursts by walking away when they occur.
   (3) Place the client in seclusion when these episodes occur.
   (4) Set limits and provide a structured, predictable environment.

41. Which of the following activities would be appropriate for the nurse to implement with a severely withdrawn client?

✓(1) art activity with a staff member
(2) board game with a small group of clients
(3) team sport in the gym
(4) avoid activity until client is ready

42. A client looks frightened and states, "The unit is wired up to the FBI, and they're taking my thoughts away." Which of the following responses by the nurse would be most therapeutic?
   (1) "These thoughts aren't real; they're part of your illness."
   ✓(2) "I don't believe this is so, but you seem scared."
   (3) "How long have you been thinking about this?"
   (4) "Let me show you that the unit is not wired."

43. A client tells a nurse, "Everyone would be better off if I weren't alive." Which of the following nursing diagnoses would be made based on this statement?
   (1) altered thought processes
   (2) ineffective individual coping.
   ✓(3) risk for violence: self-directed
   (4) impaired social interaction

44. A client was recently admitted to an inpatient psychiatric unit. The client exhibits manic behavior on the unit and wears excessive make-up as well as provocative clothes. Which of the following statements by the nurse is the most appropriate way to intervene?
   (1) "It's important to look appropriate on the clinical unit. Go change."
   ✓(2) "Let's go back to your room and I'll help you select clothing that is better for this setting."
   (3) "You are dressed like you're going to a party. I think you need to change."
   (4) " I think you would look better in more conservative clothes."

45. A client with the DSM-IV diagnosis of schizophrenia, undifferentiated type, reports that her body is stiff and like wood. Which of the following symptoms is the client is manifesting?
   (1) autism
   (2) ambivalence
   ✓(3) depersonalization
   (4) regression

46. Which of the following would the nurse consider most essential in the initial teaching of the family of a young adult recently diagnosed with schizophrenia?
   (1) A chemical imbalance in the brain is the cause of the symptoms of this disease.
   (2) Genetic history is an important factor related to the development of schizophrenia.
   (3) Schizophrenia is a serious disease affecting every aspect of a person's functioning.
   ✓(4) The distressing symptoms of this disorder can respond to treatment with medications.

47. A nurse is working with a client who has schizophrenia, paranoid type. Which of the following outcomes related to the client's delusional perceptions would the nurse establish?
   ✓(1) The client will demonstrate realistic interpretation of daily events in the unit.
   (2) The client will perform daily hygiene and grooming without assistance.
   (3) The client will take prescribed medications without difficulty.
   (4) The client will participate in unit activities.

48. A nurse working in an outpatient drug and alcohol clinic interviews an 18-year-old client referred by her school guidance counselor. The

client's history reveals she was abandoned by her father at age 4 and lives with her mother, older sister, and sister's husband, all of whom abuse both alcohol and drugs. At age 16 she was raped at a party, became pregnant, and gave the child up for adoption. Her school counselor reports frequent absences, failing grades, and suspicion of drug use. Which of the factors in this client's life would the nurse identify as the most significant for increasing the client's vulnerability for substance abuse?

(1) abandonment by father at an early age

✓(2) family history of substance abuse

(3) poor school attendance and failing grades

(4) trauma of rape and subsequent pregnancy

49. A 7-year-old child has been admitted to the inpatient psychiatric unit following aggressive behavior in school and at home. He has been in three different placements in foster care since he was 2½ years old. He has sporadic contact with his natural mother, who has a history of schizophrenia. He used a piece of glass to cut up his fingers and stated, "I want to kill myself." The diagnosis of depressive disorder, not otherwise specified, is made by the physician. The nurse would understand the most common manifestation of depression in children is

✓(1) acting-out behavior

(2) poor parental relationship

(3) school problems

(4) suicide attempts

50. A client with bipolar disorder, manic type, exhibits extreme excite-ment, delusional thinking, and command hallucinations. Which of the following is the priority nursing diagnosis?

(1) anxiety

(2) impaired social interaction

(3) sensory-perceptual alteration

✓(4) risk for violence

51. A client is admitted to an acute medical-surgical unit for treatment of multiple traumatic injuries related to a car accident. The client history indicates use of both alcohol and heroin on a regular basis. Which of the following anticipated problems would be of most concern for nursing care?

(1) client denial of alcohol and drug abuse

(2) difficulty in establishing nurse-client relationship

(3) client demonstrating active drug-seeking behavior

(4) maintenance of adequate pain control for client

52. A client who abuses alcohol and cocaine tells a nurse that he only uses substances because of his stressful marriage and difficult job. Which of the following defense mechanisms is this client using?

(1) displacement

(2) projection

(3) rationalization

(4) sublimation

53. A client has developed tolerance to CNS depressants. Which of the following is the correct interpretation of tolerance?

(1) concurrent abuse of two different substances

(2) continued use of substance despite life problems

(3) need to increase dose to obtain desired effect

(4) occurrence of physiologic symptoms when drug is discontinued

54. A nurse assesses a client for alcohol withdrawal symptoms. Which of the following would the nurse note?
(1) agitation, increased pulse rate, increased blood pressure
(2) drowsiness, decreased pulse rate, decreased blood pressure
(3) euphoria, increased energy, hostility
(4) slurred speech, incoordination, memory loss

55. A nurse is planning care for a family in which violence commonly occurs. Which of the following statements about nonvictim members of violent families is correct?
(1) These family members do not require intervention because they are not involved.
(2) These family members often experience more trauma than do actual victims.
(3) These family members should be encouraged to seek alternative living arrangements.
(4) These family members commonly experience fear and guilt from their exposure to violence.

56. An 11-year-old child diagnosed with conduct disorder is admitted to the psychiatric unit for treatment. Which of the following behaviors would be assessed by the nurse?
(1) restlessness, short attention span, hyperactivity
(2) physical aggressiveness, low stress tolerance, disregard for rights of others
(3) deterioration in social functioning, excessive anxiety and worry, bizarre behavior
(4) sadness, poor appetite and sleeplessness, loss of interest in activities

57. A mental health treatment team recommends family systems therapy for a family with a history of violence toward both adults and children in the family. The nurse understands that this treatment method is recommended for the primary purpose of
(1) allowing family members to verbalize feelings
(2) establishing responsible self-functioning of family members
(3) identifying the perpetrators of violence in the family
(4) treating child victims of abusive behaviors

58. A pregnant woman has abused heroin for the past 3 years. She is unemployed and obtains money by prostitution and stealing. Which of the following would be the most important initial nursing consideration for this client?
(1) Counsel the client about her lifestyle and needed changes.
(2) Assess one's personal attitudes about heroin addiction and prostitution.
(3) Identify the legal implications of stealing, the health risks associated with prostitution, and the effects of drugs on the fetus.
(4) Review literature on substance abuse and dependence and its impact on the health of pregnant women.

59. A nurse would understand that if a client continues to be dependent on heroin throughout her pregnancy, her baby will be at high risk for
(1) mental retardation
(2) heroin dependence
(3) addiction in adulthood
(4) psychological disturbances

60. A nurse applying psychodynamic theory to understand sexual abuse knows which of the following factors are associated with this problem?
(1) personal history of abuse for the abuser, diminished ego strength

(2) observation of incest in child-hood, poor adult role models

(3) overcoming internal controls to abuse

(4) a belief that women and chil-dren are property

61. Which of the following factors would a nurse identify as least important in the decision regarding whether a victim of family violence can safely remain in the home?

(1) the availability of appropriate community shelters

(2) the ability of the nonabusing caretaker to intervene on the client's behalf

(3) the client's possible response to relocation

✓ (4) the family's socioeconomic status

62. A family member of a client with schizophrenia questions the nurse about the cause of this disorder. Which of the following would be the most accurate response by the nurse?

(1) The disorder is thought to result from disturbed family relations and communication problems.

(2) The disorder is thought to be caused by brain alterations in the frontal lobe.

✓ (3) The disorder is thought to be caused by a combination of bio-logic, genetic, and psychosocial factors.

(4) The disorder is thought to be caused by altered dopamine transmission in the brain.

63. A psychiatric nurse generalist works with a support group of individuals who have experienced the death of a spouse. The primary purpose of this group would be

(1) to focus on problems in group living and encourage coping strategies

(2) to help members improve inter-action and plan enjoyable activ-ities

✓ (3) to provide empathy for members and reinforce existing strengths

(4) to provide educational informa-tion and encourage self-man-agement

64. A nurse is working with a group of clients on an inpatient unit. Which of the following would the nurse do when conflict occurs among mem-bers?

(1) Discuss the situation privately with the individual client(s) involved in the conflict.

✓ (2) Encourage an open discussion among group members.

(3) Ignore the situation unless it becomes a group problem.

(4) Provide specific information on how to resolve the conflict.

65. In which of the following areas would a nurse expect a client with early Alzheimer's disease to have problems?

✓ (1) balancing a checkbook

(2) self-care measures

(3) relating to family members

(4) remembering his or her own name

66. A nurse would differentiate the cog-nitive impairment disorders of delir-ium and dementia in which of the following ways?

(1) Delirium occurs slowly and responds to treatment.

✓ (2) Delirium has a rapid onset and may be reversed.

(3) Dementia has a rapid onset and can be reversed.

(4) Dementia occurs slowly and may improve rapidly.

67. A client with a history of multiple suicide attempts is admitted to the inpatient unit with a diagnosis of major depression, recurrent, with

psychotic features. All of the following medications are ordered. Which of these is ordered for the purpose of decreasing irrational thinking?
- **(1)** lorazepam (Ativan) 1 mg p.o., q.6h., p.r.n.
- **(2)** clonazepam (Klonopin), 0.5 mg p.o., daily at 5 PM
- **(3)** sertraline (Zoloft), 50 mg p.o., daily at h.s.
- **(4)** olanzapine (Zyprexa), 5 mg p.o., b.i.d.

68. Which of the following would a nurse implement for a client with Alzheimer's disease who has frequent episodes of emotional lability?
- **(1)** Attempt humor to alter mood.
- **(2)** Explore reasons for altered mood.
- **(3)** Reduce environmental stimuli to redirect attention.
- **(4)** Use logic in order to point out reality aspects.

69. Which of the following neurotransmitters has been implicated in the process of Alzheimer's disease?
- **(1)** acetylcholine
- **(2)** dopamine
- **(3)** epinephrine
- **(4)** serotonin

70. The daughter of a client with Alzheimer's disease reports feeling chronic fatigue and mild depression. Further assessment reveals that this daughter has been responsible for feeding, cleaning, and doing laundry for her parent while maintaining a full-time job and caring for two teenagers. Which of the following nursing diagnoses does the nurse establish for the client's daughter?
- **(1)** Altered family process
- **(2)** Ineffective family coping
- **(3)** Caregiver role strain
- **(4)** Social isolation

71. Which of the following assessments is most essential for a nurse to make when using a crisis intervention method of treatment?
- **(1)** communication and coping skills
- **(2)** level of anxiety and expression of feelings
- **(3)** perception of event and situational supports
- **(4)** use of reality testing and level of depression

72. A seriously ill client dies much sooner than expected. Family members are called and when they arrive, are told about the death. At this time, the nurse can expect family members to
- **(1)** demonstrate shock and disbelief
- **(2)** exhibit helplessness and withdrawal
- **(3)** share fond memories about the deceased
- **(4)** state how much they miss their family member

73. The nurse evaluates a client's response to crisis intervention as favorable if the client
- **(1)** changes coping skills and behavioral patterns
- **(2)** develops insight into reasons why crisis occurred
- **(3)** learns to relate better to others
- **(4)** returns to previous level of functioning

74. Two nurses are co-leading group therapy for seven clients in the psychiatric unit. The leaders observe that the group members are anxious and look to them for answers. Which of the following phases of development is this group in?
- **(1)** conflict resolution phase
- **(2)** initiation phase
- **(3)** working phase
- **(4)** termination phase

75. A nurse is leading a therapeutic social skills group and tells the members, "This is our group and the purpose of meeting is to learn different ways of talking to people. It is important that we practice listening. Our group is designed to help with talking and listening." These statements by the nurse are

(1) nontherapeutic because group spontaneity will be restricted

(2) therapeutic because group cohesiveness will be enhanced

(3) nontherapeutic because group norms are not addressed

(4) therapeutic because group conflict will be prevented

76. The nurse responsible for leading a therapy group evaluates the group as being in the working phase if the members

(1) begin to comment on their behaviors

(2) ask the nurse for advice regarding problems

(3) talk about someone outside the group

(4) focus on their past relationships

77. Group members have worked very hard, and the nurse reminds them that termination is approaching. Termination is considered successful if group members

(1) decide to continue

(2) evaluate group progress

(3) focus on positive experiences

(4) stop attending prior to termination

78. A nurse is assessing a family's communication skills. Which of the following data validate good communication skills?

(1) evidence that children accept and adopt parental value system

(2) family members who express agreement on issues and problems

(3) open and clear discussion of issues and feelings among members

(4) parents who state that they have no problems communicating with children

79. A nurse is providing care for an adolescent hospitalized for depression. The nurse is asked by the parents to encourage the adolescent to attend college. The nurse can intervene most therapeutically by

(1) encouraging each family member to discuss his or her feelings on this issue

(2) explaining to the parents that the adolescent can make the decision about college

(3) talking to the adolescent about the advantages of an education

(4) refusing to get involved in this issue, which is unrelated to treatment

80. A client hospitalized with a diagnosis of schizophrenia recently started taking oral trifluoperazine (Stelazine), 2 mg three times daily. The client complains of progressively stiff, painful, and tense neck muscles. Given this data, the nurse suspects that the client is experiencing

(1) increased tension related to the illness

(2) an acute dystonic reaction

(3) symptoms of pseudoparkinsonism

(4) neuroleptic malignant syndrome

81. A nurse is teaching a group of clients about the mood-stabilizing medication lithium carbonate. Teaching these clients would include telling them to avoid which of the following medications that may increase the risk of lithium toxicity?

(1) antacids

(2) antibiotics

✓ **(3)** diuretics

(4) hypoglycemic agents

82. A client has been taking haloperidol (Haldol), 5 mg three times daily, to treat schizophrenia. The nurse routinely assesses for extrapyramidal side effects. Which of the following would *not* be an extrapyramidal side effect?

✓ **(1)** dry mouth and urine retention

(2) eyes rolling upward uncontrollably

(3) excessive motor restlessness

(4) tremors and shuffling gait

83. A nurse is analyzing the functioning of healthy family systems. Which of the following situations would not be expected to increase stress on a healthy family system?

(1) an adolescent going away to college

(2) birth of a child

(3) death of a grandparent

✓ **(4)** parental disagreement

84. A client with generalized anxiety disorder has been taking diazepam (Valium), 5 mg three times daily, for the past 2 weeks. At the outpatient clinic, the nurse assesses the client's knowledge about this drug. Which of the following statements indicates the need for further instruction for the client?

(1) "I know this drug can be addicting."

(2) "I understand that when I no longer need this drug, I'll gradually have to stop taking it."

(3) "I won't drink alcohol while I'm taking this drug."

✓ **(4)** "I will take this drug only when I'm feeling upset."

85. Prior to administering the medication chlorpromazine (Thorazine), 50 mg intramuscularly, to a client who is agitated, the nurse should

(1) assess skin color and sclera

(2) obtain radial pulse

✓ **(3)** take blood pressure

(4) ask the client to void

86. The nurse evaluates the effectiveness of the neuroleptic medication, olanzapine (Zyprexa) by noting which of the following expected client outcomes?

✓ **(1)** increased motivation and improved social interaction

(2) decreased level of anxiety and normal sleep patterns

(3) increased withdrawal and decreased interest in activities

(4) decreased excitement and fewer episodes of panic

87. A client taking the MAOI antidepressant isocarboxazid (Marplan) is instructed by the nurse to avoid which of the following foods and beverages?

(1) aged cheese and red wine

(2) milk and green leafy vegetables

(3) carbonated beverages and tomato products

(4) lean red meats and fruit juices

88. A client who has been taking amitriptyline (Elavil) for depression for the past 7 days reports no improvement in her mood and asks if the drug should be discontinued. The nurse's response (ie, to tell the client to continue the medication) would be based on which of the following data?

(1) The drug's onset of action is 24 to 48 hours.

✓ **(2)** The drug's onset of action is 2 to 3 weeks.

(3) The drug's effect may be diminished in major depression.

(4) The drug's effect may not always be readily observed by the client.

89. The nurse understands that the primary role of electroconvulsive ther-

apy in psychiatric care is for the treatment of

(1) anxiety disorders

✓**(2)** depression

(3) mania

(4) schizophrenia

90. The nurse administering a typical antipsychotic medication, such as fluphenazine (Prolixin), by the oral route would know that this drug should be given

—**(1)** at least 2 hours after eating

(2) at mealtimes or with milk

(3) with plenty of water

(4) without regard to meals

91. Which of the following atypical antipsychotic medications requires weekly testing of white blood cell counts for the first 6 months of treatment?

(1) clozapine (Clozaril)

(2) pimozide (Orap)

(3) olanzapine (Zyprexa)

(4) sertindole (Serlect)

92. A nurse would expect that an elderly client would have which of the following tests prior to initiation of therapy with tricyclic antidepressants?

(1) electroencephalogram

✓**(2)** baseline electrocardiogram

—**(3)** liver function studies

(4) serum electrolytes

93. A client taking the MAOI phenelzine (Nardil) tells the nurse that he routinely takes each of the following medications. Which of these medications would cause the nurse to express concern and therefore initiate further teaching?

(1) acetaminophen (Tylenol)

✓**(2)** diphenhydramine (Benadryl)

(3) furosemide (Lasix)

(4) isosorbide dinitrate (Isordil)

94. Bupropion (Zyban) has been prescribed for a client as an aid in smoking cessation. Which of the following medical problems would contraindicate the use of this drug?

(1) angina pectoris

(2) food allergies

(3) rheumatoid arthritis

—**(4)** seizure disorder

95. A nurse is administering a psychotropic medication to an elderly client who has a history of benign prostatic hypertrophy. Which of the following would the nurse teach this client?

(1) to add fiber to diet

(2) to exercise on a regular basis

(3) to report incomplete bladder emptying

(4) to take prescribed dose at bedtime

96. A client is admitted with major depressive disorder, not otherwise specified, following the recent divorce from his wife. He complains of sleep disturbance, poor energy level, and feeling helpless and hopeless. The nursing diagnosis is *Ineffective individual coping* related to response to loss secondary to recent divorce. Which of the following is the most appropriate client outcome for this diagnosis?

(1) The client will contact his wife and request a reconciliation.

—**(2)** The client will identify three strategies to use to handle his feelings related to the divorce.

(3) The client will list the stressors that contributed to the marital problems.

(4) The client will verbalize his thoughts and feelings of hopelessness.

97. When a nurse suspects a client is experiencing either neuroleptic malignant syndrome or serotonin syndrome, which of the following is the priority action?

(1) ensuring adequate fluids
(2) maintaining bed rest
(3) monitoring client frequently
(4) withholding further drug doses

98. A nurse teaches a client taking the benzodiazepine oxazepam (Serax) to avoid excessive intake of
    (1) cheese
    (2) coffee
    (3) sugar
    (4) shellfish

99. A nurse refers a client who describes a 20-year history of alcohol abuse to Alcoholics Anonymous. The primary function of this group is
    (1) to encourage the use of a 12-step program
    (2) to help members maintain sobriety

    (3) to provide fellowship among members
    (4) to teach positive coping mechanisms

100. A nurse works in a setting using a therapeutic community approach to psychiatric treatment. Which of the following client outcomes would be most appropriately achieved in this setting?
    (1) achievement of activities of daily living and learning about crafts
    (2) prevention of aggression and monitoring medications
    (3) promotion of self-reliance and social adaptation
    (4) relief of anxiety and learning about symptoms

Answer Key

1. The answer is (4). An interpreter will enable the nurse to better assess the client's problems and concerns. Nonverbal communication is important; however, for the nurse to fully assess the client's problems and concerns, the assistance of an interpreter is essential. The use of symbolic pictures and universal phrases may assist the nurse in understanding the basic needs of the client; however, these are insufficient to assess the client with a psychiatric problem.

2. The answer is (2). The client's request is congruent with cultural beliefs and should be honored. The nurse can help by acting as the client's advocate. Telling the client that having a special healer is inappropriate in the hospital setting is a value judgment on the nurse's part; it is inappropriate for the nurse to say this to the client. Reflecting that the client is seeking magical healing is an interpretative response based on the nurse's belief system and does not reflect the client's culture. A nurse who provides culturally sensitive nursing care would facilitate the request rather than referring this to the physician. The client has the right to practice religious and cultural beliefs.

3. The answer is (4). Termination is an important phase in the therapeutic relationship. The nurse and the client reassess the client's progress, evaluate goal attainment, and explore how the therapeutic relationship was experienced. It is also important to deal with feelings about termination during this phase. Assessment is an ongoing part of the therapeutic relationship and occurs in all phases. The therapeutic relationship is also characterized by establishing trust (orientation) and planning outcomes and interventions to assist the client to meet goals (working).

4. The answer is (3). When a client makes vague, global statements, the therapeutic approach is to seek clarification. Seeking clarification helps the client become more aware of thoughts, feelings, and ideas. In the responses of answer choices **(1)** and **(2)**, the nurse is making assumptions about the meaning of the client's statement and replying in such a way that further exploration of this client's concern is cut off. In answer choice **(4)**, the nurse is challenging the client to explain behaviors and validating that the client's belief is correct.

5. The answer is (1). The behavioral framework is based on the premise that maladaptive behaviors are learned and can be changed by altering the environment that reinforces these behaviors. Techniques such as establishing a behavioral contract can be a form of operant conditioning in which the individual agrees to modify behavior according to specific rewards. Although the client is learning to change behaviors, there is not an established educational framework. Neither an interpersonal nor a psychodynamic framework utilizes a system in which specific behaviors are targeted for change by use of rewards.

6. The answer is (4). Psychoanalytic theory is based on Freud's beliefs regarding the importance of unconscious motivation for behavior and the role of the id and superego in opposition to each other. Behavioral, educational, and interpersonal theories do not emphasize unconscious conflicts as the basis for symptomatic behavior.

7. The answer is (2). The client has the basic right to make decisions in areas affecting the client's life; this is the principle of autonomy. Managing funds is an example of one area in which the client exercises the right of autonomy. Unless a court declares the client incompetent, the family is legally unable to exert control in this area. Although the ANA Code of Ethics guides the nurse's practice, the legal principle operative in this situation is autonomy. Confidentiality refers to client's right to control disclosure of information related to health status and treatment. Commitment is the legal process governing psychiatric admission.

8. The answer is (2). The principle of beneficence requires the nurse to act in ways that benefit the client. Offering other treatment options demonstrates the commitment of the nurse to promote client choice. Answer choices **(1)** and **(3)** reflect a lack of understanding on the nurse's part of the legal issues of psychiatric nursing regarding the client's right and the commitment process. Finally, the family cannot provide the consent because the client is competent until judged otherwise by a court.

9. The answer is (1). The ANA's Standards of Psychiatric and Mental Health Practice call for peer review as a mechanism for maintaining quality care. In the situation described, it would be better if a formal peer review system were in place to evaluate the nurse's performance. However, the colleagues are correct in expressing their concerns to the supervisor. The remaining answer choices do not address the nurses' responsibilities for upholding professional standards of practice.

10. The answer is (2). Cognitive framework focuses on the client's misperceptions about self, others, and the world that impact functioning and contribute to symptoms. Using medications to alter neurotransmitter activity is a psychobiologic approach to treatment. The other answer choices are frameworks for care, but they are not applicable to this situation.

11. The answer is (3). The concept that behavior is motivated and has meaning comes from the psychodynamic framework. According to this perspective, behavior arises from internal wishes or needs. Much of what motivates behavior comes from the unconscious. The remaining responses do not address the internal forces thought to motivate behavior.

12. The answer is (2). Sullivan believed that a child develops a sense of self from the appraisal received from significant others. According to Sullivan, the infant will internalize the mother's increased anxiety levels. The other therorists do not place emphasis on the relationship process.

13. The answer is (3). The client is demonstrating faulty thought processes that are negative and that govern his behavior in reference to the work situation. Cognitive theory describes the effect of faulty thinking on behavior. Answer choice **(1)** represents behavior theory. Answer choice **(2)** represents psychoanalytic theory. Answer choice **(4)** is incorrect, because there is no evidence in this situation that the client has conflictual relationships in the work environment.

14. The answer is (4). Selye's general adaptation theory describes how the body responds to stress. There are three stages: the first stage is the alarm reaction, the second is resistance, and the third is exhaustion if the stress continues. The other answer choices are actions of the nurse in a stress management program for clients.

15. The answer is (4). The nurse acknowledges the behavior observed and then asks the client to express his or her feelings. This approach will assist the client in becoming aware of anxious feelings. In answer choice **(1)**, the nurse is offering an interpretation that may or may not be accurate; the nurse is also asking a question that may be answered by a "yes" or "no" response. In answer choice **(2)**, the nurse is intervening before accurately assessing the problem. Answer choice **(3)**, which the client can answer with a "yes" or "no" response, does not encourage the client to focus on anxiety.

16. The answer is (1). Flashbacks and nightmares from past experiences are common in patients with post-traumatic stress disorder. Clients with this disorder respond with intense fear to these events. The data are insufficient to establish the nursing diagnoses of answer choices **(2)** and **(4)**. Answer choice **(3)** is incorrect, because the fear is known in post-traumatic stress disorder and is directly related to the traumatic events precipitating this disorder.

17. The answer is (2). The fear of having a serious disease is the essential feature of a person with hypochondriasis. The statement in answer choice **(1)** may be a symptom of a somatoform disorder but is not the most typical of hypochondriasis. The statements in answer choices **(3)** and **(4)** could apply to many psychiatric disorders.

18. The answer is (4). Anxiety is a response to a threat arising from internal or external stimuli. The remaining answer choices are incorrect.

19. The answer is (1). Systematic desensitization is a behavioral therapy technique that helps clients with irrational fears and avoidance behavior to face the thing they fear without anxiety. There is no attempt to promote insight with this procedure, and the client will not be taught to substitute one fear for another. The client's anxiety may decrease with successful confrontation of irrational fears. However, the purpose of the procedure is specifically related to performing activities that typically are avoided as part of the phobic response.

20. The answer is (1). The client with obsessive-compulsive behavior uses this behavior to decrease anxiety. The nurse accepts this behavior as the client's attempt to feel secure. When a specific treatment plan is developed, other nursing responses may also be acceptable. The remaining answer choices will increase anxiety for the client and therefore are inappropriate.

21. The answer is (4). Restlessness, sleep disturbance, and difficulty concentrating are all characteristics of generalized anxiety disorder as defined in the DSM-IV. The remaining answer choices are not symptoms of generalized anxiety disorder.

22. The answer is (1). Education and work history would have the least significance in relation to the client's sexual problem. Age, health status, physical attributes, and relationship issues have great influence in sexual expression.

23. The answer is (3). The nurse would plan to maintain a calm, matter-of-fact response to avoid increasing client anxiety levels that are elevated during emotional outbursts. This response by the nurse would help to defuse client anger. Ignoring emotions would not help the client gain control of outbursts. Isolating a client with borderline personality disorder will increase anxiety, because clients with this disorder are fearful of being alone. The client would monopolize a group situation, because narcissism is another characteristic of the person with this personality disorder. The group setting may also increase client anxiety because of the increased stimuli.

24. The answer is (2). The client with an antisocial personality disorder demonstrates frequent episodes of acting impulsively with poor ability to delay self-gratification. Decreased frequency of impulsive behaviors would be evidence of improvement. Charming behavior when around authority figures and statements indicating no remorse are examples of symptoms that would be typical of the client with this disorder and would not indicate successful treatment. Self-satisfaction could be a positive change if the client was expressing low self-esteem; however, this would not be typical of a client with an antisocial personality disorder.

25. The answer is (4). In autoimmune disorders, stress and the response to stress can exacerbate symptoms. Stress management techniques will help the client reduce the psychological response to stress. This in turn will help reduce the physiologic stress response. The client will experience an increased sense of control over symptoms, which are exacerbated by stress. The remaining answer choices are all areas in which the nurse may teach the client and the client will gain knowledge about the disease and treatment of the disease. However, stress management will provide the client with specific ways to control the response to stress and therefore will help control symptoms.

26. The answer is (1). The client with anorexia nervosa will demonstrate decreased heart rate due to decreased metabolic rate, as well as possible loss of heart muscle due to starvation. Lanugo occurs as a result of loss of subcutaneous tissue. Amenorrhea occurs as a result of losing fatty tissue in which estrogen is stored. Weight less than 85% of the norm for age and height is also important to establish diagnosis. The remaining symptoms are not typical of the physical manifestations related to malnutrition, which is the basis for the physiologic changes in the client with anorexia.

27. The answer is (4). The client with anorexia usually feels little control over any aspect of life besides eating behavior. Often, parental expectations and standards are quite high and lead to the client's sense of guilt over not measuring up.

28. The answer is (3). Treatment of a client with anorexia in an inpatient unit focuses first on the establishment of a plan for refeeding to combat the effects of self-induced starvation. Behavioral therapy uses a system of rewards and reinforcements to assist in establishing weight restoration. Emphasizing nutrition and teaching the client about the long-term physical consequences of anorexia may be appropriate at a later time in the treatment program. The nurse needs to assess the client's mealtime behavior continually to evaluate treatment effectiveness.

29. The answer is (2). The nurse should avoid reinforcing any secondary gains that the client with a somatoform disorder may get from physical symptoms. Physical complaints need to be evaluated by the nurse, because organic pathology may be possible with this client. Limiting manipulative behavior and teaching relaxation techniques would be helpful to the client with a somatoform disorder and would be appropriate nursing care.

30. The answer is (1). One of the essential issues in the family of a client with anorexia is the issue of control. When the client can make independent decisions and the parents can accept this, family intervention has been successful. The remaining responses may occur during the process of therapy, but would not indicate successful outcome; the central family issues of dependence and independence are not addressed in these responses.

31. The answer is (4). The client with a somatoform disorder displaces anxiety onto physical symptoms. The ability to express anxiety verbally indicates a positive change toward improved health. The remaining responses do not indicate any positive change toward increased coping with anxiety.

32. The answer is (4). Disregard for established rules of society is the most common characteristic of a client with an antisocial personality disorder. Attention to detail and order is characteristic of a client with obsessive-compulsive disorder. Bizarre mannerisms and thoughts are characteristic of a client with schizoid or schizotypal disorder. Submissive and dependent behaviors are characteristic of a client with a dependent personality.

33. The answer is (2). Behavioral changes often are subtle in persons with personality disorders. Withdrawn behavior is not typical, nor does improvement occur rapidly with these clients. A nurse may allow personal feelings to overrule professional judgment. However, this is a problem for the entire nurse-client relationship, not just the evaluation phase.

34. The answer is (3). Physiologic changes expected with depression include significant decrease or increase in appetite as well as insomnia or hypersomnia. The remaining physiologic changes are not typical for a client with a diagnosis of major depression.

35. The answer is (3). Directly questioning the client about suicide is important to determine suicide risk. The client may not bring up this subject for several reasons: guilt regarding suicide; wish not to be discovered; and lack of trust in staff. Behavioral cues are important but direct questioning is essential to determine suicide risk. Indirect questions convey to the client that the nurse is not comfortable with the subject of suicide and therefore the client may be reluctant to discuss this.

36. The answer is (2). The use of cognitive techniques means that the nurse will attempt to assist the client to recognize that negative beliefs may be distortions and that it is possible to change a negative belief to one that is more realistic as well as hopeful. Agreeing with the client's feelings and presenting a cheerful attitude are not consistent with a cognitive approach and would not be helpful to this client. Denying the client's feelings is belittling to the client and may convey that the nurse does not understand the depth of the client's distress.

37. The answer is (3). Flight of ideas occurs when the client's speech flow is continuous and the client jumps from one topic to another. The client who can speak in coherent sentences shows that concentration has improved and thoughts are no longer racing. The remaining answer choice options do not relate directly to the stated nursing diagnosis.

38. The answer is (1). Art therapy provides a nonthreatening vehicle for the expression of feelings. Use of a small group will help the client become comfortable with peers in a group setting. Basketball is a game that requires energy and is competitive; the client with major depression will not likely participate in this activity. Recommending that the client read a self-help book may increase rather than decrease the client's isolation. Watching a movie with a peer group does not guarantee that interaction will occur, and therefore the client may maintain isolation.

39. The answer is (3). Day treatment programs provide clients with chronic persistent mental illness training in social skills, such as meeting and greeting people, asking questions or directions, placing an order in a restaurant, and taking turns in a group setting or activity. Although management of hallucinations and medication teaching may also be part of the program offered in day treatment, the nurse is referring the client described in the situation because of the need for socialization skills. Vocational training generally takes place in a rehabilitation facility; the client described in this situation would not be a candidate for this service. The social skills training would be an important first step.

40. The answer is (4). Firm, nonpunitive limit setting and a structured environment are the best approach to a verbally hostile client. Answer choices **(1)** and **(3)** are too severe, considering that the outbursts are brief and there is no escalation to physical violence. Walking away when the outbursts occur would not be as useful as setting a clear limit on inappropriate behavior.

41. The answer is (1). The best approach with a withdrawn client is to initiate brief, nondemanding activities on a one-to-one basis. This approach gives the nurse an opportunity to establish a trusting relationship with the client. A board game with a group of clients or playing a team sport in the gym may overwhelm a severely withdrawn client.

42. The answer is (2). The best approach to delusional ideas is to avoid arguing with them while simultaneously acknowledging reality. It is also important to respond to the underlying message or the predominant feeling of the client. In this case, the client is frightened, so the nurse addresses this by saying she believes that the client is safe here. Answer choice **(1)** would be premature; when the client has some improvement, it may be possible to discuss delusions as part of the illness. Answer choices **(3)** and **(4)** place too much emphasis on the delusions.

43. The answer is (3). The nurse should take any statements indicating suicidal thoughts seriously and further assess for other risk factors. The remaining diagnoses fail to address the seriousness of the client's statement.

44. The answer is (2). The nurse handles the inappropriate dress in such a way that the client's dignity is preserved. The nurse also offers to assist the client in selecting clothes that are more appropriate. Answer choice **(1)** is incorrect because the client may believe that she is dressed in an appropriate manner. A client who has mania has distorted perceptions of reality. Answer choice **(3)** would embarrass the client and does not provide any specific direction for more appropriate clothing. Answer choice **(4)** is vague; the client may not understand what the nurse means by "more conservative clothes."

45. The answer is (3). Depersonalization is a feeling of strangeness or unreality about one's own body or body parts. Autism is a focus inward; the individual may create a fantasy world. Ambivalence is having strong opposing emotions about a person or situation. Regression is a defense mechanism whereby the individual returns to an earlier, more comfortable form of behavior.

46. The answer is (4). This statement is true and it can provide a focus for hope for the family who has just received this diagnosis for a member. Although the remaining statements are true, they will not provide an empathetic understanding of the family response to this diagnosis. These facts can become part of the ongoing teaching but would not be most essential initially.

47. The answer is (1). A client with schizophrenia, paranoid type, will distort perceptions and view events in the environment as related to people or institutions plotting against him. The outcome related to a realistic interpretation of daily events would establish improvement in the client's perceptual ability. Hygiene and grooming skills are not necessarily impaired when a client distorts the environment. Although taking medications and participating in unit activities may be appropriate outcomes for nursing intervention, these responses are not related to client perceptions.

48. The answer is (2). Family history presents the most significant stressor for vulnerability for substance abuse. Genetic theory and cognitive-behavioral theory have both established this factor as highly significant. Abandonment by the father and the trauma of the rape and subsequent pregnancy are stressors that are significant in terms of affecting the client's normal growth and development and may increase susceptibility to either depressive illness or post-traumatic stress disorder. Poor school attendance and failing grades represent the response of the client to significant problem areas.

49. The answer is (1). In children, depression is often manifested by acting-out behaviors (in contrast to an adult in which behavior is often withdrawal from interaction with others). Excessive sadness, hopelessness, and helplessness may also be seen in a child with depression. A poor parental relationship is a factor that would increase the child's vulnerability to depressive illness. School problems may be associated with multiple psychiatric problems in children and are not specific to depression. Although suicide attempt is a sign of depressive illness, it is not commonly seen in a young child. The fact that this child has demonstrated this would lead to the decision to hospitalize in order to provide a safe environment and decrease the risk of suicide.

50. The answer is (4). A client with these symptoms would have poor impulse control and therefore would be prone to acting-out behavior that may be harmful to either self or others. All of the remaining nursing diagnoses may apply to the client with mania; however, the priority diagnosis would be risk for violence.

51. The answer is (4). A client who has a history of substance abuse will have cross-tolerance to the medications used for analgesia. In this situation, in which the client has traumatic injuries, pain control will be a priority concern for nursing care. The client history already has documented use of abusive substance; the client's denial of this would be a defense mechanism and would not be of priority concern. Difficulty establishing a nurse-client relationship may or may not occur with this client; it would not be of priority concern. Drug-seeking behaviors would be anticipated; however, this client has multiple traumatic injuries, and therefore pain control would be a priority concern.

52. The answer is (3). Rationalization is the defense mechanism that involves offering excuses for behavior. The client is defending his substance abuse by providing reasons related to life stressors. This is a common defense mechanism used by clients with substance abuse problems. None of the remaining defense mechanisms involve making excuses for behaviors.

53. The answer is (3). Tolerance is the need for increased amounts of substance to obtain a desired effect. It is one of the characteristics of substance dependence. Concurrent abuse of two different substances is polydrug use. Continued use of substance despite life problems would be the criterion for substance dependence. Occurrence of physiologic symptoms when the drug is discontinued is the phenomenon of withdrawal.

54. The answer is (1). Alcohol withdrawal is characterized by CNS excitation, including increased vital signs. Drowsiness, decreased pulse rate, decreased blood pressure, euphoria, increased energy, and hostility do not occur in alcohol withdrawal. Slurred speech, incoordination, and memory loss would occur in alcohol intoxication rather than withdrawal.

55. The answer is (4). Observers are affected by dysfunction in family systems and often require help in coping with their emotional responses. Nonvictims are involved passively and can assist in resolving family difficulties. Available data do not support the assumption that nonvictims are more traumatized. Encouraging the nonvictim family member to seek alternative living arrangements supports family alienation and is not indicated.

56. The answer is (2). Physical aggressiveness, low stress tolerance, and a disregard for the rights of others are common behaviors in clients with conduct disorders. Restlessness, short attention span, and hyperactivity are typical behaviors in a client with attention deficit-hyperactivity disorder. Deterioration in social functioning, excessive anxiety and worry, and bizarre behaviors are typical in schizophrenic disorders. Sadness, poor appetite, sleeplessness, and loss of interest in activities are typical behaviors in depressive disorders.

57. The answer is (2). Family systems therapy as a treatment method works toward promotion of responsible self-functioning in families in which there are blurred generational boundaries and evidence of undifferentiated family ego mass. Family members may be encouraged to verbalize; however this is not the primary purpose of treatment. Members who have perpetrated violence will be identified as part of assessment, but this is not the primary purpose. The child victims of abuse will be helped by the adult members developing more responsible self-functioning.

58. The answer is (2). The nurse's attitudes can impact on the treatment of the client. Negative attitudes can be indirectly communicated and can damage the client's self-esteem. Neither counseling the client about her life-style and needed changes nor identifying the legal implications, health risks, and drug effects on her fetus because of her behavior should be the first intervention; these interventions should be done only when the nurse can demonstrate respect and a nonjudgmental attitude. Reviewing literature on substance abuse and its impact on pregnant women is incorrect as the first intervention, although it may prove helpful for the nurse who lacks information about female addicts.

59. The answer is (2). Babies born to heroin-dependent women are also heroin-dependent and need to go through withdrawal. There is no evidence to support any of the remaining answer choices.

60. The answer is (1). Psychodynamic theories identify the need to resolve conflicts associated with a history of abuse and impaired impulse control as predisposing factors for abusive behavior. Social learning theory stresses impaired learning resulting from dysfunctional examples. Overcoming internal controls to abuse and believing that women and children are property are not factors in psychodynamic theory.

61. The answer is (4). Socioeconomic status is not a reliable predictor of abuse in the home and so would be the least important consideration in deciding issues of safety for the victim of family violence. The availability of appropriate community shelters and the ability of the nonabusing caretaker to intervene on the client's behalf are important factors when making the decision regarding safety. The response of the client (if the client is a competent adult) would be the most important factor; the client is empowered by being treated as a competent person.

62. The answer is (3). As with many psychiatric disorders, a combination of factors (including biologic, genetic, and psychosocial factors) contributes to the causation. Answer choice **(1)** has not been demonstrated to be true on the basis of research findings. Answer choices **(2)** and **(4)** have been implicated in causation; however, it is the combination of factors that is most accepted as the cause of schizophrenia.

63. The answer is (3). A support group functions to provide empathy for members who have experienced similar problems and also focuses on reinforcing existing strengths. Answer choice **(1)** would be appropriate for a community living group, such as an inpatient unit. Answer choice **(2)** would be more appropriate for a socialization group. Answer choice **(4)** would be appropriate for an educational group.

64. The answer is (2). Open and honest discussion of conflict will promote healthy interaction and the ability of members to tolerate differences and negotiate solutions. Discussing the situation privately with the individual clients involved and providing specific information on how to resolve the conflict are not appropriate interventions, because the nurse is solving the problem rather than encouraging the group process to handle and resolve conflict. If the nurse ignores the existence of conflict in a group, the group loses the opportunity for learning how to resolve differences.

65. The answer is (1). In the early stage of Alzheimer's disease, complex tasks such as balancing a checkbook would be the first cognitive deficit to occur. The loss of self-care ability, relating to family members, and remembering one's own name are all areas of cognitive decline that occur later in the disease process.

66. The answer is (2). Delirium is an acute cognitive impairment with rapid onset, which may be reversible with prompt treatment. Dementia is a chronic cognitive impairment with slow, insidious onset. Treatment is difficult and often the most that can be achieved is to slow the progression of the disorder.

67. The answer is (4). Olanzapine is an antipsychotic (atypical) or neuroleptic that is used to decrease psychiatric or irrational thinking. Lorazepam is a benzodiazepine, or antianxiety agent, ordered for anxiety on an as-needed basis. Clonazepam is a benzodiazepine ordered to decrease anxiety. Sertraline is an antidepressant used to decrease depressive symptoms.

68. The answer is (3). The client with Alzheimer's disease can have frequent episodes of labile mood, which can best be handled by decreasing a stimulating environment and redirecting the client's attention. An overstimulating environment may cause the labile mood, which will be difficult for the client to understand. The client with Alzheimer's disease loses the cognitive ability to respond to either humor or logic. The client lacks any insight into his or her own behavior and therefore will be unaware of any causative factors.

69. The answer is (1). A relative deficiency of acetylcholine is associated with this disorder. The drugs used in the early stages of Alzheimer's disease will act to increase available acetylcholine in the brain. The remaining neurotransmitters have not been implicated in Alzheimer's disease.

70. The answer is (3). The client's daughter is identifying characteristics typical of a caretaker who is becoming overwhelmed with this role. Feelings of stress in the relationship with the care receiver, depression, and possibly anger are related to the long-term role of caretaker. Although the family may be experiencing altered processes and ineffective coping, the caregiver is currently identifying self-feelings of being overwhelmed. There is no evidence that the caregiver is socially isolated in this situation.

71. The answer is (3). The client's perception of the crisis event is essential for nursing assessment. The available support, such as family, friends, and the ability to provide for basic needs is the next most essential. The other areas may be assessed by the nurse, but the two most essential would be client perception and client support systems.

72. The answer is (1). The first stage of grieving consists of shock and disbelief. In this phase, the family tries to realize that their loved one is dead. Exhibiting helplessness and withdrawal are more typical of the second phases of grief. Sharing fond memories about the deceased and stating how much they miss their family member typically occur after grief is resolved.

73. The answer is (4). Crisis intervention is based on the idea that a crisis is a disturbance in a steady state. The goal is to help the person return to a previous level of equilibrium in functioning. The remaining answer choices are not considered the primary outcome of crisis intervention, although they may occur as a side benefit.

74. The answer is (2). Increased anxiety and uncertainty characterize the initiation phases. Group members are more self-reliant in the working phase, conflict resolution phase, and termination phase.

75. The answer is (2). The use of the pronouns "our" and "we" enhances the sense of the group as a viable unit. The nurse is also clarifying the purpose of the group, which will not restrict spontaneity. Her statements address group norms. The purpose of group therapy is not to prevent conflict, but to work on resolving problem areas.

76. The answer is (1). As the group progresses into the working phase, group members assume more responsibility for the group. The leader becomes more of a facilitator. Comments about behavior in a group are good indicators that the group is active and involved. The remaining answer choices would indicate the group progress has not advanced to the working phase.

77. The answer is (2). During the termination phase, group members need to evaluate the progress of the group and themselves. Deciding to continue or stopping attending before termination are actions that would fail to handle the issue of termination by denying and avoiding it, respectively. Focusing on positive experiences would fail to deal with all the issues of termination (ie, both negative and positive experiences are to be reviewed).

78. The answer is (3). In good family communication, family members openly encourage clear, direct discussions of issues and feelings. Members identify their feelings and thoughts as important and valued and they are able to initiate discussion. Evidence of the children accepting and adopting the parental value system may not validate that good communication is present. Children may adopt the parental value system in a family where communication is maladaptive. Agreement among family members may indicate good communication; but members may be enmeshed, in which case individuals are not free to express differences. Parents may feel that they communicate to their children; however, good communication requires feedback. The nurse must further assess whether children can communicate freely to the parents.

79. The answer is (1). The nurse working with families needs to remain neutral and avoid taking sides. Encouraging each family member to discuss this issue will promote communication among members and allow for clarification of members' feelings. Answer choices **(2)** and **(3)** indicate that the nurse has chosen to agree with either the adolescent or the parents on this issue. Answer choice **(4)** would be avoiding an issue and missing an opportunity to encourage family communication.

80. The answer is (2). These are classic symptoms of dystonia. The specificity of symptoms is more definitive of dystonia than of tension. Parkinsonian symptoms include akinesia or generalized rigidity, drooling, and pill rolling. Neuroleptic malignant syndrome is rare, and high fever, muscle rigidity, hypertension, and diaphoresis characterize the symptoms.

81. The answer is (3). The use of diuretics would cause sodium and water excretion, which would increase risk of lithium toxicity. Clients taking lithium carbonate should be taught to increase their fluid intake and maintain normal intake of sodium. There is no information indicating any increased risk of toxicity with concurrent use of the remaining medications.

82. The answer is (1). Dry mouth and urinary retention are symptoms indicative of anticholinergic side effects of a neuroleptic medication, not an extrapyramidal effect. The remaining answer choices are all part of the effects on the extrapyramidal system and would be assessed by the nurse on a routine basis.

83. The answer is (4). In a functional family, parents are not expected to agree on all issues and problems. Open discussion of thoughts and feelings is healthy, and parental disagreement should not be expected to cause system stress. The remaining answer choices are life transitions and are expected to increase stress on the family system.

84. The answer is (4). This statement is incorrect and would cause the nurse to question the client's ability to take the medication as prescribed. Further teaching is needed. The remaining statements are correct and provide evidence that the client has an understanding of the medication.

85. The answer is (3). Chlorpromazine (Thorazine) can cause a significant hypotensive effect. Blood pressure (lying, sitting, and standing) should be assessed before administering this drug. Although jaundice can be a side effect of this drug, the information in this question does not indicate that the client has had this drug before. This drug (which may cause tachycardia) can affect pulse rate; however, blood pressure evaluation would be the essential implementation because postural blood pressure changes can lead to client injury. This drug can cause urine retention, but asking the client to void will not alter this anticholinergic effect.

86. The answer is (1). This atypical antipsychotic is especially effective for the negative as well as the positive symptoms of schizophrenia. Therefore an expected outcome would be increased motivation and improvement in social interaction. This medication is not used to decrease anxiety levels or to normalize sleep. Increased withdrawal and decreased interest in activities would indicate a worsening of the negative symptoms of schizophrenia and would not be the expected outcome of this drug. This medication is not used for either excitation or panic responses.

87. The answer is (1). Aged cheese and red wines contain the substance tyramine which, when taken with an MAOI, can precipitate a hypertensive crisis. The other foods and beverages do not contain significant amounts of tyramine and, therefore, are not restricted.

88. The answer is (2). The onset of action of the tricyclic antidepressant amitriptyline occurs around 3 to 4 weeks after drug therapy begins. Therefore a client will seldom notice improvement before this time. Continuing to take the drug is important for this client.

89. The answer is (2). Electroconvulsive therapy is used primarily in the treatment of depression, generally when a client has not responded to antidepressant medications. Electroconvulsive therapy is not used for anxiety disorders, mania, or schizophrenia.

90. The answer is (1). Oral absorption of the typical antipsychotic medications are significantly affected by food and stomach acidity level. Therefore these agents should be taken at least 2 hours after eating and not used concurrently with antacids or histamine$_2$ blocking agents.

91. The answer is (1). This medication has been associated with a 1% to 2% incidence of agranulocytosis; therefore, the FDA mandates white blood count testing as described. The remaining atypical agents are not associated with agranulocytosis, and therefore weekly white blood count testing is not required.

92. The answer is (2). Tricyclic antidepressants are associated with an increased risk of cardiovascular effects, especially in elderly clients; therefore, baseline electrocardiogram is expected. The remaining studies would not be expected prior to therapy with these drugs in elderly clients.

93. The answer is (2). Over-the-counter medications used for allergies and cold symptoms are contraindicated because they will increase the sympathomimetic effects of the MAOIs and may cause hypertensive crisis. None of the remaining medications will increase the sympathomimetic response and therefore are not contraindicated.

94. The answer is (4). Bupropion increases the risk of seizures; therefore, a client with a history of a seizure disorder would not be able to take bupropion. None of the remaining medical problems would constitute a problem for a client taking bupropion.

95. The answer is (3). Urinary retention is a common anticholinergic side effect of psychotic medications, and the client with benign prostatic hypertrophy would have increased risk for this problem. Adding fiber to one's diet and exercising regularly are measures to counteract another anticholinergic effect, constipation. Depending on the specific medication and how it is prescribed, taking the medication at night may or may not be important. However, it would have nothing to do with urinary retention in this client.

96. The answer is (2). The client is not coping effectively currently and, with intervention, would be expected to be able to identify strategies that would improve coping ability. Contacting the wife and requesting reconciliation would not be an expected outcome, because it is not addressing the reality of the client's problem, which is adjusting to the divorce. Listing stressors that contributed to the marital problems and verbalizing thoughts and feelings of hopelessness would be appropriate as initial steps in gathering data related to the client's problem.

97. The answer is (4). Both neuroleptic malignant syndrome and serotonin syndrome are life-threatening complications of psychotropic medications. Neuroleptic malignant syndrome may occur with neuroleptic medications, whereas serotonin syndrome may occur with antidepressant medications. In either case, any further doses of the medications would be contraindicated. All of the remaining measures may be used, but the priority is avoiding further doses of the offending medications.

98. The answer is (2). Coffee contains caffeine, which has a stimulating effect on the central nervous system and would therefore counteract the effect of the antianxiety medication, oxazepam. None of the remaining foods is contraindicated.

99. The answer is (2). The primary purpose of Alcoholics Anonymous is to help members to achieve and maintain sobriety. Although each of the remaining answer choices may be an outcome of attendance at Alcoholics Anonymous, the primary purpose is directed toward sobriety of members.

100. The answer is (3). A therapeutic community is designed to help individuals assume responsibility for self, to learn how to respect and communicate with others, and to interact in a positive manner. The remaining answer choices may be outcomes of psychiatric treatment, but the use of a therapeutic community approach is concerned with promotion of self-reliance and cooperative adaptation to being with others.

Bibliography

Agency for Health Care Policy and Research—Depression Guideline Panel. (1993). *Depression in primary care: Detection, diagnosis and treatment. Technical report no. 5.* Rockville, MD: U.S. Department of Health and Human Services, Agency for Health Care Policy and Research.

Aguilera, D.C. (1998). *Crisis intervention: Theory and methodology* (8th ed.). St. Louis: Mosby.

American Nurses Association (1994). *A statement on psychiatric-mental health clinical nursing practice and standards of psychiatric-mental health clinical nursing practice.* Washington, D.C.: American Nurses Publishing.

American Psychiatric Association (1994). *Diagnostic and statistical manual of mental disorders (DSM-IV)* (4th ed.). Washington, D.C.: American Psychiatric Association.

Andrews, M.M., & Boyle, J.S. (1994). *Transcultural concepts in nursing care* (3rd ed.). Philadelphia: Lippincott.

Antai-Otong, D. (1995a). Helping the alcoholic patient recover. *American Journal of Nursing, 95*(9), 22–29.

Antai-Otong, D. (1995b). *Psychiatric nursing: Biological and behavioral concepts.* Philadelphia: W.B. Saunders.

Baier, M., & Murray, R.L.E. (1999). A descriptive study of insight into illness reported by persons with schizophrenia. *Journal of Psychosocial Nursing and Mental Health Services, 37*(1), 14–21.

Bain, L.J. (1998). Defining the basis of manic depression. *NARSAD Research Newsletter, 10*(4), 14.

Berlinger, J. (1998). Why don't you just leave him? *Nursing 98, 28*(4), 34–39.

Bonnel, W.B. (1996). Not gone and not forgotten: A spouse's experience of late-stage Alzheimer's disease. *Journal of Psychosocial Nursing and Mental Health Services, 34*(8), 23–27.

Bowen, M. (1978). *Family therapy in clinical practice.* New York: Jason Aranson.

Bradley, K., Boyd-Wickizer, J., Powell, S., & Burman, M. (1998). Alcohol screening questionnaires in women. *JAMA, 280*(2), 166–171.

Brightman, H. (1998). Manic and depressive recurrences: Search for mechanisms and treatments. *NARSAD Research Newsletter, 10*(2), 14.

Brown, A., & Lempa, M. (1996). Update on potential causes and new treatments for anxiety disorders. *NARSAD Research Newsletter, 8*(2), 13–18.

Brown, A., & Weaver R. (1998). How related are autism and childhood schizophrenia? *NARSAD Research Newsletter, 10*(3), 13–19.

Brown, S.W., Griep, A.Z., Buckley, S., et al. (1998). Process-oriented critical pathways in inpatient psychiatry: Our first year. *Journal of Psychosocial Nursing and Mental Health Services, 36*(6), 31–36.

Burgess, A.W. (1997). *Psychiatric nursing: Promoting mental health.* Stanford, CT: Appleton and Lange.

Burkhardt, M., & Nathaniel, A. (1998). *Ethics and issues in contemporary nursing.* Albany, NY: Delmar.

Chez, N. (1994). Helping the victim of domestic violence. *American Journal of Nursing, 94*(5), 33–38.

Connections. (1998). *Alzheimer's Disease Education and Referral Center, 7*(2), 3–4.

Deglin, J.W., & Hazard-Vallerand, A. (1997). *Davis's drug guide for nurses* (5th ed.). Philadelphia: F.A. Davis.

Department of Health and Human Services. (1996). Report to Congress. Referenced in *Journal of Psychosocial Nursing and Mental Health Services, 36*(12).

Evans, B. (1999). Complementary therapies and HIV infection. *American Journal of Nursing, 99*(2), 42–45.

Fine, J.I., Rouse-Bane, S. (1995). Using validation techniques to improve communication with cognitively impaired older adults. *Journal of Gerontological Nursing, 21*(6), 39–45.

Fingeld, D. (1999). Use of brief interventions to treat individuals with drinking problems. *Journal of Psychosocial Nursing and Mental Health Services, 37*(4), 23–30.

Fontaine, K.L., & Fletcher, J.S. (1999). *Psychiatric mental health nursing.* Albany, NY. Delmar.

Frisch, N., & Frisch, L. (1998). *Psychiatric mental health nursing.* Albany, NY: Delmar.

Fuime, TJ. (1997). Treatment of addiction [unpublished paper].

Glod, C. (1998). *Contemporary psychiatric-mental health nursing: The brain–behavior connection.* Philadelphia: F.A. Davis.

Greenwald, J. (1998). Herbal healing. *Time Magazine, 98*(11), 60–69.

Haber, J. et al. (1997). *Comprehensive psychiatric nursing* (5th ed.). St. Louis: Mosby.

Haggerty, B.M. (1995). Advances in understanding major depressive disorder. *Journal of Psychosocial Nursing and Mental Health Services, 33*(11), 27–34.

Hobbs, H., Wilson, J.H., & Archie, S. (1999). The alumni program: Redefining continuity of care in psychiatry. *Journal of Psychosocial Nursing and Mental Health Nursing, 37*(1), 23–29.

Johnson, B.S. (1997). *Psychiatric-mental health nursing* (4th ed.). Philadelphia: Lippincott-Raven.

Johnson, B.S. (1998). The 5 R's of becoming a psychiatric nurse practitioner: Rationale, readying, roles, rules and reality. *Journal of Psychosocial Nursing and Mental Health Services, 38*(9), 20–24.

Jones, J.E. (1994). Chronic anxiety and the adrenocortical response, and differentiation. *Family Systems: Journal of Natural Systems Thinking in Psychiatry and the Sciences, 1*(2), 30–38.

Keltner, N., Folks, D., Palmer, C.A., & Sowers, R. (1998). *Psychobiological foundation of psychiatric care*. St. Louis: Mosby-Year Book.

Keltner, N.L., & Schwecke, L.H. (1999). *Psychiatric nursing* (3rd ed.). St. Louis: Mosby.

Kerr, M. (1997). A systems model for disease. In Bowen, M. *Theory and practice*. Washington, D.C.: Georgetown Family Center.

Keys, S.G., Bemak, F., & Lockhart, E.J. (1998). Transforming school counseling to serve mental health needs of at-risk youth. *Journal of Counseling and Development, Fall 76*(2), 381–387.

Lesseig, D.Z. (1998). Pharmacotherapy for long-term care residents with dementia-associated behavioral disturbance. *Journal of Psychosocial Nursing and Mental Health Services, 36*(2), 27–31.

Mayfield, D.G., McCleod, G., & Hall, D. (1974). The C.A.G.E. questionnaire. *American Journal of Psychiatry, 131,* 1121–1123.

Mendlewicz, J. (1998). Genetic vulnerability. *NARSAD Research Newsletter, 10*(4), 11–13.

Minuchin, S. (1974). *Families and family therapy*. Cambridge, MA: Harvard University Press.

Mohr, W.K. (1998). Cross-ethnic variations in care of psychiatric patients: A review of contributing factors and practice considerations. *Journal of Psychosocial Nursing and Mental Health Services, 36*(5), 16–21.

Mohr, W.K. (1998). Updating what we know about depression in adolescents. *Journal of Psychosocial Nursing and Mental Health Services, 36*(9), 12–18.

Morse, J.M. (1992). Exploring empathy: A conceptual fit for nursing practice. *Image: Journal of Nursing Scholarship, 24*(4), 275.

Mynatt, S. (1996). A model of contributing risk factors to chemical dependency in nurses. *Journal of Psychosocial Nursing and Mental Health Services, 34,* 13–22.

NARSAD (National Alliance for Research on Schizophrenia and Depression) (1997). *NARSAD Research Newsletter, 9*(34).

NARSAD (1998). *NARSAD Research Newsletter, 10*(2).

NARSAD (1998). *NARSAD Research Newsletter, 10*(4).

National Institute on Drug Abuse (NIDA) (1999). NIDA Infofax–nationwide trends. Bethesda, MD: U.S. Department of Health and Human Services.

Nemeroff, C.B. (1998). Neurobiology of depression. *Scientific American, 698*(6), 42.

Newman, C.F. (1999). Cognitive therapy with depressed and suicidal adolescents. *Healing Magazine, 4*(1), 24–27.

Nugent, E. (1995). Try to remember: Reminiscence as a nursing intervention. *Journal of Psychosocial Nursing and Mental Health Services, 3*(11), 7–11.

Papero, D. (1997). Responsibility for self. In Brown, M. *Theory and practice* (pp. 123–132). Washington, D.C.: Georgetown Family Center.

Poliafico, F. (1999). Abstinence is not the only answer. *RN, 62*(1), 58–60.

Post, R.M. (1997). Molecular biology of behavior. *Archives of General Psychiatry,* 607.

Richman, D. (1998). To restrain or not to restrain? *RN, 61*(7), 55–58.

Satir, V. (1964). *Conjoint family therapy*. Palo Alto, CA: Science and Behavior Books.

Shea, C., Mahoney, M., & Lacey, J. (1997). Breaking through the barriers to domestic violence intervention. *American Journal of Nursing, 97*(6), 26–33.

Spencer, V. (1996). Combined therapy in O.C.D. *Journal of Psychosocial Nursing and Mental Health Services, 34*(7), 37–40.

Staff (1998). Childhood sexual abuse: Understanding the journey of survival. *Journal of Psychosocial Nursing and Mental Health Services, 36*(12), 13–17.

Townsend, M. (1999). *Essentials of psychiatric/mental health nursing.* Philadelphia: F.A. Davis.

Wakefield, M., & Pallister, R. (1997). Cognitive-behavioral approaches to panic disorder. *Journal of Psychosocial Nursing and Mental Health Services, 35*(3), 12–20.

Walker, G., & Scott, P.S. (1998). Impact of child sexual abuse on addiction severity: An analysis of trauma processing. *Journal of Psychosocial Nursing and Mental Health Services, 36*(3), 10–18.

Wilson, J., & Hobbs, H. (1999). The family educator: A professional resource for families. *Journal of Psychosocial Nursing and Mental Health Services, 37*(6), 22–27.

Wolfe, S. (1998). Look for signs of abuse. *RN, 61*(8), 48–54.

Wong, D. (1997). *Whaley and Wong's essentials of pediatric nursing* (5th ed.). St. Louis: Mosby.

Yalom, I. (1985). *The theory and practice of group psychotherapy* (3rd ed.). New York: Basic Books.

Yesavage, J.A., & Brink, T.L. (1983). Development and validation of a Geriatric Depression Screening Scale: A preliminary report. *Journal of Psychiatric Research, 17,* 37–49.

Zanarini, M.C., Williams, A.A., Lewis, R.E., et al. (1997). Reported pathological childhood experiences associated with development of borderline personality disorders. *American Journal of Psychiatry, 154*(8), 10–37.

Zook, R. (1996). Take action before anger builds. *RN, 59*(4), 46–50.

Index

Note: Page numbers followed by f refer to figures; those followed by t refer to tables; and those followed by b refer to boxed material.

A

Abstraction, selective, 29t
  with eating disorders, 66
Abuse, 161–172
  behavioral and psychological
    signs of, 165t
  and borderline personality
    disorder, 83
  child
    assessment of, 168t
    behavioral and psychological
      signs of, 165t
    and childhood psychiatric
      disorders, 184
    legal issues in, 163
    nursing process for, 170–171
    physical signs of, 164t
    sexual, 162, 164t, 165t
    statistics on, 162
  cycles of, 163
  defined, 161
  and dissociative disorders, 49
  economic, 161
  of elderly
    assessment of, 168t
    behavioral and psychological
      signs of, 165t
    legal issues in, 163
    nursing process for, 171
    physical signs of, 164t
    statistics on, 162
  etiology of, 166
  family characteristics with,
    163–164
  legal issues with, 163
  management of, 166–167
  nursing process for, 167–172
    assessment in, 167–169, 168t
    implementation in, 170–172
    nursing diagnoses in, 169–170
    outcome evaluation in, 172
    planning and outcome
      identification in, 170
  physical, 161
  physical signs of, 164t
  prevention of, 167
  psychological, 161
  sexual, 161, 162, 163
    assessment of, 168–169
  of children, 162, 164t, 165t
  statistics on, 162
  types of, 161
  of women
    assessment of, 168t
    behavioral and psychological
      signs of, 165t
    crisis intervention services for,
      167
    legal issues in, 163
    nursing process for, 171
    physical signs of, 164t
    remaining in relationship with,
      164–166
    statistics on, 162
Abuser
  characteristics of, 165b
  defined, 161
  implementation of nursing plan
    for, 171–172
  nursing diagnoses for, 169–170
  planning and outcome
    identification for, 170
Acamprosate, 151t
Acetylcholine, 21, 249
Acquired immunodeficiency
    syndrome (AIDS) dementia
    complex, 201
Acquisition, 27
Activities of daily living (ADL), 203,
    207
Activity groups, 230
Acupuncture, 62t
Acute dystonic reaction, 254t
Addiction, 138
ADHD (attention deficit-hyperactivity
    disorder), 181, 182t, 186t,
    190–191
Admission, voluntary, 10
Adolescent(s), of substance abusers,
    141
Adolescent psychiatric disorders. See
    Childhood psychiatric
    disorders
Adult day care services, 202
Advanced practice RN (APN, APRN),
    4
Adventitious crisis, 215, 216t
Affective flattening, 119

Agitation
  in children, 186t
  in dementia, 203t
  in schizophrenia, 130
Agnosia, 197
Agoraphobia, panic disorder with,
    44
Agranulocytosis, due to
    psychotropic medications,
    255t
AIDS (acquired immunodeficiency
    syndrome) dementia
    complex, 201
Akathisia, 254t
Alarm reaction, 37, 38t, 39f
Alcohol abuse, 139t, 142. See also
    Substance-related disorders
  assessment of, 150–151
  blood alcohol level in, 142
  chronic, 142
  genetic predisposition to, 148
  immediate effects of, 142
  medications for, 150, 151t
  statistics on, 140, 148
  withdrawal from, 142, 144t
Alexithymia, 63
All-or-nothing thinking, 104t
Alogia, 119
Alprazolam (Xanax), 45t, 266t
Alternative(s), examination of, 8
Alternative family, 237
Alternative settings, 2–3
Alternative therapies, 13
  for mind-body disorders, 61, 62t
Aluminum, in dementia, Alzheimer's
    type, 201
Alzheimer's Association, 202
Alzheimer's type dementia
  epidemiology of, 199
  etiology of, 201
  home care for, 208b
  management of, 201–202, 202t,
    203t
  nursing process for, 203–209
    analysis in, 205
    assessment in, 203–204, 204t,
      205t
    implementation in, 206–207,
      207t, 208b

Alzheimer's type dementia, nursing
    process for, *(continued)*
  nursing diagnoses in, 205
  outcome evaluation in, 209
  planning and outcome
    identification in, 206
  prevention of caregiver burnout
    for, 208b
  stages of, 199t
  symptoms of, 197–198, 199t
Ambien (zolpidem), 266t
Ambivalence, 119
American Nurses Association (ANA),
    3–4
  Code of Ethics for Nurses with
    Interpretive Statements of,
    12
  Standards of Psychiatric-Mental
    Health Clinical Practice of,
    12
Americans with Disabilities Act
    (1990), 3, 11
Amitriptyline (Elavil), 105t, 257t
Amnesia
  antegrade, from alcohol abuse,
    142
  dissociative, 49b
  fugue, 49b
Amnestic disorders
  classification of, 190–199
  defined, 197
  diagnosis of, 200
  epidemiology of, 199–200
  etiology of, 201
  management of, 202
  nursing process for, 203–209
    analysis in, 205
    assessment in, 203–204, 204t,
      205t
    implementation in, 206–207,
      207t, 208b
    nursing diagnoses in, 205
  outcome evaluation in, 209
  planning and outcome
    identification in, 206
  onset and course of, 200
  substance-induced, 142, 198
  symptoms of, 198
Amoxapine (Ascendin), 257t
Amphetamines, abuse of, 139t, 144t,
    145–146
Amyloid plaques, 201
ANA (American Nurses Association),
    3–4
  Code of Ethics for Nurses with
    Interpretive Statements of,
    12
  Standards of Psychiatric-Mental
    Health Clinical Practice of,
    12
Anafranil. *See* Clomipramine
    (Anafranil)
Analgesics, narcotic, abuse of, 138,
    139t, 143–145, 144t
Anal stage, 25t
Angry client, crisis intervention for,
    220–221
Anhedonia
  in depression, 99–100
  in schizophrenia, 120

Anorexia nervosa, 66–69, 67t–69t
  nursing process for, 70–72, 70b,
    71t
Antabuse (disulfiram), 151t
Antegrade amnesia, from alcohol
    abuse, 142
Antianxiety medications, 45t,
    265–269, 266t–268t
  abuse of, 139t, 143, 144t
  for dementia, 203t
  for generalized anxiety disorder,
    44
  for obsessive compulsive disorder,
    47
  for panic disorder, 46
  for post-traumatic stress disorder,
    48
Anticholinergic toxicity, 259t
Anticholinesterase drugs, 202t,
    270–271, 270t
Anticonvulsants
  for dementia, 203t
  for mood disorders, 105t, 263t,
    264–265
Antidepressants, 256–262, 257t
  for anxiety disorders, 45t
  atypical, 257t, 262
  for children, 186t
  for dementia, 203t
  for eating disorders, 69t
  monoamine oxidase inhibitors,
    257t, 259–260, 260t
  for mood disorders, 105t
  nontricyclic selective
    norepinephrine reuptake
    inhibitors, 262
  selective serotonin reuptake
    inhibitors, 257t, 260–261,
    261t
  tricyclic, 256–259, 257t, 259t
Antihistamines, 266t, 267–268
Antimanic agents, 105t
Antioxidants, 202t
Antipsychotics, 124t, 250–254, 251t
  atypical, 251t, 252–254
  for children, 186t
  contraindications to, 251–252
  for dementia, 203t
  indications for, 250
  interactions with, 252
  mechanism of action of, 250, 252
  pharmacokinetics of, 250, 254
  side effects of, 126, 252,
    253t–256t, 254
  standard, 250–252, 251t, 253t–256t
  use across lifespan of, 251
Antisocial personality disorder, 82
  etiology of, 83, 84
  nursing assessment of, 86
  nursing diagnosis for, 87t
Anxiety
  defined, 37
  with dementia, 203t
  with eating disorders, 67
  effects of, 40f
  in Freudian theory, 23
  levels of, 40f
  nursing process for, 41–43, 43b
  psychobiologic aspects of, 38–40
  psychosocial theories of, 41

  responses to, 37–38
  separation, 180t, 182, 186t
  Sullivan's theory of, 24
Anxiety-related disorders, 43–52
  in children, 180t, 182, 186t, 191
  dissociative disorders, 49–50, 49b
  education for, 43b
  generalized, 44, 45t, 46b
    in children, 180t, 182
    nursing process for, 50–52, 51t
  medications for, 44, 45t
  nursing process for, 50–52, 51t
  obsessive compulsive disorder,
    47, 47b
    in children, 47, 47b
  overview of, 43–44
  panic disorder, 44–46, 46b
  phobic disorder, 48, 48b
    in children, 182
  post-traumatic stress disorder,
    48–49, 49b
Anxiolytics. *See* Antianxiety
    medications
Anxious personality disorders, 82,
    87t, 89
Aphasia, 197
APN (advanced practice RN), 4
Apraxia, 197
APRN (advanced practice RN), 4
Arbitrary inference, 29t
Aricept (donepezil), 202t, 270, 270t
Ascendin (amoxapine), 257t
Assertiveness training, 28
Associations, loose, 119, 120t
Atarax (hydroxyzine), 266t
Atenolol (Tenormin), 45t
Ativan (lorazepam), 266t
  for anxiety disorders, 45t
  for dementia, 203t
Attention deficit-hyperactivity
    disorder (ADHD), 181, 182t,
    186t, 190–191
Authoritarian leadership, 229t
Autism, 180, 181t
Autoimmune disorders, 59, 60t
Autonomy, 12, 13
  vs. shame and doubt, 25t
Aversive therapy, 28
Avoidant personality disorder, 82,
    86, 87t
Avolition, 119
Awareness, levels of, 22
Ayurveda, 62t
Azapirones, 45t

B
"Bad-me," 24
"Bad trip," 147
Baily, Harriet, 3
BAL (blood alcohol level), 142
Barbiturates, abuse of, 139t, 143,
    144t
Battered women
  behavioral and psychological
    signs in, 165t
  crisis intervention services for,
    167
  legal issues with, 163
  nursing process for, 171
  physical signs in, 164t

remaining in relationship of, 164–166
statistics on, 162
Beck, Aaron, 29
Beck's cognitive therapy, 29
Beck's theory, of depression, 103
Behavioral contracting, for eating disorders, 69
Behavioral responses, in children, 188
Behavioral theory, 27–28
of personality disorders, 83
of stress and anxiety, 41
Behavior modification, 27–28
Belief systems, in family, 240t
Benadryl (diphenhydramine), 266t
for acute dystonic reaction, 254t
Beneficence, 12, 13
Benzodiazepines (BZAs), 265–267, 266t
for anxiety disorders, 45t
anxiolytic, 266t
contraindications to, 266–267
for dementia, 203t
indications for, 265
interactions with, 267
mechanism of action of, 266
overdose of, 268t
pharmacokinetics of, 266
safe use of, 267t
sedative-hypnotic, 266t
side effects of, 267, 267t, 268t
use across lifespan of, 266
Benztropine (Cogentin), for acute dystonic reaction, 254t
Beta blockers, for anxiety disorders, 45t
Binge eating, 67t
Biofeedback, 28
Biogenic amine theory, 102
Biologic vulnerability
to eating disorders, 66–67
to generalized anxiety disorder, 44
to obsessive compulsive disorder, 47
to panic disorder, 44
to sexual disorders, 65
Bipolar disorder
characteristics of, 100
in children, 183
on continuum of mood disorders, 98f
defined, 97
genetic predisposition to, 102
nursing assessment of, 107t, 108t
prevalence of, 99
types I and II, 100
Bizarre behavior, in schizophrenia, 128
Blackouts, from alcohol abuse, 142
Blended family, 237
Blocker, in group, 228
Blood alcohol level (BAL), 142
Blunted affect, 119
Body dysmorphic disorder, 63
Body image, distorted, with eating disorders, 67
Borderline personality disorder, 82
etiology of, 83, 84

management of, 84
nursing assessment of, 85
nursing diagnosis for, 87t
Boundaries, 5
in family, 237, 240t
Brain structure abnormalities
in childhood psychiatric disorders, 184
in dementia, 201
in schizophrenia, 123
Bulimia, 66–69, 67t–69t
nursing process for, 70–72, 70b, 71t
Buprenorphine (Buprenex), 151t
Bupropion (Wellbutrin), 105t, 257t, 262
Buspirone (BuSpar), 266t, 268–269
for anxiety disorders, 45t
for dementia, 203t
BZAs. *See* Benzodiazepines (BZAs)

C
Caffeine, 139t, 146
Cannabinoids, abuse of, 138–140, 139t, 144t, 147–148
Carbamazepine (Tegretol), 263t, 265
for dementia, 203t
for mood disorders, 105t
Caregiver, for client with cognitive impairment disorder, 203–204, 206, 208b
Care maps, 2
Case finding, for mood disorders, 106
Case law, 11
Case management approach, 2
to schizophrenia, 124
Catastrophic reactions, 197, 207
Catatonic excitement, 121
Catatonic schizophrenia, 121
Catatonic stupor, 121
Cathexis, 22
Central nervous system (CNS) depressants, abuse of, 138, 139t, 142–145, 144t
Central nervous system (CNS) stimulants, abuse of, 138, 139t, 144t, 145–147
Centrax (prazepam), 266t
Cerebral hemispheres, 20
Cerebrum, 20
Certification, 4
Chemical dependence. *See* Substance-related disorders
Chemical dependency units, 149
Child(ren)
crisis intervention for, 217
of substance abusers, 141
Child abuse
assessment of, 168t
behavioral and psychological signs of, 165t
and childhood psychiatric disorders, 184
legal issues in, 163
nursing process for, 170–171
physical signs of, 164t
sexual, 162, 164t, 165t
statistics on, 162

Childhood psychiatric disorders, 179–191
ADHD, 181, 182t, 186t, 190–191
agitation, 186t
anxiety disorders, 180t, 182, 186t, 191
autism, 180, 181t
conduct disorder, 181, 191
developmental theory and, 179
diagnosis of, 179
education in, 185, 190b
etiology of, 184–185
hyperactivity, 181, 182t, 186t
impulsiveness, 186t
management of, 185–187, 186t
mental retardation, 179–180
mood disorders, 98, 180t, 183, 186t, 191
nursing process for, 187–191
assessment in, 187–188, 187t
implementation in, 189–191, 190b
nursing diagnoses in, 188–189
outcome evaluation in, 191
planning and outcome identification in, 189
obsessive-compulsive disorder, 182
onset of, 179
oppositional defiant disorder, 182, 191
pervasive developmental disorders, 179–181, 181t, 190
prevention of, 185
psychotic, 186t
schizophrenia, 182, 186t
statistics on, 179
substance abuse disorder, 183–184, 191
suicide, 183, 183b
symptoms of, 179, 180t
types of, 179–184, 181t, 182b, 183b
Child welfare agencies, for family violence, 167
Chinese medicine, traditional, 62t
Chiropractic, 62t
Chlordiazepoxide (Librium), 45t, 266t
Chlorpromazine (Thorazine), 251t
for schizophrenia, 124t
childhood, 186t
Chlorprothixene (Taractan), 251t
CID. *See* Cognitive impairment disorders (CID)
Circadian rhythm changes, in mood disorders, 102
Clang association, 120t
Clarification, 8
Classical conditioning, 27
Client-centered therapy, 30
Client-identifying data, 7t
Clinical nurse specialist (CNS), 4
Clomipramine (Anafranil), 257t
for anxiety disorders, 45t
for children, 186t
for mood disorders, 105t
Clonazepam (Klonopin), 45t, 266t
Clorazepate (Tranxene), 266t

Closed boundaries, 237
Clozapine (Clozaril), 124t, 251t
Clubhouse programs, 3
CNS (clinical nurse specialist), 4
CNS (central nervous system)
  depressants, abuse of, 138,
    139t, 142–145, 144t
CNS (central nervous system)
  stimulants, abuse of, 138,
    139t, 144t, 145–147
Coalitions, in family, 238
Cocaine, abuse of, 140, 144t,
    146–147
Codependence, 138, 141
Cogentin (benztropine), for acute
    dystonic reaction, 254t
Cognex (tacrine), 202t, 270, 270t
Cognitions, negative, 103, 104t
Cognitive-behavioral theory
  of eating disorders, 67
  of family violence, 166
  of mood disorders, 103, 104t
  of sexual disorders, 65
  of somatoform disorders, 63
  of substance abuse, 148
Cognitive-behavioral therapy
  for eating disorders, 69
  for generalized anxiety disorder,
    44
  for mood disorders, 106
  for obsessive compulsive disorder,
    47
  for panic disorder, 46
  for phobic disorder, 48
  for post traumatic stress disorder,
    48
  for sexual disorders, 66
Cognitive framework, for psychiatric
    care, 28–30, 29t
Cognitive impairment disorders
    (CID), 197–209
  in children, 188
  defined, 197
  diagnosis of, 200
  with eating disorders, 66
  education for, 208b
  epidemiology of, 199–200
  etiology of, 200–201
  home care for, 208b
  management of, 201–202, 202t,
    203t
  nursing process for, 203–209
    analysis in, 205
    assessment in, 203–204, 204t,
      205t
    implementation in, 206–207,
      207t, 208b
    nursing diagnoses in, 205
    outcome evaluation in, 209
    planning and outcome
      identification in, 206
  onset and course of, 200
  prevention of caregiver burnout
    for, 208b
  symptoms of, 197–198
  types of, 198–199, 199t
Cognitive restructuring, 29
  for phobic disorder, 48
Cognitive theory, 25t, 26–27
  of stress and anxiety, 41

Combative behavior, with dementia,
    203t
Commentator, in group, 228
Commitment
  involuntary, 11
  state laws on, 10–11
Communication
  in family, 240t, 243
  in schizophrenia, 121–122, 128,
    128b
  therapeutic, 6–8
Community-based treatment
  for childhood psychiatric
    disorders, 185
  for cognitive impairment
    disorders, 202
  for eating disorders, 69
  for mood disorders, 106
  for schizophrenia, 124–125
  for sexual disorders, 65
  for substance abuse, 149, 150t
Community care, population-based,
    2
Community meeting groups, 230
Community Mental Health Centers
    Act (1963), 1
Community social service agencies,
    for family violence, 167
Complementary therapies, 13
  for mind-body disorders, 61, 62t
Compulsions, 47, 47b
Conceptual framework(s), 19–31
  behavioral, 27–28
  cognitive, 28–30, 29t
  defined, 19
  developmental, 22–27, 23t, 25t
  examples of, 19
  function of, 19
  humanistic, 30–31
  psychobiology as, 19–22
Concrete operations stage, 25t
Concrete thinking, in schizophrenia,
    120
Conditioned response, 27
  in phobic disorder, 48
Conditioning
  classical, 27
  operant, 27, 28
Conduct disorder, 181, 191
Confabulation, 197
Conference Group on Psychiatric
    Nursing, 3
Confidentiality, 5, 11, 12
Conscious, 22
Consent, informed, 11
Consultation, 1
Consumer movement, 3
Continuity of care, for
    schizophrenia, 123–124
Contract
  behavioral, for eating disorders,
    69
  in therapeutic relationship, 5
Control, and stress response, 40
Controlled response pattern, to
    sexual assault, 163
Conversion disorder, 63
Coordinator, in group, 228
Coping strategies, 41, 41b
Cost containment, 2

Countertransference, 24
Crack cocaine, 140
Crisis(es)
  adventitious, 215, 216t
  balancing factors with, 215–216
  defined, 215
  developmental, 215, 216t
  in emergency nursing, 217
  general considerations for,
    215–216
  in gerontologic nursing, 217
  in maternal-child nursing, 217
  in medical-surgical nursing, 217
  in pediatric nursing, 217
  in psychiatric nursing, 217
  situational, 215, 216t
  symptoms in individuals
    experiencing, 216t
  types of, 215, 216t
Crisis development, sequence of,
    216, 216t
Crisis intervention, 215–221
  assistance in, 217
  defined, 215
  for family violence, 167
  general considerations with,
    215–216, 216t
  nursing process in, 218–221, 219t
  principles of, 217–218
  role of nurse in, 217
  for suicidal behavior, 106
Crisis intervention worker, 218
Crisis resolution, 215
Critical incident stress debriefing,
    217
Critical pathways, 2
Cross-tolerance, 138
Cultural data, 7t
Cultural diversity, 9
Cultural factors
  in alcohol use, 140
  in eating disorders, 67
  in major depressive disorder, 98
  in mood disorders, 99
  in psychiatric nursing, 8–10, 13
  in somatoform disorders, 63
Culturally competent nursing, 9–10
Culture, 8
Current problem, 7t
Cyclothymia
  characteristics of, 100
  on continuum of mood disorders,
    98f
Cylert (pemoline), for ADHD, 186t,
    269t

D
Dalmane (flurazepam), 266t
DAT. *See* Dementia, Alzheimer's type
Day treatment programs, for
    schizophrenia, 125
Defense mechanisms, 23, 23t
  with substance-related disorders,
    141
Delirium
  classification of, 198
  defined, 197
  vs. depression, 203, 204t
  diagnosis of, 200
  epidemiology of, 199–200

etiology of, 200
management of, 201
nursing process for, 203–209
  analysis in, 205
  assessment in, 203–204, 204t,
    205t
  implementation in, 206–207,
    207t, 208b
  nursing diagnoses in, 205
  outcome evaluation in, 209
  planning and outcome
    identification in, 206
onset and course of, 200
substance-induced, 198
symptoms of, 198
Delirium tremens, 142
Delusions, 119, 120b
nursing process for, 129–130,
  129b
Dementia
Alzheimer's type
  epidemiology of, 199
  etiology of, 201
  stages of, 199t
  symptoms of, 199t
classification of, 198
defined, 197
vs. depression, 203, 204t
diagnosis of, 200
epidemiology of, 199–200
etiology of, 200–201
home care for, 208b
management of, 201–202, 202t,
  203t
nursing process for, 203–209
  analysis in, 205
  assessment in, 203–204, 204t,
    205t
  implementation in, 206–207,
    207t, 208b
  nursing diagnoses in, 205
  outcome evaluation in, 209
  planning and outcome
    identification in, 206
onset and course of, 200
prevention of caregiver burnout
  for, 208b
symptoms of, 197–198, 199t
vascular (multi-infarct), 198, 200
Democratic leadership, 229t
Denial, 23t
with substance-related disorders,
  141
Depakene. *See* Valproic acid
  (divalproex, Depakene,
  Depakote)
Depakote. *See* Valproic acid
  (divalproex, Depakene,
  Depakote)
Dependence
co-, 138
substance, 137
Dependent personality disorder, 82,
  86, 87t
Depersonalization, 49b
in schizophrenia, 119
Depression
vs. cognitive impairment disorder,
  203, 204t
defined, 97

with dementia, 203t
major
  characteristics of, 99–100
  in children, 180t, 183, 186t
  on continuum of mood
    disorders, 98f
  episodes of, 99
  etiology of, 101–103
  prevalence and incidence of,
    98–99
  medications used in treatment of,
    105t
  nursing assessment of, 107t, 108t
  postpartum, 100
  unipolar, 97
Derealization, 119
Desensitization, systematic, 28
  for phobic disorder, 48
Desipramine (Norpramin), 257t
  for eating disorders, 69t
  for mood disorders, 105t
Despair, integrity *vs.,* 25t
Desyrel (trazodone), 105t, 257t, 262
Detoxification
  defined, 138
  hospitalization for, 149
Developmental crisis, 215, 216t
Developmental disorders, pervasive,
  179–181, 181t, 190
Developmental stages, of family,
  238
Developmental tasks, 26
Developmental theories, 22–27, 23t,
  25t
  of childhood psychiatric
    disorders, 179
  of personality disorders, 83
  of schizophrenia, 123
  of substance abuse, 148
Dextroamphetamine (Dexedrine),
  269t
Diazepam (Valium), 266t
Dichotomous thinking, 29t
  with eating disorders, 66
Diencephalon, 20
Differentiation, in family, 238, 240t
Diffuse boundaries, 237
Diphenhydramine (Benadryl), 266t
  for acute dystonic reaction, 254t
Disaster response teams, 217
Disengagement, in family, 238
Disorganized schizophrenia, 121
Disorientation, 197
Displacement, 23t
Dissociative amnesia, 49b
Dissociative disorders, 49–50, 49b
  nursing process for, 50–52, 51t
Dissociative fugue, 49b
Dissociative identity disorder, 49b
Distress, in mind-body disorders, 59
Disulfiram (Antabuse), 151t
Divalprolex. *See* Valproic acid
  (divalprolex, Depakene,
  Depakote)
Dolophine (methadone), 150, 151t
Donepezil (Aricept), 202t, 270, 270t
Dopamine, in schizophrenia, 20,
  123, 249
Doubt, autonomy *vs.,* 25t
Doxepin (Sinequan), 257t

Dramatic personality disorders, 82,
  87t, 88
Drives, 23
Driving under the influence (DUI),
  142
Drug(s). *See* Medications
Drug abuse. *See* Substance-related
  disorders
Dual diagnosis, 137
Duty to warn, 11
Dysfunctional family system, 184,
  239, 240t
Dysthymia
  characteristics of, 100
  on continuum of mood disorders,
    98f
  incidence of, 98
Dystonic reaction, acute, 254t

E
Eating disorders, 66–69, 67t–69t, 70b
  nursing process for, 70–73, 70b,
    71t
Eccentric personality disorders,
  81–82, 87t, 88
Echolalia, 120t
Echopraxia, 120, 120t
Economic abuse, 161. *See also*
  Abuse
ECT (electroconvulsive therapy),
  249–250, 271–273
Education, 1
  for anxiety disorder, 43b
  for childhood psychiatric
    disorders, 185, 190b
  for cognitive impairment
    disorders, 208b
  for family, 243
  for mind-body disorders, 61
  for mood disorders, 110, 110b
  for personality disorders, 89, 89t
  for schizophrenia, 125, 131b
  for somatoform disorders, 64,
    70b
  stress, 61
  for substance-related disorders,
    149–150, 152, 153b, 155
Education groups, 230
Effexor (venlafaxine), 105t, 257t, 262
Ego, 22
Ego-dystonic disorder, 66
Ego syntonic disorders, 62, 66
Elaboration, 8
Elavil (amitriptyline), 105t, 257t
Elderly
  abuse of
    assessment of, 168t
    behavioral and psychological
      signs of, 165t
    legal issues in, 163
    nursing process for, 171
    physical signs of, 164t
    statistics on, 162
  crisis intervention for, 217
  mood disorders in, 98
  pseudodementia in, 101
Electroconvulsive therapy (ECT),
  249–250, 271–273
Ellis, Albert, 29
Emergency care, 1

Emergency room (ER) treatment, of
  abuse victims, 166–167
Emergency shelter, for battered
  women, 167
Emotional brain, 20
Emotional personality disorders, 82,
  87t, 88
Empathic nurse behaviors, 5, 6t
ENA-713 (Exelon), 202t
Encephalopathy, HIV, 201
Encourager, in group, 228
Enculturation, 8
Enmeshment, 238
Environment, 21
Environmental theories
  of childhood psychiatric
    disorders, 184–185
  of family violence, 166
  of mood disorders, 103
  of substance abuse, 148
EPS (extrapyramidal symptoms),
  126, 254t
Erikson's theory, 25t, 26
Erratic personality disorders, 82, 87t,
  88
ER (emergency room) treatment, of
  abuse victims, 166–167
Eskalith (lithium carbonate), for
  mood disorders, 105t,
  262–264, 263t, 264t
Ethical issues, in nursing practice,
  12–13
Ethnic differences, 9. *See also*
  Cultural factors
Ethnic groups, 9
Ethnicity, 9
Evaluation phase, of therapeutic
  relationship, 6
Evaluator, in group, 228
Exelon (ENA-713), 202t
Exhaustion stage, in adaptation to
  stress, 37
Existential therapy, 30
Expressed response pattern, to
  sexual assault, 163
Extended family, 237
External influences, delusions of,
  120b
External locus of control, 28
Extinction, 27
Extrapyramidal symptoms (EPS),
  126, 254t

F
Family
  of abuse victim, 169, 170, 172
  alternative, 237
  blended, 237
  characteristics of, 239, 240t
  of child with psychiatric disorder,
    188, 190b
  of client with cognitive
    impairment disorder, 202,
    203–204, 205, 208b
  of client with mind-body disorder,
    69, 70b
  of client with mood disorder, 99,
    110, 110b
  of client with personality disorder,
    89, 89b

  of client with schizophrenia, 122,
    126, 127–128, 130, 131b
  communication in, 240t, 243
  defined, 237
  developmental stages of, 238
  differentiation in, 238
  dysfunctional, 184, 239, 240t
  extended, 237
  functional, 239, 240t
  members of, 237–238
  nuclear, 237
  relationships within, 238
  single-parent, 237
  substance abuse and, 141
  tasks of, 239
Family data, 7t
Family genogram, 239, 241f
Family history. *See* Genetic
  predisposition
Family support, for substance abuse,
  150
Family systems, 237–239, 240t
Family systems therapy, 239
Family theories
  of childhood psychiatric
    disorders, 184, 185
  of eating disorders, 68
  of family violence, 166
  of personality disorders, 84
  of schizophrenia, 123
  of substance abuse, 148
Family therapy, 237–243
  for childhood psychiatric
    disorders, 185
  concepts in, 237–239, 240t
  definition of terms in, 237
  for eating disorders, 69
  for family violence, 167
  goal of, 239
  nursing process for, 241–243, 242t
  objectives of, 239, 241f
  role of nurse in, 241
  for substance abuse, 150
  types of, 239–241
Family violence
  cycles of, 163
  defined, 161
  etiology of, 166
  family characteristics with,
    163–164
  legal issues with, 163
  management of, 166–167
  nursing process for, 167–172
    assessment in, 167–169, 168t
    implementation in, 170–172
    nursing diagnoses in, 169–170
    outcome evaluation in, 172
    planning and outcome
      identification in, 170
  prevention of, 167
  statistics on, 162
Fearful personality disorders, 82,
  87t, 89
Federal legislation, 11
Feedback, 6
Fetal alcohol syndrome (FAS), 142
Fetal exposure
  to cocaine, 147
  to opioids, 145
Fidelity, 12

"Fight or flight" response, 37, 38t,
  39f
Flashbacks, with hallucinogens, 147
Fluoxetine (Prozac), 257t
  for anxiety disorders, 45t
  for children, 186t
  for eating disorders, 69t
  for mood disorders, 105t
Fluphenazine (Prolixin), 124t, 251t
Flurazepam (Dalmane), 266t
Fluvoxamine (Luvox), 257t
  for anxiety disorders, 45t
  for children, 186t
  for mood disorders, 105t
Focusing, 8
Formal operations stage, 25t
Fortune telling, 104t
Freudian theory, 22–24, 23t, 25t
  of depression, 103
Frontal lobe, 20
Functional family system, 239, 240t
Fusion, in family, 238

G
Gain, primary and secondary, 62
Gamma-aminobutyric acid (GABA),
  21, 249
  in stress and anxiety, 38
Gatekeeper, in group, 228
Gender identity, 64
Gender identity disturbance, 65
General adaptation syndrome, 37,
  38t, 39f
Generalization, over-, 29t
  with eating disorders, 66
  with mood disorders, 104t
Generalized anxiety disorder, 44,
  45t, 46b
  in children, 180t, 182
  nursing process for, 50–52, 51t
Generativity, *vs* stagnation, 25t
Genetic predisposition
  to anxiety-related disorders, 40
  to childhood psychiatric disorders,
    184
  to dementia, Alzheimer's type, 201
  to eating disorders, 67
  to family violence, 166
  to mood disorders, 101–102
  to obsessive compulsive disorder,
    47
  to panic disorder, 46
  to phobic disorder, 48
  to schizophrenia, 122, 123
  to substance abuse, 148
Genetics, 21
Genital stage, 25t
Genogram, 239, 241f
Gestalt therapy, 29
Ginkgo biloba, 250
"Good-me," 24
Grandiose delusions, 120b
Grief, defined, 97
Grief resolution, 97
Grief response, maladaptive, 97
Grieving, acute, 97
Group(s)
  activity, 230
  community meeting, 230
  curative factors in, 227, 228t

defined, 227
development of, 228, 231–232
education, 230
leadership of, 229, 229t
reality-orientation, 230
self-help, 230
  for somatoform disorders, 64
  for substance abuse, 149, 150t
socialization, 230
stages of, 228, 231–232
support, 229–230
  for dissociative disorders, 50
  for mood disorders, 106
  for post-traumatic stress
    disorder, 49
  for substance abuse, 149, 150,
    150t
therapeutic, 227, 229–230
Group dynamics, 227–229, 228t,
  229t
Group norms, 228
Group process, 227
Group psychotherapy, 227
Group roles, 228
Group therapy, 227–232
  definitions for, 227
  group dynamics in, 227–229, 228t,
    229t
  nursing process for, 230–232
  for personality disorders, 84
  role of nurse in, 229
  setting for, 229
  types of, 229–230
Guilt, initiative *vs.*, 25t

H
Halcion (Triazolam), 266t
Hallucinations
  in dementia, 203t
  in schizophrenia, 119, 129–130
Hallucinogens, abuse of, 138, 139t,
  144t, 147
Haloperidol (Haldol), 251t
  for dementia, 203t
  for schizophrenia, 124t
    childhood, 186t
Harmonizer, in group, 228
Health maintenance organizations
  (HMOs), 2
HEE (high expressed emotion), 123
Hepatotoxicity, of psychotropic
  medications, 255t
Herbal therapy, 62t, 250
  for mood disorders, 105t
Heroin abuse, 140, 143–145
  medications for, 150, 151t
High expressed emotion (HEE), 123
Histrionic personality disorder, 82,
  85, 87t
HIV (human immunodeficiency
  virus) encephalopathy, 201
HMOs (health maintenance
  organizations), 2
Holistic theory, 59, 61
Home care, for dementia, 208b
Home health visits, for cognitive
  impairment disorders, 202
Homelessness, and childhood
  psychiatric disorders, 185
Homeopathic medicine, 62t

Homeostasis, 237
Hormonal influences, 21
Hospitalization
  for borderline personality
    disorder, 84
  for childhood psychiatric
    disorders, 185–186
  for eating disorders, 69
  for mood disorders, 103–106
  partial, 1
    for childhood psychiatric
      disorders, 185
    for substance abuse, 149
  for schizophrenia, 124
  for substance abuse, 149
Hostility, in schizophrenia, 128–129
HPA
  (hypothalamic-pituitary-adren
  al) axis, in depression, 21,
  102
Human immunodeficiency virus
  (HIV) encephalopathy, 201
Humanistic theory, 30–31
  of stress and anxiety, 41
Hydroxyzine (Atarax, Vistaril), 266t
Hyperactivity, 181, 182t, 186t,
  190–191
Hypericum perforatum (St. John's
  Wort), 105t, 250
Hyperorality, 197
Hypertensive crisis, due to MAOIs,
  260, 260t
Hypochondriasis, 63
Hypomania, 100
  on continuum of mood disorders,
  98f
Hypothalamic-pituitary-adrenal
  (HPA) axis, in depression, 21,
  102
Hypothalamus, 20
Hypothyroidism, depression due to,
  21, 102

I
Id, 22
Identification, 23t
Identity, *vs.* role diffusion, 25t
Identity disorder, dissociative, 49b
Illogical thinking, 120t
Illusions, 119
Imipramine (Tofranil), 257t
  for anxiety disorders, 45t
  for children, 186t
  for eating disorders, 69t
Impulsiveness, in children, 186t
Inappropriate affect, 119
Incompetence, 12
Independent practice organizations,
  2
Inderal (propranolol), for anxiety
  disorders, 45t
Individuation conflicts
  with borderline personality
    disorder, 83
  with eating disorders, 67
Industry, *vs.* inferiority, 25t
Inference, arbitrary, 29t
Inferiority, industry *vs.*, 25t
Information, giving of, 8
Information seeker, in group, 228

Informed consent, 11
Inhalants, abuse of, 139t, 140, 145
Initiative, *vs.* guilt, 25t
Initiator, in group, 228
Instincts, 23
Integrity, *vs.* despair, 25t
Intellectualization, 23t
Interactional therapy, 240–241
Internal locus of control, 28
Interpersonal theory, 24–26, 25t
  of stress and anxiety, 41
Intimacy, *vs.* isolation, 25t
Intoxication, defined, 137
Intuitive stage, 25t
Involuntary commitment, 11
Isocarboxazid (Marplan), 105t, 257t
Isolation
  defense mechanism of, 23t
  intimacy *vs.*, 25t
  in schizophrenia, 128

J
Justice, 12

K
Kindling theory, of mood disorders,
  21, 102
Kinetics, 7
Klonopin (clonazepam), 45t, 266t
Korsakoff's syndrome, 142

L
LAAM (levomethadyl acetate), for
  heroin dependence, 151t
Labeling, 104t
La belle indifference, 63
Lactate sensitivity, panic disorder
  with, 45
Laissez-faire leadership, 229t
Latency stage, 25t
Leadership, of group, 229, 229t
Legal issues
  in family violence, 163
  in psychiatric practice, 10–12
Levomethadyl acetate (LAAM), for
  heroin dependence, 151t
Librium (chlordiazepoxide), 45t,
  266t
Limbic system, 20
Lithium carbonate (Eskalith,
  Lithobid, Lithonate), 105t,
  262–264, 263t, 264t
Locus of control, 28
Loose associations, 119, 120t
Lorazepam (Ativan), 266t
  for anxiety disorders, 45t
  for dementia, 203t
Loxapine (Loxitane), 251t
LSD, 144t, 147
Ludiomil (maprotiline), 257t
Luvox. *See* Fluvoxamine (Luvox)

M
Magnification, 29t
  with eating disorders, 66
Major depressive disorder
  characteristics of, 99–100
  in children, 180t, 183, 186t
  on continuum of mood disorders,
  98f

Major depressive disorder *(continued)*
   episodes of, 99
   etiology of, 101–103
   medications used in treatment of,
      105t
   nursing assessment of, 107t, 108t
   prevalence and incidence of,
      98–99
Maladaptive behaviors, 27
Managed care, 2, 13
Manerix (moclobemide), 257t
Mania. *See also* Bipolar disorder
   on continuum of mood disorders,
      98f
   defined, 97
   medications used in treatment of,
      105t
   nursing assessment of, 107t, 108t
MAOIs. *See* Monoamine oxidase
      inhibitors (MAOIs)
Maprotiline (Ludiomil), 257t
Marijuana, 138–140, 139t, 144t,
      147–148
Marplan (isocarboxazid), 105t, 257t
Maslow's hierarchy of needs, 30
   in crisis intervention, 218
Medical conditions, mood disorders
      due to, 103
Medical detoxification units, 149
Medical history, 7t
Medications, 249–273
   abuse of. *See* Substance-related
      disorders
   antianxiety (anxiolytic), 45t,
      265–269, 266t–268t
   anticholinesterase, 270–271, 270t
   antidepressant, 256–262, 257t,
      259t–261t
   antipsychotic (neuroleptic),
      250–254, 251t, 253t–256t
   for childhood psychiatric
      disorders, 186–187, 186t
   delirium due to, 200
   for dementia, 202, 202t, 203t
   for eating disorders, 69t
   mood disorders due to, 102–103
   mood stabilizing, 105t, 262–265,
      263t, 264t
   nursing process for, 271–273
   overview of, 249
   psychostimulant, 269–270, 269t
   psychotropic (psychoactive), 249
   for schizophrenia, 124t
   sedative-hypnotic, 266t
   for substance-related disorders,
      150, 151t
Melancholic features, of major
      depressive disorder, 99–100
Mellaril (thioridazine), 124t, 251t
Memory losses, 197
Mental health nursing. *See*
      Psychiatric nursing
Mental health services, for family
      violence, 167
Mental health treatment, evolution
      of, 1–3
Mental retardation, 179–180
Mental status examination, 7t
Mesoridazine (Serentil), 251t
Message, 6

Methadone (Dolophine), 150, 151t
Mind-body disorders, 59–73
   defined, 59
   eating disorders, 66–69, 67t–69t,
      70b
   education for, 61
   etiology of, 60–61
   key concepts of, 59–60, 60t
   management of, 61, 62t
   nursing process for, 70–73, 71t
   overview of, 59–61, 60t, 62t
   sexual disorders, 64–66
   somatoform disorders, 62–64
Mind reading, 104t
Minimization, 29t
Mirtazapine (Remeron), 105t, 257t
Mistrust, trust *vs.*, 25t
Mitral valve prolapse, panic disorder
      with, 46
Mobile crisis teams, 217
Moclobemide (Manerix), 257t
Modeling, 27
Molindone (Moban), 124t, 251t
Monoamine oxidase inhibitors
      (MAOIs), 257t, 259–260
   for anxiety disorders, 45t
   interactions with, 259–260, 260t
   for mood disorders, 105t
Monopolizer, in group, 228
Mood disorders, 97–112
   case finding for, 106
   in children, 183, 188, 191
   cognitive-behavior therapy for,
      106
   continuum of, 97, 98f
   crisis intervention services for,
      106
   cultural considerations with, 99
   definitions of, 97, 98f
   education for, 110, 110b
   effect on family of, 99
   etiology of, 101–103, 104t
   hospitalization for, 103–106
   impact of, 98
   medications used in treatment of,
      105t
   nursing management of, 103–106,
      105t
   nursing process for, 106–112
      analysis and nursing diagnosis
         in, 108–109
      assessment in, 106–108, 107t,
         108t, 109b
      implementation in, 110–112
      outcome evaluation in, 112
      planning and outcome
         identification in,
         109–110, 110b
   prevalence and incidence of,
      98–99
   primary prevention of, 106
   resources for, 106
   risk factors for, 101t, 106
   suicidal behavior, 97, 101t,
      107–108, 109b
   types of, 99–101
Mood reactivity, in major depressive
      disorder, 100
Mood stabilizers, 105t, 262–265,
      263t, 264t

Multidisciplinary team approach, to
      dementia, 201–202
Multi-infarct dementia, 198, 200
Mutual respect, in family, 238

N
Naloxone (Narcan), 145
Naltrexone (ReVia), 151t
Narcissistic personality disorder, 82,
      86, 87t
Narcotic analgesics, abuse of, 138,
      139t, 143–145, 144t
Nardil (phenelzine), 257t
   for anxiety disorders, 45t
   for mood disorders, 105t
National Alliance for the Mentally
      Ill, 3, 106
National Depressive and Manic
      Depressive Association, 106
National League for Nursing (NLN),
      3
Naturopathic medicine, 62t
Navane (thiothixene), 124t, 251t
Needs
   Maslow's hierarchy of, 30
      in crisis intervention, 218
   Sullivan's theory of, 24
Nefazodone (Serzone), 257t, 262
   for dementia, 203t
   for mood disorders, 105t
Negative cognitions, 103, 104t
Negative punishment, 27
Negative reinforcement, 27
Negative symptoms, of
      schizophrenia, 120, 126t
Neglect, 161. *See also* Abuse
Neologism, 120t
Neuroanatomy, 20
Neurochemical imbalances, in
      schizophrenia, 123
Neurodevelopmental abnormalities,
      in schizophrenia, 122–123
Neuroendocrine dysregulation, in
      mood disorders, 102
Neurofibrillary tangles, 201
Neuroleptic(s). *See* Antipsychotics
Neuroleptic malignant syndrome
      (NMS), 256t
Neurotransmitters, 20–21, 249
   in dementia, Alzheimer type, 201
   in mood disorders, 102
   in schizophrenia, 123
   in stress and anxiety, 38–39
Newborns
   cocaine withdrawal in, 147
   opioid withdrawal in, 145
Nicotine, 139t, 146
Nightingale, Florence, 3
NLN (National League for Nursing),
      3
NMS (neuroleptic malignant
      syndrome), 256t
Nonmaleficence, 12
Nonverbal behaviors
   empathic, 6t
   in therapeutic relationship, 7–8
Norepinephrine, 20, 249
   in stress and anxiety, 39
Norepinephrine reuptake inhibitors,
      selective, 262

Norms, group, 228
Norpramin (desipramine), 257t
    for eating disorders, 69t
    for mood disorders, 105t
Nortriptyline (Aventyl, Pamelor),
    257t
    for mood disorders, 105t
"Not-me," 24
Nuclear family, 237
Nurse(s), substance-related disorders
    in, 140–141
Nurse Practice Acts, 12
Nursing assessment, of psychiatric
    client, 7t

O
Obsessions, 47, 47b
Obsessive compulsive disorder
    (OCD), 47, 47b
    in children, 182, 186t
    nursing process for, 50–52, 51t
Obsessive-compulsive personality
    disorder, 82, 86, 87t
Occipital lobe, 20
Odd personality disorders, 81–82,
    87t, 88
Offering oneself, 8
Olanzapine (Zyprexa), 251t
    for schizophrenia, 124t
    childhood, 186t
Open boundaries, 237
Open-ended questions, 8
Opening remarks, 8
Operant conditioning, 27, 28
Opioids, abuse of, 138, 139t,
    143–145, 144t
Oppositional defiant disorder, 182,
    191
Oral stage, 25t
Orap (pimozide), 251t
Orgasmic disorders, 64
Orientation phase
    of groups, 228, 231
    of therapeutic relationship, 5, 7t
Outpatient care, 1
Outpatient counseling, for substance
    abuse, 149
Outreach services, for
    schizophrenia, 125
Overdose
    of benzodiazepines, 268t
    of CNS depressants, 143
    of opioids, 145
    of tricyclic antidepressants, 259t
Overgeneralization, 29t
    with eating disorders, 66
    with mood disorders, 104t
Oxazepam (Serax), 266t

P
Pain disorder, 63
Panic disorder, 44–46, 46b
    nursing process for, 50–52, 51t
Panic reactions, from hallucinogens,
    147
Paralanguage, 8
Paralogical thinking, 120t
Paranoid personality disorder, 81,
    85, 87t
Paranoid schizophrenia, 120

Paraphilias, 65
Parietal lobe, 20
Parnate (tranylcypromine), 105t,
    257t
Paroxetine (Paxil), 257t
    for anxiety disorders, 45t
    for mood disorders, 105t
Partial hospitalization, 1
    for childhood psychiatric
        disorders, 185
    for substance abuse, 149
Patient education. *See* Education
Patient's Bill of Rights, 11
Pavlov's theory, 27
PCP (phencyclidine), 138, 144t,
    147
Pedophilia, 65
Pemoline (Cylert), for ADHD, 186t,
    269t
Peplau, Hildegarde, 3, 26
Perception, and stress response, 40
Perls, Fritz, 29
Perpetrator
    sexual, 163
    violence
        characteristics of, 165b
        defined, 161
        implementation of nursing plan
            for, 171–172
        nursing diagnoses for, 169–170
        planning and outcome
            identification for, 170
Perphenazine (Trilafon), 251t
Persecution, delusions of, 120b
Perseveration phenomenon, 197
Personality
    Freudian theory of, 22
    Sullivan's theory of, 24–26
Personality disorder(s), 81–90
    antisocial, 82, 83, 84, 86, 87t
    anxious, fearful, 82, 87t, 89
    avoidant, 82, 86, 87t
    borderline, 82, 83, 84, 85, 87t
    characteristics of, 81
    classification of, 81
    defined, 81
    dependent, 82, 86, 87t
    dramatic, emotional, erratic, 82,
        87t, 88
    education for, 89, 89t
    etiology of, 83–84
    functioning with, 81
    histrionic, 82, 85, 87t
    management of, 84
    narcissistic, 82, 86, 87t
    nursing process for, 84–90
        assessment in, 84–86, 85t
        implementation in, 88–89, 89b
        nursing diagnoses in, 86–87, 87t
        outcome evaluation in, 89–90
        planning and outcome
            identification in, 87–88
    obsessive-compulsive, 82, 86, 87t
    odd, eccentric, 81–82, 87t, 88
    paranoid, 81, 85, 87t
    schizoid, 81, 85, 87t
    schizotypal, 82, 85, 87t
    self-perception with, 81
    treatment-seeking behavior with,
        81

Personality traits, with
    substance-related disorders,
    141
Pervasive developmental disorders,
    179–181, 181t, 190
Phallic stage, 25t
Pharmacotherapy. *See* Medications
Phencyclidine (PCP), 138, 144t, 147
Phenelzine (Nardil), 257t
    for anxiety disorders, 45t
    for mood disorders, 105t
Phobic disorder, 48, 48b
    in children, 182
    nursing process for, 50–52, 51t
Physical abuse, 161. *See also* Abuse
Physical assessment, 7t
Piaget's theory, 25t, 26–27
Pimozide (Orap), 251t
Polysubstance abuse, 137
Population-based community care, 2
Positive punishment, 27
Positive reinforcement, 27
Positive symptoms, of
    schizophrenia, 120, 126t
Postpartum depression, 100
Post-traumatic stress disorder
    (PTSD), 48–49, 49b
    nursing process for, 50–52, 51t
Poverty, and childhood psychiatric
    disorders, 184
Prazepam (Centrax), 266t
Preconceptual stage, 25t
Preconscious, 22
Predictability, and stress response,
    40
Preferred provider organizations, 2
Prenatal influences, on childhood
    psychiatric disorders, 184
Primary gain, 62
Prion disease, 201
Problem resolution, in family, 240t
Problem-solving approach, in crisis
    intervention, 218
Projection, 23t
    in borderline personality disorder,
        82
    in substance-related disorders,
        141
Prolixin (fluphenazine), 124t, 251t
Propranolol (Inderal), for anxiety
    disorders, 45t
Protriptyline (Vivactil), 257t
Proxemics, 7
Prozac. *See* Fluoxetine (Prozac)
Pseudodementia, 101
Pseudoparkinsonism, 254t
Psychiatric history, 7t
Psychiatric-Mental Health Nurse
    Generalist, 4
Psychiatric-Mental Health Nurse
    Specialist, 4–5
Psychiatric nurse practitioner, 4
Psychiatric nursing
    crisis intervention in, 217
    cultural considerations in, 8–10
    current practice in, 4–5
    ethical issues in, 12–13
    history of, 3–4
    legal issues in, 10–12
Psychic energy, 22

Psychoactive medications. *See also*
  Medications
  abuse of, 137
  defined, 249
  side effects of, 253t–256t
Psychoactive substances, defined,
  137
Psychoanalytic theory
  of eating disorders, 67
  of mood disorders, 103
  of personality disorders, 83
  of somatoform disorders, 63
Psychobiologic theory, 19–22
  of childhood psychiatric
    disorders, 184
  of family violence, 166
  of personality disorders, 83
  of somatoform disorders, 63
  of stress and anxiety, 38–40
  of substance abuse, 148
Psychodynamic theories, 22–24, 23t
  of mood disorders, 103
  of stress and anxiety, 41
  of substance abuse, 148
Psychological abuse, 161. *See also*
  Abuse
Psychological factors, affecting
  general medical conditions,
  60, 72
Psychoneuroimmunology, 59
Psychopharmacology. *See*
  Medications
Psychosexual theory, 25t
Psychosocial rehabilitation, for
  schizophrenia, 125
Psychosocial stressors, 37
Psychosocial theories, 25t, 26
  of family violence, 166
  of generalized anxiety disorder,
    44
  of mood disorders, 103
  of panic disorder, 46
  of stress and anxiety, 41
  of substance abuse, 148
Psychostimulants, 186t, 269–270,
  269t
Psychotherapy
  for dissociative disorders, 50
  for eating disorders, 69
  group, 227
  for personality disorders, 84
  for somatoform disorders, 64
Psychotic disorders, in children,
  186t
Psychotic features, of major
  depressive disorder, 100
Psychotropic medications. *See also*
  Medications
  abuse of, 137
  defined, 249
  side effects of, 253t–256t
PTSD (post-traumatic stress
  disorder), 48–49, 49b
  nursing process for, 50–52, 51t
Public child welfare agencies, for
  family violence, 167
Punishment
  negative, 27
  positive, 27
Purging, 67t

Q
Questions, open-ended, 8
Quetiapine (Seroquel), 124t, 251t

R
Rape, assessment of, 168–169
Rational-emotive therapy, 29
Rationalization, 23t
  with substance-related disorders,
    141
Reaction formation, 23t
Reality orientation, 207t
Reality-orientation groups, 230
Receiver, 6
Receptor sites, 21, 249
  in schizophrenia, 123
Recognition seeker, in group, 228
Reference, delusions of, 120b
Reflecting, 8
Regressive behavior, in
  schizophrenia, 128
Reinforcement
  negative, 27
  positive, 27
Relaxation techniques, 28, 41b
Remeron (mirtazapine), 105t, 257t
Repression, 23t
Residential treatment programs, 3
  for cognitive impairment
    disorders, 202
Residual schizophrenia, 121
Resistance stages, in adaptation to
  stress, 37
Respect, mutual, in family, 238
Response
  conditioned, 27
    in phobic disorder, 48
  unconditioned, 27
Restating, 8
Restoril (temazepam), 266t
Restraints, 12, 13
  for childhood psychiatric
    disorders, 186
Restructuring, cognitive, 29
ReVia (naltrexone), 151t
Right to refuse treatment, 11
Risperidone (Risperdal), 251t
  for dementia, 203t
  for schizophrenia, 124t
    childhood, 186t
Ritalin (methylphenidate), 186t, 269t
Rogers, Carl, 30
Role definitions, in family, 240t
Role diffusion, identity *vs.,* 25t

S
SAD (seasonal affective disorder),
  100
Safe house, for battered women,
  167
Safety, with cognitive impairment
  disorder, 206
Schismatic parental relationship, 238
Schizoid personality disorder, 81, 85,
  87t
Schizophrenia, 119–131
  agitated behavior in, 130
  catatonic, 121
  childhood, 182, 186t
  classification of, 120

communication patterns in,
  121–122, 128, 128b
defined, 119
delusions in, 119, 120b, 129–130,
  129b
disorganized, 121
DSM-IV criteria for, 119
education for, 125, 131b
etiology of, 122–123
family of client with, 122, 126,
  127–128, 130, 131b
hallucinations in, 119, 129–130
highly suspicious or hostile clients
  with, 128–129, 129b
interpersonal relationships in, 122
management of, 123–125, 124t
nursing process for, 125–131
  assessment in, 125–126, 125t,
    126t
  implementation in, 128–130,
    128b, 129b, 131b
  nursing diagnoses in, 126–127
  outcome evaluation in, 130–131
  planning and outcome
    identification in, 127–128
onset and course of, 121
paranoid, 120
perception of reality in, 121–122
regressive or unusual behaviors
  in, 128
residual, 121
statistics on, 121
symptoms of, 119–120, 120b,
  120t, 126t
  positive and negative, 120, 126t
types of, 120–121
undifferentiated, 121
violence potential with, 130
withdrawal and isolation in, 128
Schizotypal personality disorder, 82,
  85, 87t
Seasonal affective disorder (SAD),
  100
Seclusion, 11
  for childhood psychiatric
    disorders, 186
Secondary gain, 62
Sedative/hypnotics, 266t
  abuse of, 139t, 143, 144t
Seizures, due to psychotropic
  medications, 255t
Selective abstraction, 29t
  with eating disorders, 66
Selective norepinephrine reuptake
  inhibitors (SNRIs), 262
Selective serotonin reuptake
  inhibitors (SSRIs), 257t,
  260–261
  for anxiety disorders, 45t
  for children, 186t
  for eating disorders, 69t
  for mood disorders, 105t
  side effects of, 261t
Self-confessor, in group, 228
Self-help groups, 230
  for somatoform disorders, 64
  for substance abuse, 149, 150t
Self-system, 24
Self-talk, for schizophrenia, 130
Selye's theory, 37, 38t, 39f

Sender, 6
Sensorimotor stage, 25t
Separation anxiety disorder, 180t, 182, 186t
Separation-individuation conflicts with borderline personality disorder, 83
with eating disorders, 67
Serax (oxazepam), 266t
Serentil (mesoridazine), 251t
Seroquel (quetiapine), 124t, 251t
Serotonin, 20
in stress and anxiety, 39
Serotonin reuptake inhibitors, selective. *See* Selective serotonin reuptake inhibitors (SSRIs)
Serotonin syndrome (SS), 256t, 259
Sertindole (Serlect), 124t, 251t
Sertraline (Zoloft), 257t
for anxiety disorders, 45t
for children, 186t
for mood disorders, 105t
Serzone (nefazodone), 257t, 262
for dementia, 203t
for mood disorders, 105t
Sex therapy, 66
Sexual abuse. *See also* Abuse
assessment of, 168–169
of children, 162, 164t, 165t
defined, 161
Sexual arousal disorders, 64
Sexual assault, 163
Sexual behavior, normal, 64
Sexual desire disorders, 64
Sexual disorders, 64–66
nursing process for, 70–73, 70b, 71t
Sexual dysfunctions, 64–65
Sexual expression, 64
Sexual health, 64
Sexuality, 64
Sexual pain disorders, 64
Sexual perpetrator, 163
Sexual response cycle, 64
"Shakes, the," 142
Shame, autonomy *vs.*, 25t
Should statements, 104t
Silence, in therapeutic communication, 8
Sinequan (doxepin), 257t
Single-parent family, 237
Situational crisis, 215, 216t
Skewed parental relationship, 238
Skilled nursing facilities, for cognitive impairment disorders, 202
Skinner's theory, 27
SNRIs (selective norepinephrine reuptake inhibitors), 262
Socialization groups, 230
Social phobia, 48
Social Security Act (1993), 11
Social services agencies, for family violence, 167
Sociocultural theory
of eating disorders, 67
of family violence, 166
of major depressive disorder, 98
of personality disorders, 83

of somatoform disorders, 63
of substance abuse, 148
Socioeconomic status, 9
and schizophrenia, 123
Sodium lactate, panic disorder with, 45
Somatic delusions, 120b
Somatic therapies, 22. *See also* Electroconvulsive therapy (ECT); Medications
Somatization disorder, 63
Somatoform disorders, 62–64
education for, 64, 70b
nursing process for, 70–73, 70b, 71t
Spirituality, 12–13
Splitting, in borderline personality disorder, 82
SS (serotonin syndrome), 256t, 259
SSRIs. *See* Selective serotonin reuptake inhibitors (SSRIs)
St. John's Wort (hypericum perforatum), 105t, 250
Stagnation, generativity *vs.*, 25t
State commitment laws, 10–11
Stelazine (trifluoperazine), 124t, 251t
Stereotyping, 9
Stimulants, 186t, 269–270, 269t
Stimulus, 27
Stress
adaptation to, 37, 38t, 39f
defined, 37
in mind-body disorders, 59, 60–61, 60t
nursing process for, 41–43, 43b
positive and negative sources of, 37
post-traumatic, 48–49, 49b
psychobiologic aspects of, 38–40
psychosocial theories of, 41
ranking scale for, 37
Stress education interventions, 61
Stressors, 7t, 37
and mood disorders, 103
Stress reduction, coping strategies for, 41b
Stress response, 21
components of, 37–38, 38t, 39f
psychological influences on, 40–41
sustained, 40f
Stress-vulnerability model, of schizophrenia, 123
Striatum dysfunction theory, of obsessive-compulsive disorder, 47
Structural therapy, 240
Sublimation, 23t
Substance abuse
assessment of, 7t
defined, 137
poly-, 137
Substance dependence, defined, 137
Substance intoxication, defined, 137
Substance-related disorders, 137–155
in adolescents and children, 183–184, 191
with alcohol, 140, 142
amnestic disorders due to, 142, 198

with amphetamines, 145–146
with cannabinoids, 137–139, 138t, 147–148
classification of, 138–140, 139t
with CNS depressants, 138, 139t, 142–143
with CNS stimulants, 138, 139t, 145–147
with cocaine, 146–147
cultural differences in, 140
defense mechanisms with, 141
definitions in, 137–138
delirium due to, 198
education for, 149–150, 152, 153b, 155
etiology of, 148
and family, 141
with hallucinogens, 138, 139t, 147
with inhalants, 139t, 140, 145
laboratory testing for, 141
management of, 149–150, 150t, 151t
nursing process for, 150–155
assessment in, 150–152, 152t
education in, 153b
implementation in, 154–155
nursing diagnoses in, 152–154
outcome evaluation in, 155
planning and outcome identification in, 154
in nursing profession, 140–141
with opioids, 138, 139t, 143–145
personality traits with, 141
prevention of, 149–150
statistics on, 140, 148
types of, 142–148
withdrawal in, 144t
in women, 140
Subsystem, 237
Suffocation alarm theory, 46
Suicidal attempt, 97
Suicidal behavior
in children and adolescents, 183, 183b
crisis intervention for, 106, 220
defined, 97
hospitalization for, 103–106
nursing assessment of, 107–108, 109b
risk factors for, 101t, 107–108, 109b
substance abuse and, 140
Suicidal gesture, 97
Suicidal threat, 97
Sullivan's theory, 24–26, 25t
Summarizing, 8
Sundown syndrome, 197
Superego, 22
Superstitious thinking, with eating disorders, 66
Support groups, 229–230
for dissociative disorders, 50
for mood disorders, 106
for post-traumatic stress disorder, 49
for substance abuse, 149, 150, 150t
Supportive housing, for schizophrenia, 124

Supportive therapy, for schizophrenia, 125
Supra system, 237
Surmontil (trimipramine), 257t
Suspicion, in schizophrenia, 128–129, 129b
Sustained-stress response, 39f
Synapse, 20
System(s)
  defined, 237
  family, 237–239, 240t
  sub-, 237
  supra, 237
Systematic desensitization, 28
  for phobic disorder, 48
Systems theory, 59
  of sexual disorders, 65

T
Tacrine (Cognex), 202t, 270, 270t
Taractan (chlorprothixene), 251t
Tarasoff case, 11
Tardive dyskinesia, 254t
TCAs. *See* Tricyclic antidepressants (TCAs)
Teaching. *See* Education
Tegretol (carbamazepine), 263t, 265
  for dementia, 203t
  for mood disorders, 105t
Temazepam (Restoril), 266t
Temporal lobe, 20
Tenormin (atenolol), 45t
Termination phase
  of group, 228, 231–232
  of therapeutic relationship, 6
Tetrahydrocannabinol (THC), 147
Thalamus, 20
Therapeutic communication, 6–8
Therapeutic groups, 227, 229–230
Therapeutic nurse behaviors, 5, 6t
Therapeutic relationships, 5–6, 6t, 7t
Therapeutic Touch, 62t
Thioridazine (Mellaril), 124t, 251t
Thiothixene (Navane), 124t, 251t
Thorazine (chlorpromazine), 251t
  for schizophrenia, 124t
  childhood, 186t
Thought patterns, 29t
Thought stopping, 29
  for schizophrenia, 130
Thyroid gland, depression due to, 21, 102
Tofranil. *See* Imipramine (Tofranil)
Token economy, 28
Tolerance
  cross-, 138
  defined, 137
Touch
  Therapeutic, 62t
  in therapeutic communication, 7–8

Toxin model, of dementia, Alzheimer's type, 201
Traditional Chinese medicine, 62t
Transference, 24
Tranxene (clorazepate), 266t
Tranylcypromine (Parnate), 105t, 257t
Trauma
  dissociative disorders due to, 49
  post-traumatic stress disorder due to, 48–49, 49b
  nursing process for, 50–52, 51t
Trazodone (Desyrel), 105t, 257t, 262
Treatment, right to refuse, 11
Triangling, 84, 238
Triazolam (Halcion), 266t
Tricyclic antidepressants (TCAs), 256–259, 257t
  for anxiety disorders, 45t
  for children, 186t
  contraindications to, 258
  for eating disorders, 69t
  indications for, 256
  interactions with, 258
  mechanism of action of, 256
  for mood disorders, 105t
  overdose of, 259t
  pharmacokinetics of, 258
  side effects of, 258–259, 259t
  use across lifespan of, 258
Trifluoperazine (Stelazine), 124t, 251t
Trilafon (perphenazine), 251t
Trimipramine (Surmontil), 257t
Trust, *vs.* mistrust, 25t
24-hour inpatient care, 1

U
Unconditioned response, 27
Unconscious, 22
Undifferentiated schizophrenia, 121

V
Validation therapy, 207t
Valium (diazepam), 266t
Valproic acid (divalproex, Depakene, Depakote), 263t, 265
  for dementia, 203t
  for mood disorders, 105t
Value differences, 13
Vascular dementia, 198, 200
Venlafaxine (Effexor), 105t, 257t, 262
Veracity, 12
Verbal behaviors, empathic, 6t
Violence. *See also* Abuse
  crisis intervention for, 220–221
  defined, 161
  family. *See* Family violence
  in schizophrenia, 130

Violence perpetrator
  characteristics of, 165b
  defined, 161
  implementation of nursing plan for, 171–172
  nursing diagnoses for, 169–170
  planning and outcome identification for, 170
Vistaril (hydroxyzine), 266t
Vitamin E, for dementia, 202t
Vivactil (protriptyline), 257t
Voluntary admission, 10

W
Wellbutrin (bupropion), 105t, 257t, 262
Wernicke's syndrome, 142
Withdrawal
  from alcohol, 142, 144t
  from amphetamines, 144t, 146
  from cannabinoids, 140, 144t, 148
  from CNS depressants, 138, 143, 144t
  from CNS stimulants, 138, 144t, 146
  from cocaine, 144t, 147
  defined, 137
  from hallucinogens, 138, 144t, 147
  from inhalants, 140, 145
  from opioids, 138, 144t, 145
  in schizophrenia, 128
  treatment of, 144t
Women
  abuse of
    assessment of, 168t
    behavioral and psychological signs of, 165t
    crisis intervention services for, 167
    legal issues in, 163
    nursing process for, 171
    physical signs of, 164t
    remaining in relationship with, 164–166
    statistics on, 162
  substance abuse in, 140
Word salad, 120t
Working phase
  of groups, 228, 231
  of therapeutic relationship, 5–6

X
Xanax (alprazolam), 45t, 266t

Z
Ziprasidone (Zeldox), for schizophrenia, 124t
Zoloft. *See* Sertraline (Zoloft)
Zolpidem (Ambien), 266t
Zyprexa (olanzapine), 251t
  for schizophrenia, 124t
  childhood, 186t

Lippincott's Review Series CD-ROMs provide a convenient way to assess readiness for academic tests and licensure exams. One hundred carefully selected, multiple-choice questions are provided for study and simulated testing. In Study Mode, correct and incorrect feedback with rationale is provided following each question. In Test Mode, questions are scored with feedback available for review at the conclusion of the test.

System Requirements
Windows 95 or higher
486/66 Processor or higher
16 MB RAM
6 MB Free Hard Disk Space
CD-ROM Drive
640 x 480 Color Monitor or higher
256 Colors or higher

Installation
Insert the CD-ROM into your CD-ROM drive.
Click on the **Start** button, and then click **Run**.
At the command line, type **D:\setup.exe**. (Note: The letter D represents the CD-ROM drive. If your drive is designated by a different letter, use your drive letter instead.)
Click **OK**.
Follow the online instructions.

Technical Support
If you experience difficulty viewing the text, it may be the result of the color settings on your system. Should you need assistance or you have any questions regarding the use or content of this CD-ROM, please contact our Technical Support department by telephone at **800-638-3030** or **410-528-4532**, by fax at 410-528-4422, or by email at techsupp@LWW.com. Technical Support is available from 8:30 am to 5:00 pm (EST), Monday through Friday.